STATISTICS

for **Professional Courses**

in

Agriculture
Allied Health Sciences
Basic Sciences
Biology
Biotechnology
Dentistry
Environmental Sciences
Economics
Health Sciences
Life Sciences
Management
Medicine
Nursing
Pharmacy
Public Health
Research
Veterinary Sciences

χ^2

B. L. AGARWAL

Other CBS Titles by the same Author

- **Theory and Analysis of Experimental Designs**
- **Statistics for Senior Secondary$^{9,\ 10+2}$ Students**

STATISTICS

for **Professional Courses**

in

• Agriculture • Allied Health Sciences • Basic Sciences
• Biology • Biotechnology • Dentistry
• Environmental Sciences • Economics • Health Sciences
• Life Sciences • Management • Medicine • Nursing
• Pharmacy • Public Health • Research • Veterinary Sciences

B.L. Agarwal MSc (maths) MStat PhD

Ex-Professor of Statistics and
University Head
Department of Statistics and Mathematics
Rajasthan Agricultural University
RCA Campus, Udaipur
Rajasthan

CBS

CBS Publishers & Distributors Pvt Ltd

New Delhi • Bengaluru • Pune • Kochi • Chennai

ISBN : 978-81-239-1981-2 (Soft Cover)
ISBN : 978-81-239-1982-9 (Hard Cover)

First Edition : 2011
Reprint : 2011

Published by Satish Kumar Jain and produced by V.K. Jain for
CBS Publishers & Distributors Pvt. Ltd.,
CBS Plaza, 4819/XI Prahlad Street, 24 Ansari Road, Daryaganj,
New Delhi - 110002, India. • Website: www.cbspd.com
e-mail: delhi@cbspd.com, cbspubs@airtelmail.in
Ph.: 23289259, 23266861, 23266867 • Fax: 011-23243014

Branches:

- ***Bengaluru:*** Seema House, 2975, 17th Cross, K.R. Road, Bansankari 2nd Stage, Bengaluru - 560070 Ph.: +91-80-26771678/79 Fax: +91-80-26771680 • E-mail: cbsbng@gmail.com, bangalore@cbspd.com
- ***Pune:*** Bhuruk Prestige, Sr. No. 52/12/2+1+3/2, Narhe, Haveli (Near Katraj-Dehu Road By-pass), Pune - 411051 Ph.: +91-20-64704058/59, 32342277 • E-mail: pune@cbspd.com
- ***Kochi:*** 36/14, Kalluvilakam, Lissie Hospital Road, Kochi - 682018, Kerala • Ph.: +91-484-4059061-65 Fax: +91-484-4059065 • E-mail: cochin@cbspd.com
- ***Chennai:*** 20, West Park Road, Shenoy Nagar, Chennai - 600030 Ph.: +91-44-26260666, 26208620 • Fax: +91-44-42032115 E-mail: chennai@cbspd.com

Printed at :
India Binding House, Noida (UP)

to

Dr Suresh C. Goyal

Professor of Paediatrics
RNT Medical College
Udaipur

Preface

STATISTICS is an applied science which deals with quantitative data. Application of statistics has become ubiquitous in all streams of science like biotechnology, biology, ecology, medicine, health, agricultural sciences, as well as in economics, business management, marketing, advertising, etc. Statistics in various disciplines is included as a secondary course. All institutions and universities are keen to impart workable knowledge of statistics to their students of professional and applied science courses. This requires a composed applied book on statistics.

The present book **STATISTICS for Professional Courses** written for courses of various disciplines fully meets this requirement. The material given in this book, presented in a lucid and simple manner, is enough for the beginners.

Probability theory dealt with dexterity, divided into four chapters, is its peculiarity. Further, statistical inferences are based on sample studies. To draw conclusions about population from sample studies, estimation and testing of hypothesis are two strong tools. These have been presented expositive in Chapter 14.

Theory supported by a large number of solved numerical examples from a variety of areas of application makes the statistical concepts absolutely clear. This will enable the students to solve numerical problems correctly and independently in minimum time.

An adequate number of objective type questions given at the end of each chapter will further develop insight into the subject matter.

On the whole, this book on statistics will prove to be a boon to the readers of all professional and applied courses.

Study it and succeed.

Basant Lal Agarwal

Acknowledgements

I gratefully acknowledge the help given by Dr SP Agarwal, Ex-Professor, College of Veterinary Sciences, CS Haryana Agricultural University, Hissar. I am thankful to Dr Bhawna Agarwal, Assistant Professor, Quantitative Methods and Operations Research, IILM, Lodi Road, New Delhi, for assisting him along the way.

I also wish to thank my suave colleagues Dr B Upadhaya and Dr HK Jain, Assistant Professor, Department of Agricultural Statistics, RCA, MPUAT, Udaipur.

Basant Lal Agarwal

Contents

3. Diagrammatic and Graphical Presentation of Data 21–42

4. Statistical Central Values 43–63

5. Measures of Dispersion 64–98

14. Estimation and Hypothesis Testing 213–262

χ^2

CHAPTER 1

Statistics and Collection of Data

INTRODUCTION

In day-to-day life one generally comes across the term 'statistics about all vital events expressed by way of numerical figures. The word 'statistics' for a common man is nothing more than counting of population of a country or nation. Those who know little more, consider statistics as a science of counting. They are right in their thinking to some extent because in early days, kings and rulers gathered information regarding the population of their states and revenue. Still the statistics about these two aspects are inevitable for any government or ruler. With time, the scope of statistics did not remain confined to these two aspects. It emerged as the fullfledged science in the form of applied mathematics. As a first development, people became interested in averages of certain factors of interest, e.g. the average age of people, average income per family, the average consumption of foodgrains per person, etc. In view of these facts, Prof. A.L. Bowley called statistics,

i. The science of counting.
ii. The science of averages.

When the emphasis was laid on averages, people attached a number of stories which adversely reflected on the idea of averages. A few interesting tales are given here.

1. If you put the head of a person in a refrigerator and the legs in a furnace, the average temperature will be quite cozy for the person. So he will feel comfortable. As a matter of fact, the person will hardly be able to survive.
2. Mark Twain wrote that if you beat your wife twice a day and I don't. If we take the average, it will easily be concluded that both of us beat our wives once a day.

Many more tales are available in the literature, but all of them can not be narrated here. Any science used without sense will not deliver goods. So was the case with thc above tales. Statistics is a fully developed science and is used by one and all in one way or the other.

In Webster's New World Dictionary, the word **Statistics** is defined as "facts or data of a numerical kind, assembled and classified so as to present significant information."

R.A. Fisher defined statistics in view of the fact that statistics deals with data. No matter by which method they are collected. His definition is:

"The science of statistics is essentially a branch of applied mathematics and may be regarded as mathematics applied to observational data."

ORIGIN OF STATISTICAL THEORY

The credit of development of statistical theory goes to the gamblers and mathematicians of France, Germany and England. The gamblers put forth their problems to the mathematicians like Blaise Pascal (1623–1662), James Bernoulli (1654–1705), etc. They wanted to know the most favourable batting condition in their games of dice. This gave rise to the theory of probability. Probability is the backbone of statistics. Almost all statistical techniques involve probability theory directly or indirectly.

LIMITATIONS OF STATISTICS

Statistics has a wide range of applicability in various areas of study. But it has its own limitations as given below.

i. Statistics cannot deal with a single value. It deals with aggregates only.
ii. Statistics deal with those subjects of study which are capable of being quantitatively measured or can be expressed numerically. Quantitative measurements pertain to recording of observations like weight, height, percentage of nutrients, area, length, yield of crops, etc.
iii. Statistical data and results based on data involve an element of approximation. They are not so exact as the mathematics. The element of approximation in statistics enters through probability. Another point that causes approximation is that one observes a limited number of units or individuals but draws conclusions about a large group of units or individuals usually known as population to which the units under study belong.

STATISTICAL OPERATIONS

One thing is clear from the above discussion that statistics deals with large number of numerical values, so called data, not a single figure. These figures reveal lot of information about the population of individuals. Then the question arises how to handle large scale data to arrive at right conclusions about the population from which the data have been collected. This requirement made people to think and evolve a number of statistical methods. Primarily, statistics is considered to have four operations.

1. Collection of data
2. Compilation of data
3. Analysis of data
4. Interpretation of data

Data have been categorised into two types namely,

i. Primary data
ii. Secondary data.

PRIMARY DATA

The data originally collected by the investigator for purpose of study are called **primary data**.

SECONDARY DATA

The data obtained from records for purpose of study, which were originally collected by other persons(s), are called *secondary data*. They were used for another purpose and already exist somewhere as records.

Collection of Primary Data

Various methods are evolved for collection of required information or data. But mainly five methods are in vogue namely:

a. Personal enquiry method
b. Mailed enquiry method
c. Through experiments
d. Vital statistics
e. Industrial production
f. Telephone interview

a. In **personal enquiry method**, an investigator prepares or collects a list of persons (respondents) from whom the information is to be collected. Then he contacts the respondents personally and makes queries as per the questions given in the schedule. For the knowledge of inquisitive minds, schedule is a list of questions which are relevant for the purpose of study and generally it contains possible alternative answers also. For example, enquiry is made from the houses of a colony about the number of children in the house. Alternative answers may be given as 1, 2, 3, 4, and others. This method of survey is under complete control of the investigator. But it is highly expensive and time consuming.

b. In **mailed enquiry method**, a questionnaire (a list of questions with alternative answers) is sent through mail to the respondents. They are requested to fill the questionnaire themselves and return the same to the investigator within the prescribed time. This type of enquiry is possible only in case of educated mass. This method saves lot of time and money.

Mailed enquiry method suffers with the lacuna that response in general is very poor i.e. a large number questionnaires are not returned by the respondents. In mailed enquiry, even 40 per cent response is considered as a good response.

c. Besides above survey methods, data are also generated by conducting **experiments**. Generally these data are obtained from experiments in agriculture, i.e. regarding crop and animal sciences, medical sciences, laboratory experiments in chemical sciences and electronics, etc.
d. **Vital statistics** mainly concerns data regarding births, deaths, marriages, etc.
e. Records of articles produced in industries and thereafter their consumption also generate lot of data.
f. **Telephone interview:** In the last few years, a large number of homes, shops and business houses have been well equipped with telephone facility. This amenity has led to contact people very quickly. Big companies has made tremendous use of telephone to conduct surveys. A telephonic conversation of a company's representative, the interviewer, with a respondent, the interviewee, with regard to any information, investment, etc. is called a telephonic interview. In this approach, follow up telephonic interviews are very convenient and easy.

In all, telephonic interviews are the cheapest, least time consuming, reliable and practically expedient. There are no bounds on coverage area of survey in telephonic interviews.

The data obtained under the methods (a) to (f) are known as primary data.

Sources of Secondary Data

There are two sources of secondary data,

a. internal sources
b. external sources

a. **Internal sources:** Those data which are available in the records of a company, institution or daily account of transactions, and can be used for further investigation are termed as internal sources of secondary data. For instances, salaries of workers, production of units, consumption of electricity, etc. are maintained as records by the companies. They can be suitably used as secondary data.
b. **External sources:** Lot of data are collected and published for various purposes, which can be used for extracting additional information and conclusions. Such publications are called external sources of secondary data. Such data are available in census

reports, magazines, published bulletins of various departments like agriculture, mining, fisheries, forestry, industries, Reserve Bank of India, etc. Besides published data, huge amount of data regarding various aspects of economy, commerce, industry and research are available on-line. One should be wary of using secondary data. If secondary data are inaccurate, outdated, incomplete and unreliable, then an investigator should not use secondary data. Instead he should collect primary data. The operations, compilation and analysis of data, interpretation of results are covered in the chapters ahead.

Statistical methods have a wide range of applications in the areas of economics, biological sciences, medical sciences, agricultural research, astronomy, etc. Statistics is the need of the present time and hence one should learn it as thoroughly as possible.

PRACTICE QUESTIONS AND EXERCISES

1. Write a short note on the importance of statistics.
2. Discuss the areas in which statistics is useful.
3. What was the role of statistics in ancient times?
4. What are the limitations of statistics.
5. What are various statistical operations?
6. In what way, data are collected through personal enquiry method?
7. Describe the method of collecting data by mailed questionnaire.
8. What are the methods of collecting data other than mailed and personal enquiry?
9. Why people made fun of statistics as a science of averages?
10. Who were the first to contribute to the theory of statistics?
11. Give two definitions of statistics.
12. Differentiate between primary and secondary data.
13. Is it always good to collect primary data for any investigation? Give reasons to your answer.
14. In what manner, should a researcher proceed to choose between collection of primary or secondary data?
15. How the data are generated through experiments?
16. What aspects are covered under vital statistics?
17. Distinguish between the manner in which the collection of data from industries may lead to primary data as well as secondary data?
18. What is the notion of a common man about statistics?

OBJECTIVE TYPE QUESTIONS

Select the correct alternative.

19. Statistics is a branch of:

a. Applied data b. Applied mathematics

c. Computer applications d. Revenue collection

20. Statistics is considered as a science of:
    a. Averages
    b. Counting
    c. Data analysis
    d. All of the above
21. The credit of initial development of statistics goes to:
    a. England
    b. France
    c. Germany
    d. All of the above
22. Statistics is capable to deal with:
    a. Single value
    b. Numerical data
    c. Qualitative information
    d. Whole numbers only
23. Statistical data are categorized as:
    a. Primary and secondary data
    b. Primary and stationary data
    c. Secondary and collective data
    d. Secondary and imaginary data
24. Collection, compilation and analysis of data are known as:
    a. Variations of statistics
    b. Operations of statistics
    c. Components of statistics
    d. None of the above
25. Primary data can be collected through:
    a. Personal enquiry
    b. Experiments
    c. Mailed enquiry
    d. All of the above
26. Do statistics reveals facts about:
    a. An individual
    b. Human population only
    c. Government policies
    d. Masses in general
27. Secondary data can be collected from:
    a. Census reports
    b. Discussion with people
    c. General observation
    d. Measuring instruments
28. Cheapest method of collecting primary data is:
    a. Mailed enquiry
    b. Telephonic interview
    c. Observation method
    d. None of the above
29. Data that are available in the records of a company are categorized as:
    a. External source of data
    b. Unreliable source of data
    c. Internal source of data
    d. Manipulated data
30. Which method of survey can cover an unlimited area?
    a. Mailed questionnaire method
    b. Personal interview method
    c. Telephonic interview method
    d. All of the above

CHAPTER 2

Classification and Tabulation of Data

INTRODUCTION

Compilation means to gather statistics or data in an orderly form. In quest of the same, classification and tabulation are the two best tools of compilation which are discussed in this chapter. Before discussing these two topics it is necessary to undetstand statictical terminology which will frequently be used in this chapter and throughout the book.

STATISTICAL TERMINOLOGY

Every science has terms which are commonly used in its study. So is with statistics. Their definition or meaning be learnt and understood for correct usage. There are thousands of terms in statictics which have its own meaning and application, some of the terms which the beginners should know are defined and explained below alongwith the examples.

POPULATION

Population in statistics does not mean only the human population or the population of animals. But it is an aggregate of animates or inanimates in which we are interested. As a definition, "Population is the totality of individuals, objects, items or anything coceivable pertaining to certain characteristics." The term population as defined in the dictionary of technical terms by Kendall and Buckland is,

"In statistical usuage, the term population is applied to any finite or infinite collection of individuals."

For further clarification, the examples of pupulation are:-

i. In a medical study on tuberculosis, interest lies only in persons suffering from the disease of tuberculosis(TB). Hence, the totality of all persons suffering from TB is the population. Any person not suffering from TB is not an element of population.

ii. If our interest lies in the students of a particular school, then only those students who are on the rolls of this school constitute the population and none else.

iii. If an horticulturalrist is interested to conduct a study on orange trees in an orchard, then all the orange trees in this orchard constitute the population.

iv. If one wants to study the life of electric bulbs produced in a factory on a particular day, then population comprises of all the bulbs produced on that day.

In all the above examples, populations have a countable number of units. So they are called *finite population*(s).

INFINITE POPULATION

The population generated by natural numbers leads to an infinite population. Similarly, throws of dice, tossing of a coin, drawing of cards from a pack with replacement, an unlimited number of times result into infinite populations. The populations of insects, bacteria, etc. are also considered infinite.

SAMPLING UNIT

Every population consists of a number of units or individuals from which the information is collected or on which the observation are taken. Each unit or individual of a population is known as *sampling unit*. For example, any patient of TB of a population is a sampling unit. Similarly the orange trees in an orchard, an electric bulb of a factory are sampling units.

VARIABLE

In real life, one does not study the unit or individual as a whole but some characteristics or factor(s) related to it. For instance, in case of a person, one studies certain characters like, age, height, weight, colour, blood pressure, pulse rate, etc. Each of these is a variable. Similarly, to study an orange tree, one measures its height, spread, number of fruits per tree, size of fruits, vitamin C content in the fruits, etc. These are also variables. In the study of bulbs, life of bulbs in hours is a variable. In crop experiments, yield per hectare is a variable. From these example, it is evident that a measure is taken on each individual which is either a count or has a unit of measurement. Hence, a variable may be difined as, "A factor or character, which can take different values, is called a variable". A variable is classified into two types,

i. Discrete variable

ii. Continuous variable.

Discrete Variable

A variable which takes a whole number value, a finite number of times, is called a **discrete variable.** Discrete values are generally whole numbers, e.g., test scores, family size, number of employees, number of goals in football matches, etc.

Continuous Variable

A variable which can take any numerical value within a certain range is called *continuous variable*, e.g. height or weight of persons, distance, temperature, rainfall per day, yield of a crop per hectare, etc. For example, height of persons is given as 5.76, 6.23, 5.45, inches.

FREQUENCY

Number of times a variate value occurs in a collection of data is known as *frequency* of that variate value.

Example 2.1. The age of children is recorded in a class of 15 students. There are 6 students of 5 years age and 9 students of 6 years age. Here age is a variable. 5 years age is a variate value and 6 is its frequency. Similarly the value 6 years has a frequency 9.

Example 2.2. There are 20 families in a locality out of 20 families, each of 4 families has only one child, 5 families have 2 children each, 8 families have 3 children each and 2 families are with 4 children each and 1 family has 5 children.

In this example, number of children is a variable and number of families is the frequency. The variate values (x) and their corresponding frequencies (f) can be written as follows:

No. of children (x) :	1	2	3	4	5
No. of families (f) :	4	5	8	2	1

Frequency Distribution

The manner in which the frequencies occur according to their respective variate values is called *frequency distribution.*

Example 2.2 presents the frequency distribution of number of children in the locality.

Cumulative Frequency (cf)

To obtain cf it is necessary to arrange the frequency distribution in ascending or descending order according to variate values. Ascending order means lower variate value to next higher value and descending order means higher value to next lower value till all the values are exhausted. In an ordered frequency distribution, on adding the sum of all the previous frequencies to the freqency of a variate value, one gets the cumulative frequency for that value. In case of ascending order, cumulative frequency gives the number of units which possess a value less than or equal to that value. On the contrary, in case of descending order frequency distribution, a cumulative frequency gives the number of units which are greater than or equal to that value.

Example 2.3. The cumulative frequencies of both types of ordered frequency distributions of example 2.3. are presented below.

i	ii	iii	iv	v	vi
Ascending order (less than type)			*Descending order (more than type)*		
No. of children (x)	*Freq. (f)*	*cum. freq.*	*No. of children (x)*	*Freq. (f)*	*cum. freq. c.f.*
1	4	4	5	1	1
2	5	5 + 4 = 9	4	2	2+1 = 3
3	8	8 + 9 = 17	3	8	8 + 3 = 11
4	2	2 + 17 = 19	2	5	5 + 11 = 16
5	1	1 + 19 = 20	1	4	4 + 16 = 20

In the above table, it is easy to note that cumulative frequency 9 in column (iii) shows the number of families which have two or one children. Similarly c.f. 17 in column (iii) gives the number of families having 3 children or less and so on.

Again the cumulative frequency 3 in column (vi) reveals that there are 3 families which have 4 or 5 children. Cumulative frequency 11 in column (vi) yields the information that 11 families out of 20 have 3 or more children and so on.

Note: Above frequency distribution represents discrete series.

SAMPLE

From the discussion so far, it is clear that a population consists of a large number of sampling units. Hence, the study of whole population requires too many skilled persons to carry out the investigation, huge amount of money, lot of time, etc. Also the chances of errors in collection, compilation and analysis of data are substantial. Therefore to overcome these difficulties, some sampling units are selected by a suitable method which represent the population. These selected units constitute a *sample*.

Definition of a Sample

Sample is a randomly selected part of the population studied to gain knowledge about the population.

GROUPED DATA

Many times the number of variate values is very large. If each individual value is considered, the frequency distribution becomes cumbersome and is not easily accessible or suitable for further usage. To ease out the problem, groups of variate values are formed and the number of values falling within the group is known as its frequency. Grouping of data is same as classification of data in case of quantitative data.

Classification of Data

Data collected in any manner is usually large and haphazard. It is the inability of one's mind to grasp the information contained in the raw data for any purpose. To deal with this problem, some process to condense the data is required so that the essential information contained in it can be extracted and data are fit for further treatment. Classification is one such method.

Definition

L R. Connor – Classification is the process of arranging things (either actually or notionally) in groups or classes according to their resemblaces and affinities and gives expression to the unity of attributes that may subsist amongst a divesity of individuals.

Purposes of Classification

i. To condense the data in a simple manner for better understanding and treatment.
ii. To present the data in such a form that comparisons can easily be made.
iii. To emerge the salient features of the data.
iv. To draw statistical inferences.
v. To prepare a report about the population under study.
vi It provides the basis for tabulation.

Norms for Classification

i. It should be suitable for the purpose of study.
ii. Classes should be exhaustive and nonoverlapping, i.e., all values be contained in these classes and no unit may belong to more than one class. In a continuous distribution, lower limit of class is included.
iii. Classification should be unambiguous.
iv. Number of classes should neither be large nor small.
v. Width of classes should be adequate. As far as possible, all classes should be of equal width.
vi. Classes should be continuous i.e., the upper limit (l_i) of the preceding class should be the lower limit of the following class. It is not, say it is (l_{i+1}) then it should be made continuous. For this, substract the quantity $(l_{i+1} - l_i)/2$ from the lower limit of each class and add it to the upper limit of each class. For example.

Discontinuous Classes		*Continuous Classes*
5 — 10		4.5 — 10.5
11 — 16	⟶	10.5 — 16.5
17 — 22		16.5 — 22.5

Since, $\frac{11-10}{2}=0.5$. In this process, the class interval increases by the quantity $l_{i+1}-l_i$. Here it is 1.

vii. Classes should be flexible in the sense that they may be amended according to the situation.

viii. All units in a class should be homogenous.

ix. The difference between upper limit and lower limit of a class is called its *class intervals.*

Basics of Classification

Classification is done according to four criteria as given below.

1. **Geographical:** Unit are classified according to the region or place, e.g., statewise classification of literacy rate.

Example 2.4. Classification of percentage of population in respect of literacy of five northern states of India is depicted below as per census 1991.

States	*Percentage of literates*
Punjab	57.14
Rajasthan	38.81
Haryana	55.33
Uttar Pradesh	41.71
Delhi	76.09

2. **Chronological:** Classification is done with respect to time i.e, weekly, monthly, yearly, etc. For instance, number of deaths due to road accidents per year in Delhi, number of sucides due to illenss in India per year in last ten years. Production of a crop in India in the last decade, etc.

Example 2.5. Production of rice and wheat in India from 1985 to 1992 is classified as below.

Years	*Rice (M. Tones)*	*Wheat (M. Tones)*
1985	58.3	44.1
1986	63.8	47.0
1987	60.6	44.3
1988	56.9	46.2
1989	70.5	54.1
1990	73.6	49.8
1991	74.3	55.1
1992	43.7	55.0

3. **Qualitative:** Unit or individual are classified in respect of some attributes such as sex, habits, qualification, religion, profession, etc.

Example 2.6. Classification of employees of a company according to sex can be given as follows.

Employees
500

Male 430 | Female 70

Note: Such a classification is accroding to *dichotomy*, since the division is always into two groups. It may be healthy/sick, educated/illiterate, etc.

Example 2.7. Employees of the example 2.6 may further be classified according to their qualification as well.

	Employees		
Qualifications	*Male*	*Female*	*Total*
Middle	75	36	
Secondary	256	27	
Graduate	99	7	
Total	430	70	500

Note: Such a classification is called manifold since the classification is done on the basis of more than one attribute.

4. **Quantitative:** If the units are classified or grouped according to some numerical measure of a varibale, then it is said to be a quantitative classification e.g., marks of the students of a class in a subject, monthly income of wage earners, consumption of petrol per person per month, etc. As given earlier, the data are divided into classes and the number of units belonging to classes (frequency) is written side by side. Some points related to the formation of classes are discussed further.

Example 2.8. The distribution of marks in economics according to quantitative classes can be given as follows:

Marks (Classes)	*No. of students (Frequency)*
10–25	5
25–40	21
40–55	33
55–70	24
70–85	5
85–100	2

NUMBER AND WIDTH OF CLASSES

During the process of classification, a major question arises, what should be the number of classes and their width? As a matter fact, if the number of classes is decided, width is automatically fixed and vice-versa. No hard and fast rule can be given for determining the number of classes. However, as a rule of thumb it is felt that the number of classes should not be less than 6 and more than 15. Anyhow, for a huge data it may be upto 20. Once, the number of classes 'n' is decided, then

$$\text{Class-width} = \frac{\text{largest value} - \text{smallest value}}{\text{No. of classes}} \tag{2.1}$$

This value will generally be a fractional value. But it is rounded to the nearest whole number.

Further,

$$\text{Mid-value of a class} = \frac{\text{Lower class limit} + \text{upper class limit}}{2} \tag{2.2}$$

Now the theory given so far will be elucidated by way of practical examples.

Note: Classification according to variate values is also known as *frequency distribution.*

Example 2.9. The marks of 50 students in statistics obtained out of 100 are as given below:

Marks

8	26	54	49	28	28	40	54	68	63
50	72	28	65	37	38	26	56	40	28
50	36	31	42	10	11	26	23	40	40
40	36	40	12	19	16	33	16	26	28
50	54	51	13	03	58	15	06	00	15

In the above data of marks, minimum marks are zero and maximum 72. If one considers each individual value, there are 30 values to be taken separately. This is too large a number of values. Hence, it is better to form classes (groups) with an interval of 10. In this way there shall be eight classes, the first as 0 – 10 and last 70 – 80. In every class lower limit of the class is included. Frequencies of the classes are counted with the help of tally marks.

Class of marks	*Tally marks*	*Frequency*	*Cumulative frequency*
0 — 10	||||	4	4
10 — 20	~~||||~~ ||||	9	4 + 9 = 13
20 — 30	~~||||~~ ~~||||~~	10	13 + 10 = 23
30 — 40	~~||||~~ |	6	23 + 6 = 29
40 — 50	~~||||~~ |||	8	29 + 8 = 37
50 — 60	~~||||~~ ||||	9	37 + 9 = 46
60 — 70	|||	3	46 + 3 = 49
70 — 80	|	1	49 + 1 = 50

Above classified grouped data represents a continuous frequency distribution. Cumulative frequencies in the last column are shown just for practice. Readers will come across such types of grouped data in the chapters ahead also.

Tabulation of Data

Classification is one-way presentation of data in condensed and systematic form. But many situations arise when the data are to be arranged in respect of two or more variables and/or attributes. Here the discussion will be given by considering only two variables or attributes i.e., two way tables.

DEFINITION

A table is a systematic and orderly arrangement of two related variables or attributes of data into rows and columns in a scientific manner.

FORMATION OF A TABLE

In a table, the groups of values (s) of a variable or components of an attribute are taken along rows and for the other variable or attribute along columns. Vertical and horizontal lines are drawn actually or notionally so as to create the cells which contain the properties of both. If there are p groups of X and q groups of Y, then there will be $p \times q$ cells. Each cell will have certain frequency of a variate value. This as a whole constitutes a table. First the data are classified and then tabulated.

Parts of a Table

A table consists of eight parts, namely– (1) Table number (2) Title (3) Captions (4) Stubs (5) Body (6) Headnote (7) Footnote (8) source note

1. **Table number.** This provides the identity of a table. This is given either on top or below the table.
2. **Title.** This gives fairly good information about the contents of a table. It is always given above the table.
3. **Captions.** it gives the heads of columns which level data found in the columns of a table
4. **Stubs.** The heads of an attribute or groups of a variable are given along first column which level the data found in the rows of a table.
5. **Body.** This contains numerical information in the cells, mostly frequencies or observation.
6. **Headnote.** It is a pharse or small note below the title which further elaborates information about the contents of a table. It is seldom required.
7. **Foot note.** It reveals some information about a specific item of the table which is to be high -lighted. It is placed just below the table.

8. **Source note.** The source of data given in the table is to be disclosed as a rule. This enables one to verify all facts about data. It is given below the footnote.

skeleton of a table showing various parts is displayed below.

Table No. ----------

Title ----------

Headnote ----------

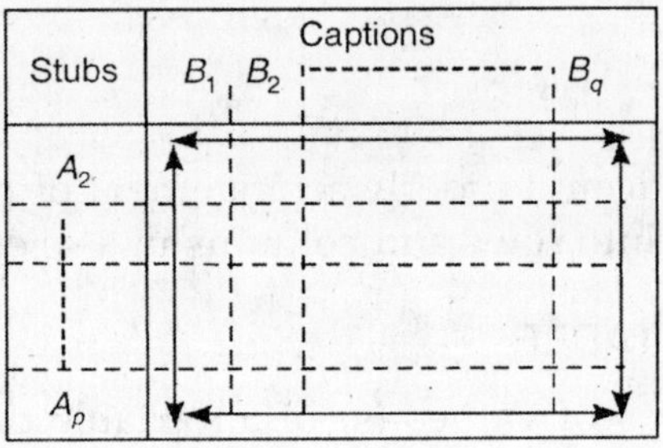

Footnote ----------

Sourcenote --------

Advantages or Purposes of Tables

1. Tables consolidate data.
2. A table presents the data in such a simple and systematic form that one can understand the values associated with the variable and/or attributes.
3. They reveal the association of a variable or attribute with the other.
4. Any errors or omissions present in the data come to the surface.
5. Comparison of one factor with the other becomes easy and reliable.
6. Diagrammatic and graphical representation of data becomes simple and accurate with the help of tables.
7. Tables portray more information in lesser space.
8. Persons are to give little time in gathering any required information, i.e. tables are time savers.
9. Tables are the basis of statistical calculations and analysis of data.
10. Tables make interpretation of data easier and better as compared to raw data.

Example 2.10. Distribution of number of women interviewed by a textile factory according to their merital status and area of experience is tabulated below.

Table 2.1: Distribution of women according ot marital status and area of experience

Marital status	*Area of experience*		*Total*
	Textile	*Non-textile*	
Marrried	180	269	449
Unmarried	120	396	516
Total	300	665	965

Foot note : Data are fictitions.
Source : An examination paper

N.B.: Table 2.1 provides information according to two atributes.

Example 2.11. Data pertaining to the heights in inches and weights in kg. of 28 married women are given below.

Height	*Weight*	*Height*	*Weight*
60	38	67	66
65	42	63	58
64	46	64	49
58	45	65	52
66	52	58	56
63	48	59	51
60	46	62	49
52	51	61	46
55	61	64	61
61	58	67	65
65	42	65	52
63	46	60	54
62	52	63	56
66	57	66	48

Two way tale of married women by height and weight can be constructed as follows:

Lowest value of height is 52 and largest 67. So form the classes of height by taking a class interval of 2 inches. The classes will be 52 - 54, 54 - 56, ..., 66 - 68. Again weight varies from 38 to 66. So it is better to take class interval of 4 kg. In this way classes will be 38 - 42, 42 - 46, ..., 66 - 70. In both the cases, lower limit of the class is included and upper limit is excluded.

Table 2.2: Distribution of married women by height and weight

<table>
<tr><th>Height</th><th colspan="8">Weight</th><th>Total</th></tr>
<tr><td></td><td>38-42</td><td>42-46</td><td>46-50</td><td>50-54</td><td>54-58</td><td>58-62</td><td>62-66</td><td>66-70</td><td></td></tr>
<tr><td>52-54</td><td></td><td></td><td></td><td>| = 1</td><td></td><td></td><td></td><td></td><td>1</td></tr>
<tr><td>54-56</td><td></td><td></td><td></td><td></td><td></td><td>| = 1</td><td></td><td></td><td>1</td></tr>
<tr><td>56-58</td><td></td><td></td><td></td><td></td><td></td><td></td><td></td><td></td><td>–</td></tr>
<tr><td>58-60</td><td></td><td>| = 1</td><td></td><td>| = 1</td><td>| = 1</td><td></td><td></td><td></td><td>3</td></tr>
<tr><td>60-62</td><td>| = 1</td><td></td><td>|| = 2</td><td></td><td>| = 1</td><td>| = 1</td><td></td><td></td><td>5</td></tr>
<tr><td>62-64</td><td></td><td></td><td>||| = 3</td><td>| = 1</td><td>| = 1</td><td>|| = 2</td><td></td><td></td><td>7</td></tr>
<tr><td>64-66</td><td></td><td>|| = 2</td><td>|| = 2</td><td>|| = 2</td><td></td><td></td><td></td><td></td><td>6</td></tr>
<tr><td>66-68</td><td></td><td></td><td>| = 1</td><td>| = 1</td><td>| = 1</td><td></td><td>| = 1</td><td>| = 1</td><td>5</td></tr>
<tr><td>Total</td><td>1</td><td>3</td><td>8</td><td>6</td><td>4</td><td>4</td><td>1</td><td>1</td><td>28</td></tr>
</table>

Footnote: Blank cells show zero or no frequency. Table 2.2 is according to two variate values.

Example 2.12. Table 2.3 shows the distribution of empolyees by age and their status in a company.

Table 2.3: Distribution of employers in respect of age and status

Age	*Status*				*Total*
	Clerical	*Supervisor*	*Officer*	*Executive*	
20–30	25	15	6	2	48
30–40	22	18	8	3	51
40–50	16	18	10	5	49
50–60	11	24	19	8	62
60–70	2	6	12	6	26
Total	76	81	55	24	236

N.B.: In the above table, stubs represent a variable, i.e. age and captions an attribute, i.e. status.

A thorough study of the matter given in this chapter will lay good foundation of compilation of data.

PRACTICE QUESTIONS AND EXERCISES

1. Define and discuss population.
2. What do you understand by a sample?
3. Explain sampling unit and give two examples.
4. Define continuous and diserete variables and give two examples of each type of variable.
5. Discuss frequency and frequency distribution.
6. What does a cumulative frequency indicate?
7. What do you understand by grouped data? Why is it so important in statistics?

8. Given the age in years of 40 males at the time of marriage, prepare a frequency distribution by choosing the classes with an interval of two years.

Age (years)

22	19	20	22	28	20	19	21	23	22
23	24	23	28	22	20	21	23	22	24
25	27	20	22	21	19	22	21	20	25
28	23	25	22	20	21	22	23	24	19

Also find the cumulative frequencies.

9. Marks of 48 students in an examination paper of chemistry of 100 marks were as follows:

Marks

16	33	16	26	28	50	54	51	13	03	58	15
06	00	15	25	32	54	37	31	51	47	54	52
23	47	16	45	36	36	34	36	46	68	41	32
25	33	05	40	55	36	36	14	45	10	71	61

a. Prepare the grouped frequency distribution taking class intervals of ten marks.

b. Construct the cumulative frequency distribution.

10. Differentiate between finite and infinite populations.
11. Distinguish between grouped and ungrouped data.
12. Define and discuss classification of data.
13. For what purposes data are classified.
14. What are the requirements for a good classification?
15. Name the basis of classification and explain them in brief.
16. Give the formula for detemining the width of classes.
17. How to get the mid-point of a class and what is its importance?
18. What is a statistical table and why is it so important in statistics?
19. What purposes are served by statistical table?
20. Give main parts of a table and what do they reveal.
21. Compare classification and tabulation.
22. Out of 4000 workers in a factory, 3500 are men and rest are women. The total number of union members in 3300, out of which 100 women. Present the data in a suitable tabular form.

OBJECTIVE TYPE QUESTIONS

23. All blinds found in India constitute:

a. A population   b. A sample

c. An infinite population   d. A finite population

24. Number of deaths per months occurring in India due to suicides are categorized as:

a. Random number   b. Continuous variable

c. Discrete variable   c. Frequency

25. Each employee of a factory can be considered as:
    a. Population unit b. Sampling unit
    c. Statistical unit d. All of the above
26. Protein content in cow milk can be classified as:
    a. Continuous variable b. Advertisement
    c. Discrete variable d. Nutrition
27. Number of units taking values less than or equal to an ordered value is known as:
    a. Frequency b. Frequency distribution
    c. Cumulative frequency d. Variable
28. Purpose of classification of data is:
    a. To highlight the salient features b. To condense the data
    c. To prepare a basis for tabulation d. All of the above
29. The manner in which the frequencies occur according to variate values is called:
    a. Cumulative frequency b. Discrete distribution
    c. Continuous distribution d. Frequency distribution
30. The term classification of data is strictly used in respect of:
    a. Qualitative data b. Quantitative data
    c. Attributes d. None of the above
31. Are grouping and classification of data synonymous?
    a. Yes b. No
    c. Cannot say d. Exchangeably used in parlance
32. The criterion of chronological classification is:
    a. Region b. Characteristic of units
    c. Time-period d. All of the above
33. Class interval in a grouped data is:
    a. The difference between highest and lowest value in a data set
    b. Half of the difference between upper and lower limits of a class
    c. Difference between upper and lower limit of a class
    d. Average of the upper and lower limit of a class.
34. A complete two way table consists of:
    a. Eight parts b. Seven parts
    c. Six parts d. Five parts
35. If the individual can be divided into two categories only, then such a classification is known as:
    a. Unique b. Dichotomous
    c. Manifold d. Multiple

CHAPTER 3

Diagramatic and Graphical Presentation of Data

DIAGRAMS

Statistics deals with numerical values which are mostly in huge number and scattered. These values are well understood by an expert. But a common man can not extract information contained in them. Even for an educated person, it is not easy to grasp the data as such. Hence, diagramatic presentation of data is a proper approach. There is an adage, "a picture is worth thousand words". So is true with diagrams. A diagram clearly depicts the existing situations. Further they are attractive, easily understandable, better memorizable and comparable. Diagams suffer from certain lacunae as given below.

1. They are meant for comparison only.
2. They give only an approximate idea.
3. Three dimensional diagrams are complicated to understand.
4. They do not reveal small differences.
5. Their construction is time consuming and costly.

Bar Diagram

This type of diagram can be used for any series of data given either for places or periods. But it is especially suitable for categorical data. For example, to show consumption of milk in different cities, to display the population of different states, to depict the production of steel in different steel plants, etc.

Following points be kept in mind while constructing a bar diagram.

1. Bar is a rectangle of small width.
2. All bars should be of equal width and should rest on the same line or axis except in some special cases.
3. For drawing a bar diagram, use of graph paper should be preferred.
4. Categories be taken on a horizontal line (x-axis) at equal distances for vertical bars and vice-versa. The distance between bars be such that no two bars should touch or overlap each other.

5. The bar should be erected by choosing a proper scale on Y-axis so as the variation is displayed most effectively.
6. The scale caption and index be given on top of the bar diagram.
7. Vertical bars be arranged from left to right in order of categories.

There are many types of bar diagrams, namely simple bar, sub-divided bar, percentage bar diagram, etc. Only first three will be described hereunder through examples.

Simple Bar Diagram

A simple bar is a one-dimensional diagram in which the height of bar represents the magnitude of a category. Bars are generally filled with colours or some patterns of line segments or dots so that the diagrams become eye catching.

Example 3.1. Production of all grains in million tonnes from 1979-80 to 1985-86, i.e. for seven years, was as follows:

Years :	1979-80	1980-81	1981-82	1982-83	1983-84	1984-85	1985-86
Production: (Mn.Tonnes)	109.7	129.6	133.3	129.5	152.4	145.5	150.5

The production data can be very well displayed by a simple bar diagram taking years on X-axis and production along Y=axis. Figure 3.1 shows a simple bar diagram taking the scale as 20 Mn.T = 1 cm.

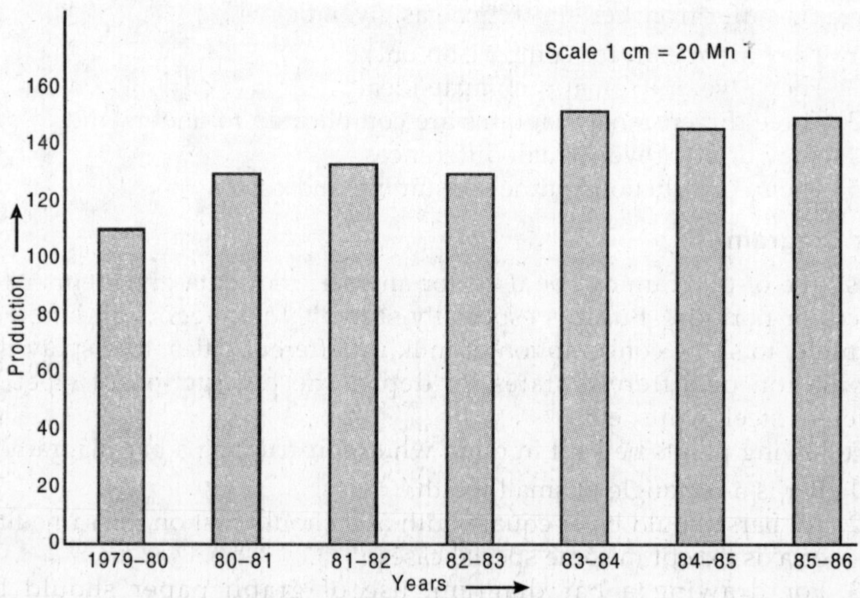

Fig. 3.1: Simple bar diagram

Figure 3.1 clearly shows that the production boosted up in the year 1980-81 and remained almost the same for three years. Again there was a jump in 1983-84. In the year 1984-85, the production went down slighly and there was a marginal increase in the subsequent year and so on.

Sub-divided bar diagram

In this type of diagram, a bar depicts information about various components of a bar itself. The height of bar is divided into sub-divisions in proportion to the magnitude of the components. It should be remembered that the same scale is to be maintained for all bars and its components and further the order of the components within all bars should remain the same. Each portion of a bar be filled with different colours or patterns to depict each component distinctly. This makes the diagram attractive as well.

Example 3.2. The data regarding rabi and kharif components of production of all food grains (Mn. Tonnes) in India are given below.

	Years						
Seasons	1979-80	80-81	81-82	82-83	83-84	84-85	85-86
Rabi food grains	46.45	51.95	53.92	59.60	63.14	61.00	64.00
Kharif food grains	63.25	77.65	79.38	69.90	89.26	84.50	86.00
Total	109.70	129.60	133.30	129.50	152.40	145.50	150.50

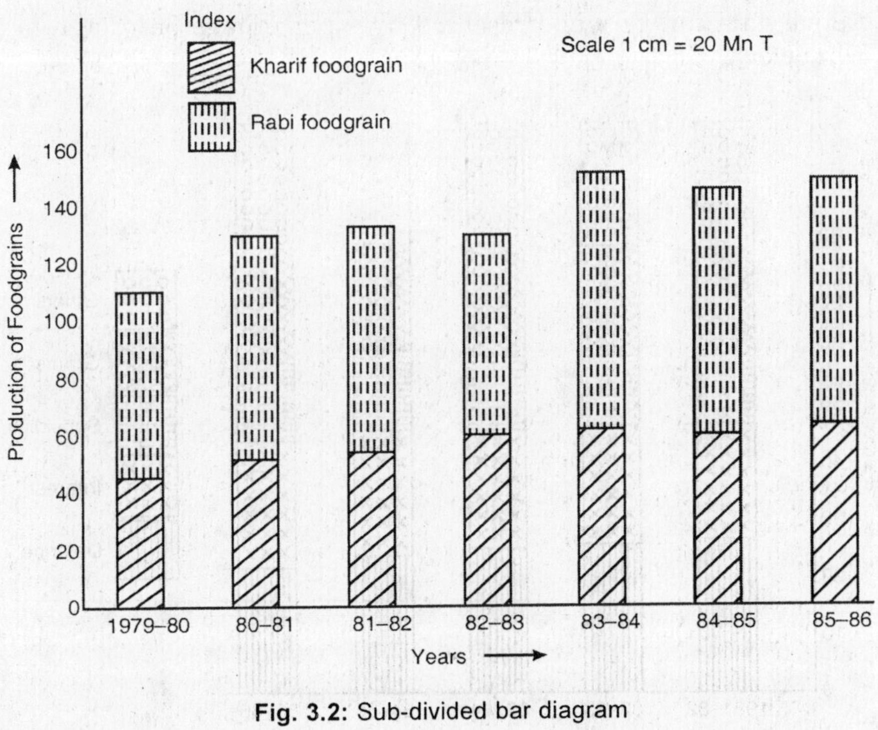

Fig. 3.2: Sub-divided bar diagram

In Fig. 3.2, it is easy to compare the food grain production of rabi and kharif reasons within years and also between years.

PERCENTAGE BAR DIAGRAM

The distribution of aggregate of a category into its components can effectively be presented on percentage basis. Such diagrams are especially useful when relative changes in the magnitudes of components are to be highlighted. A bar can be divided into any number of segments. In the example 3.2, there are only two components. But for percentage bar diagram, an example is chosen which have five components.

Example 3.3. The percentages of central goverment's revenue expenditure on five major heads were as follows.

Years	*Percentage of Expenditure*				
	Defence	*Interest*	*Subsidies*	*Grants*	*Others*
1981 – 82	27.0	20.7	12.0	18.5	21.8
1982 – 83	26.0	21.0	12.0	19.4	21.6
1983 – 84	25.6	21.7	12.4	19.9	20.4
1984 – 85	23.7	22.1	13.9	19.3	21.0
1985 – 86	22.1	21.9	14.1	21.4	20.5

Above data can be well presented by a percentage bar diagram as shown below.

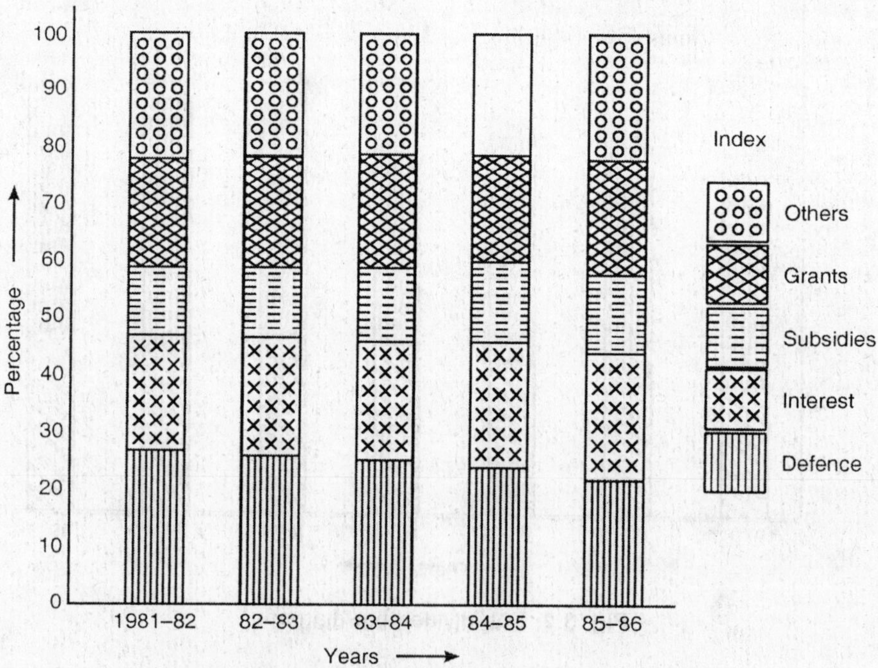

Fig. 3.3: Percentage sub-divided bar diagram

From the above diagram, percentage of expenditure under various heads are conveniently comparable.

HISTOGRAM

This type of diagram is also a kind of bar diagram and is suitable for frequency distributions with continuous class intervals. In this diagram, class intervals are taken on the X-axis (Abscissa) and the heights of bars in proportion to the frequency of the classes are taken along Y-axis (Ordinate) by choosing an appropritе scale. Histogram differs from a bar diagram in three ways.

1. In a histogram one bar touches the next bar, but never overlap each other.
2. Height of a bar represents the frequency of its class.
3. The width of the bar is equal to the class interval.

This is obvious that number of bars is equal to the number of classes. The bars are filled with colours or pattern to make the diagram fascinating.

Example 3.4. A continuous frequency distribution of marks of 50 students with a class interval of 10 marks is given below:

Classes	*Frequency*
0 – 10	4
10 – 20	9
20 – 30	10
30 – 40	6
40 – 50	8
50 – 60	9
60 – 70	3
70 – 80	1

The above distribution of marks is very well displayed through a histogram given in the Fig. 3.4 (on next page).

Histogram with varying Base Length

In a histogram, the rectangle (bars) are generally erected on bases of same width equal to the class intervals. In this situtaion, the heights of the bars are enough to compare the class frequencies. But in many cases, it is not possible to take all classes of equal width. To illustrate, consider the distribution of monthly wages of workers as given in Fig. 3.4.

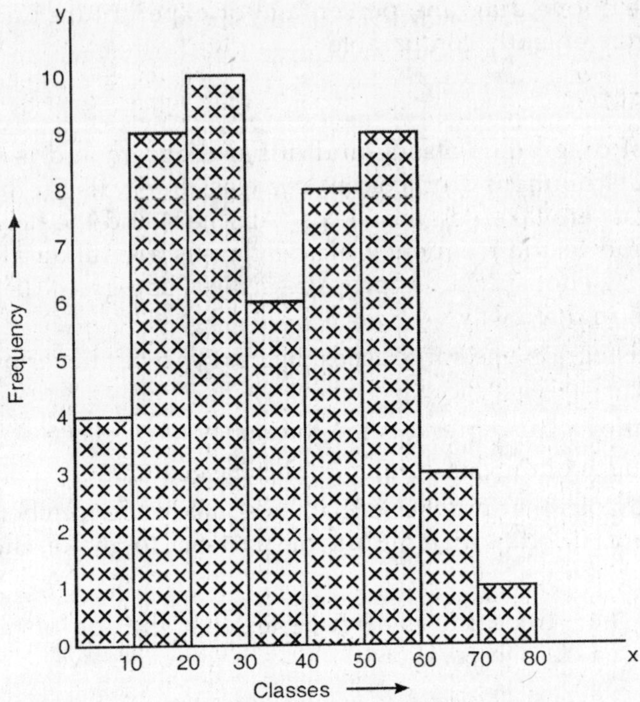

Fig. 3.4: Histogram

Wages/month	*Class width*	*No. of workers*	*Active frequencies*
75 – 100	25	8	8/25 = 0.32
100 – 125	25	12	12/25 = 0.48
125 – 150	25	25	25/25 = 1.00
150 – 175	25	30	30/25 = 1.20
175 – 225	50	8	8/50 = 0.16
225 – 300	75	4	4/75 = 0.053
300 – 400	100	3	3/100 = 0.03

Looking to the above distribution, it is easy to reckon that if one takes constant class intervals of Rs. 25 for all classes, then the classes after the wages of Rs 175, a large number of classes will have zero frequency. Therefore, it is preferable to have classes with unequal class intervals. In this case heights of bars can not be the criterion for comparison, instead the areas of the rectangle are comparable. In case of unequal classes, one has to work out the active frequencies. The formula for calculating the active frequency is,

$$\text{Active frequency} = \frac{\text{Frequency of the class}}{\text{Corresponding class width}} \qquad (3.1)$$

Active frequencies are worked out and shown in the last column of the above frequency distribution. Active frequency is often called the *density* per unit class internal.

Example 3.5. The histogram for the frequency distribution given in theory is drawn with class intervals and corresponding active frequencies. The same is displayed below.

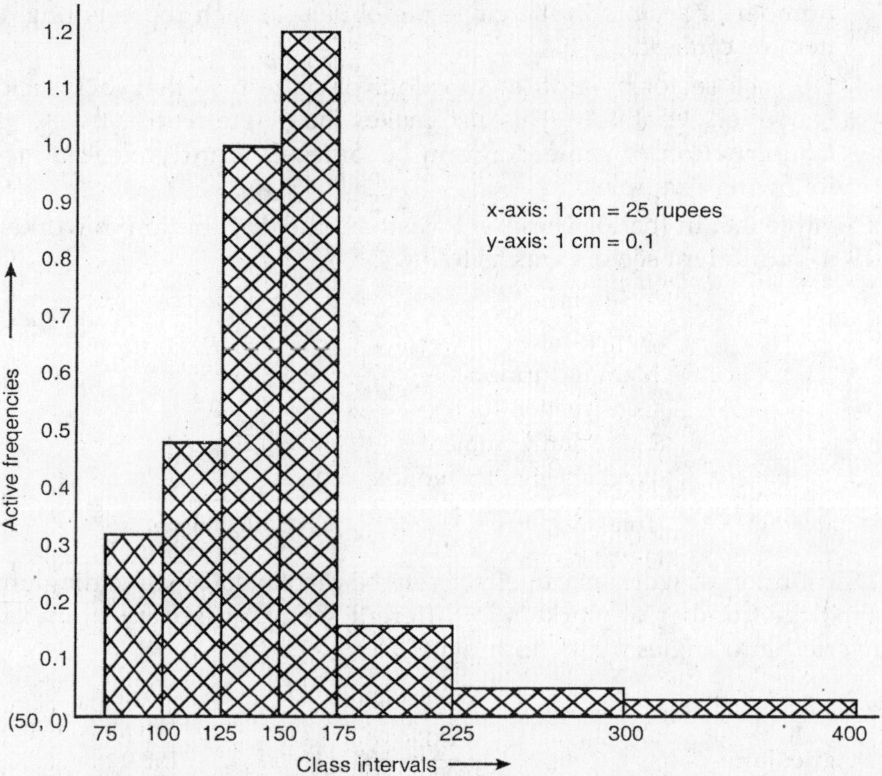

Fig. 3.5: Histogram width unequal class internals

Pie diagram

It is circular diagram. A pie diagram is also known as **angular** or **sector diagram**. In this diagram, a circle is divided into as many sectors as the number of items. So each sector represents an item. This diagram can be used for data as well as percentage.

The method of constructing a pie diagrams is as follows:

1. Draw a circle of proper size.
2. Divide 360° angle of the circle into components such that angle for each components is proportional to the value of that category to which the sector is going to represent. The formula for this is,

$$\text{(Intemized)Angle} = \frac{\text{Category value}}{\text{Sum of all values}} \times 360 \qquad (3.2)$$

or $$\text{Itemwise angle} = \frac{\text{Percentage of the item}}{100} \times 360 \qquad (3.3)$$

Note: It should always be checked that the sum of the intewise angles is 360.

3. Draw a radius in the circle. Make angles one after the other for each category starting from this radius. In this way, the required number of sectors in the circle are obtained, each representing an item or category.
4. Fill each sector by a different colour or pattern so that each sector is marked separately. This also makes the diagram attractive.

Construction of a pie-diagram becomes evidently clear by the following examples.

Example 3.6. In Jhadol Thesil of Rajasthan, the distribution of workers in 1991 in different sectors was as follows:

Sectors	*No. of workers*
Agriculture	4390
Manufacturing	1285
Construction	380
Trade and Commerce	2095
Workers in other services	1850
Total	10,000

Distribution of workers can effectively be displayed by a pie diagram.

First the number of workers in different sectors are proportionately converted into angles by the formula (3.2).

Sectors	*Calculation*	*Angle*
Agriculture	$\frac{4390}{10000} \times 360$	158.04
Manufacturing	$\frac{1285}{10000} \times 360$	46.26
Construction	$\frac{380}{10000} \times 360$	13.68
Trade and Commerce	$\frac{2095}{10000} \times 360$	75.42
Workers in other services	$\frac{1850}{10000} \times 360$	66.60
	Total	360.00

Now pie diagram from the worked out angles is constructed as per procedure and exhibited below.

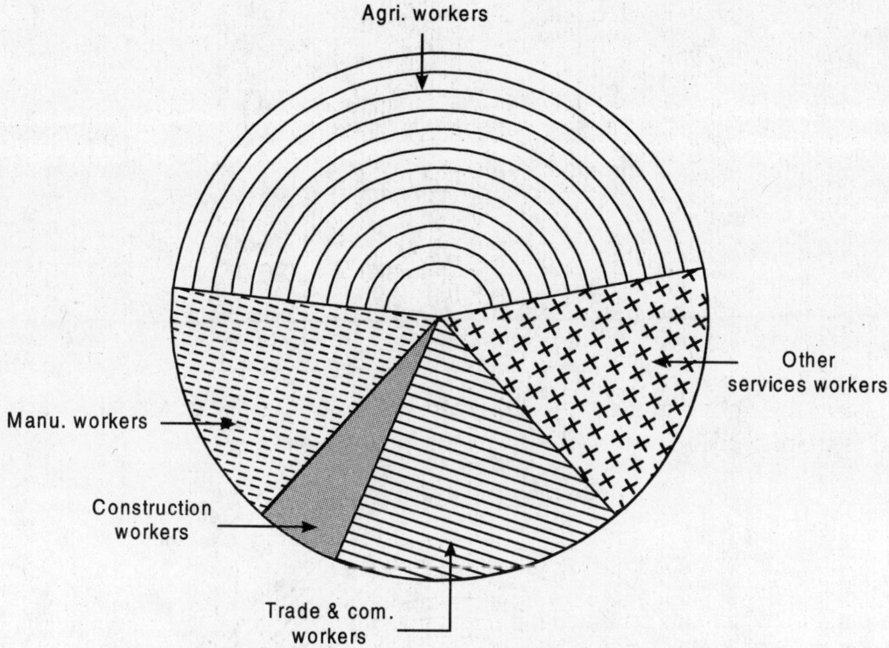

Fig. 3.6: Pie diagram for number for workers

Example 3.7. Per cent expenditure of government of India in a year on different items is as follows:

Item	*Per cent expenditure*
1. General Public Services	20.2
2. Defence	27.4
3. Education	21.7
4. Health	4.2
5. Housing	2.6
6. Economic Services	17.8
7. Others	6.1
Total	100.0

The pattern of expenditure can be displayed by a pie diagram in a nice way. First divide the percentages into angles by the formula (3.3) for each item.

Item No.	*Angles*
1.	$\frac{20.2}{100} \times 360 = 72.7$
2.	$\frac{27.4}{100} \times 360 = 98.6$
3.	$\frac{21.7}{100} \times 360 = 78.1$

4.	$\frac{4.2}{100} \times 360 =$	15.1
5.	$\frac{2.6}{100} \times 360 =$	9.4
6.	$\frac{17.8}{100} \times 360 =$	64.1
7.	$\frac{6.1}{100} \times 360 =$	22.0
	Total	360.00

Using the above angles, pie diagram is drawn by the given procedure and is displayed below.

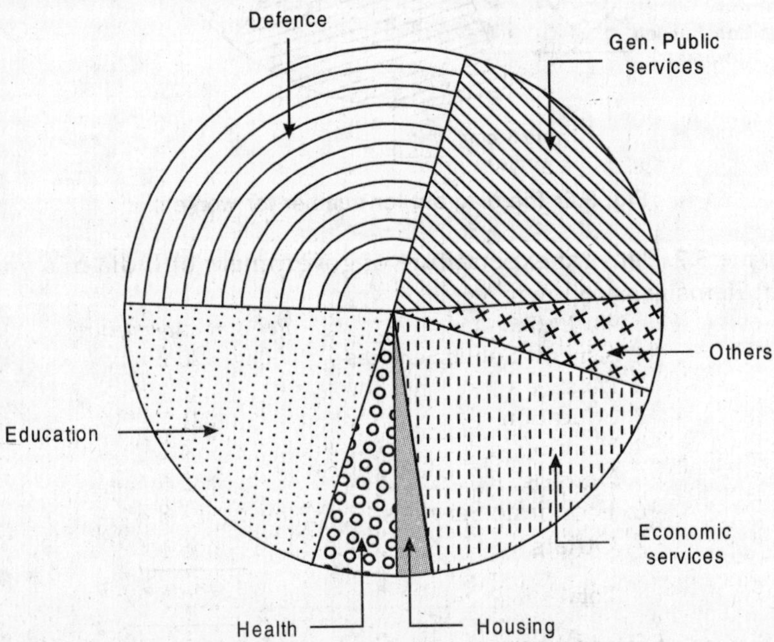

Fig. 3.7: Pie chart for percentage expenditure

GRAPHS

It is a representation of the values of a variable in relation to the values of the other variable through lines. Graphs differ from diagrams in respect of the following points.

1. Diagram can be drawn on the plain paper whereas the graphs are drawn only on graph paper.
2. Diagrams are attractive whereas graphs are not.

3. Diagrams simply show a situation whereas graphs reflect the mathematical relationship between two variables.
4. More than one graph can be drawn on the same graph paper but only one diagram can possibly be made at a time.
5. Graphs can be used for interpolation and extrapolation of vaues which is not possible in case of diagrams.

METHOD OF MAKING A GRAPH

Take a graph paper and draw two straight line which intersect each other perpendicularly almost in the middle. The point of intersection of these two lines is taken as **origin**. These two lines are called **axes**. The horizontal line is known as **X-axis** or **Abscissa** and vertical line is called **Y-axis** or **Ordinate**. All distances are measured from origin. The distances to the right side of origin on X-axis and in upward direction on Y-axis are taken to be positive. On the contrary, the distances to left of origin on X-axis and downward on Y-axis are taken to be negative. In this way, the axes divide the graph paper into four parts. Each part is known as **quadrant**. The perpendicular distance of a point in a quadrant from Y-axis is called its x-coordinate whereas from X-axis is called Y-coordinate. The location of a point is marked by the coordinates written as (x, y). x and y coordinate take positive or negative values depending on their location and vice-versa.

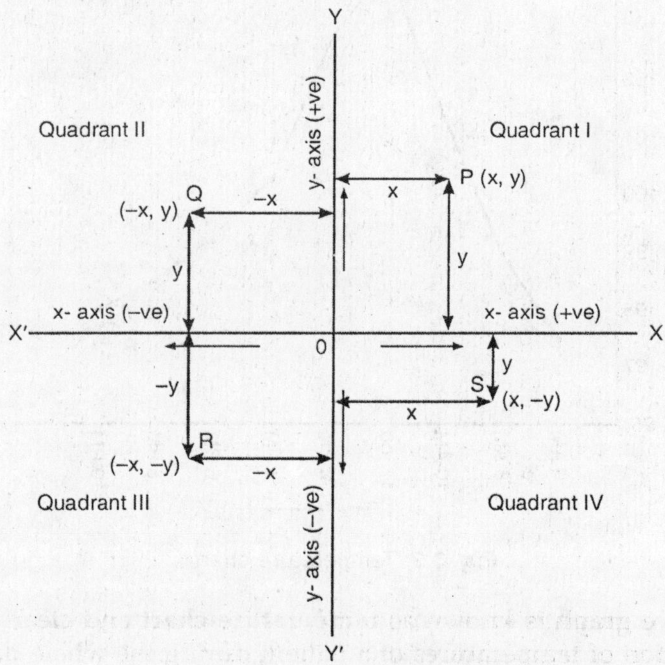

Fig. 3.8: Sketch of quadrants

For making a graph, points are plotted taking the paired values of two variables under consideration. Then these points are joined in sequence by the line segments. The resulting figure is called a graph. Four quadrants and coordinates of points in these four quadrants are shown in the Fig. 3.8.

Note: Also it is important to remember that the independent variate values are always taken along X-axis and dependent variate values along Y-axis.

Example 3.8. In a nursing home, the temperature of a typhoid patient was recorded at every two hours gap from 6 A.M. to 10 P.M. The temperature was as follows:

Time:	6 AM	8AM	10AM	12.00AM	2PM	4PM	6PM	8PM	10PM
Temperature: (°F)	97.5	99.0	101.4	104.0	102.6	100.3	99.2	98.5	98.0

In hospital system, temperatures are recorded on a graph as shown below.

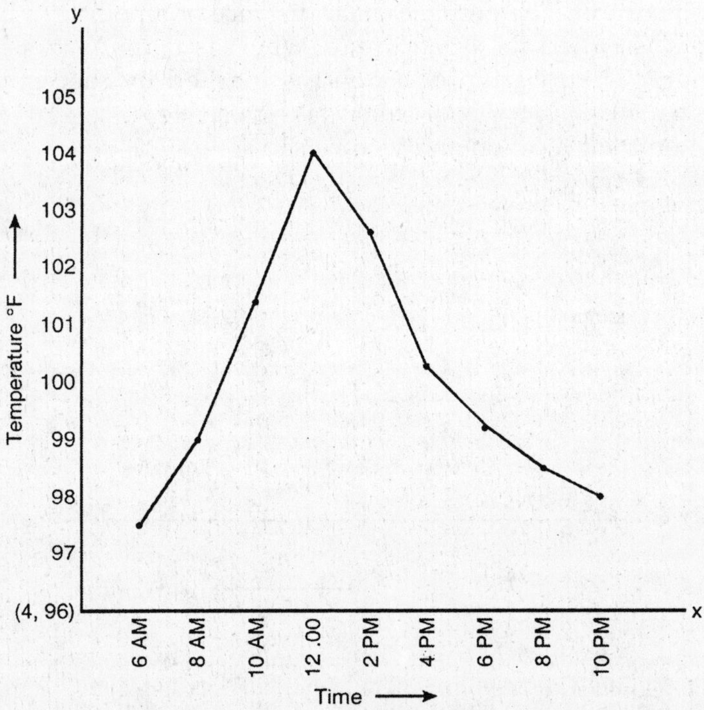

Fig. 3.9: Temperature chart

The above graph is known as **temperature chart** and clearly depicts the fluctuation of temperatures of a patient during the whole day.

Example 3.9. Infant mortality rate per thousand live births from 1982-1989 in rural and urban areas are given below.

Periods	*Rural*	*Urban*
1982	114	65
1983	114	66
1984	113	66
1985	107	59
1986	105	62
1987	104	61
1988	102	62
1989	98	58

Above data pertaining to rural and urban infant mortality can be effectively displayed on a graph paper for comparative study. Here two graphs will be drawn on the same paper with the same scale, one for mortality rate in rural areas and another in urban areas.

Taking origin as (1981, 50) and scales as 1 year = 1 cm and 10 mortalities = 1 cm, thc graph is displayed below.

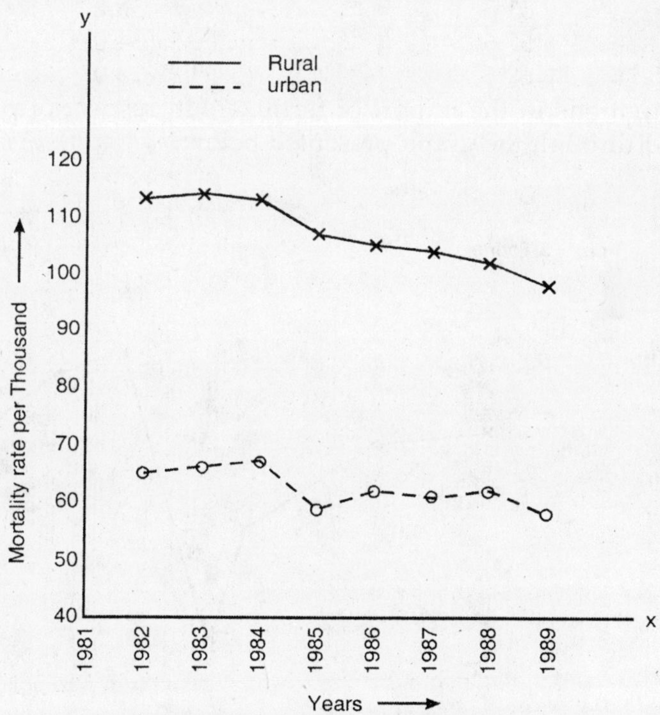

Fig. 3.10: Mortality rates in rural and urban areas

From the above graph, it is easy to conclude that

1. The mortality rate in urban area is much lower than rural areas as the whole graph for urban areas lies below the rural area graph.

2. The variation in mortality rate in all the years in both type of populations is very small.

Two factor graphs

In the preceding two examples, one factor is time and another factor is a variable. Now consider another type of graphs in which one wants to know the type of relationship between the two variables. For example, the type of relation between height and weight of person, import and export, input and output cost, birth and death rates, temperature and evaporation, etc. can be presented by a graph.

Example 3.10. The data regarding production and imports of fertilizers in lac Tonnes from 1979-80 to 1986-87 are given below.

Production (Lac Tonnes)	*Imports (Lac Tonnes)*
28.8	20.0
30.0	27.6
40.9	20.4
44.0	11.3
45.3	13.6
51.8	36.2
57.6	34.0
69.5	25.0

The fluctuations in the import of fertilizers in respect of production are depicted through the graph presented below.

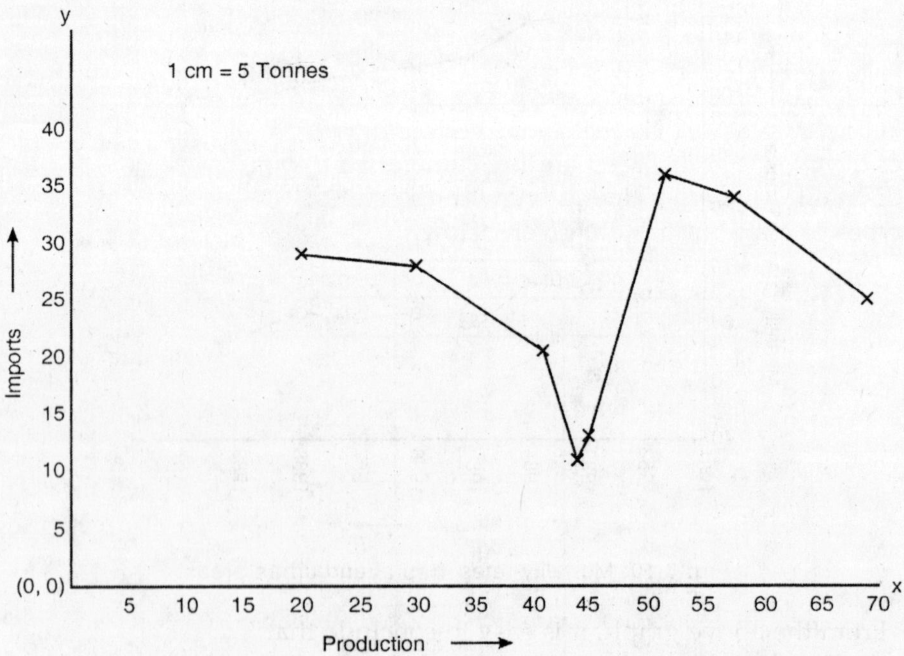

Fig. 3.11: Graph between imports and production

Cumulative frequency graph

A graph for variate values and their cumulative frequencies is a curve of elongated shape. This curve is known as **Ogive**. To construct a graph, plot the points for variate values and their corresponding cumulative frequencies. Join these points in order by free hand smooth curve. The S-shaped curve so obtained is a cumulative frequency curve. This curve can be drawn for less than type as well as more than type distributions. For a more than type distribution, the shape of the curve is that of elongated laterally inverted S, i.e. the cumulative frequency curve for less than type is of S shape.

Example 3.11. Following table gives the frequency and cumulative frequency distributions of weights of family members in a locality for more than type as well as less than type.

More than type			*Less than type*		
Weight (Kg)	*Frequency*	*Type Cumulative frequency*	*Weight (Kg)*	*Frequency*	*Cumulative Frequency*
90–100	2	2	0–10	1	1
80–90	3	5	10–20	2	3
70–80	4	9	20–30	6	9
60–70	8	17	30–40	22	31
50–60	20	37	40–50	31	62
40–50	31	68	50–60	20	82
30–40	22	90	60–70	8	90
20–30	6	96	70–80	4	94
10–20	2	98	80–90	3	97
0–10	1	99	90–100	2	99

The cumulative frequency curves are drawn by taking the mid-points of the classes and corresponding cumulative frequencies of both types of distributions. Mid-values alongwith the cumulative frequencies for both types of distributions are given below.

More than type		*Less than type*	
Mid-points	*cu.freq.*	*Mid-points*	*cu. freq*
95	2	5	1
85	5	15	3
75	9	25	9
65	17	35	31
55	37	45	62
45	68	55	82
35	90	65	90
25	96	75	94
15	98	85	97
5	99	95	99

Graph is drawn by taking the variate values on the X-axis and cumulative frequencies along Y-axis and presented below.

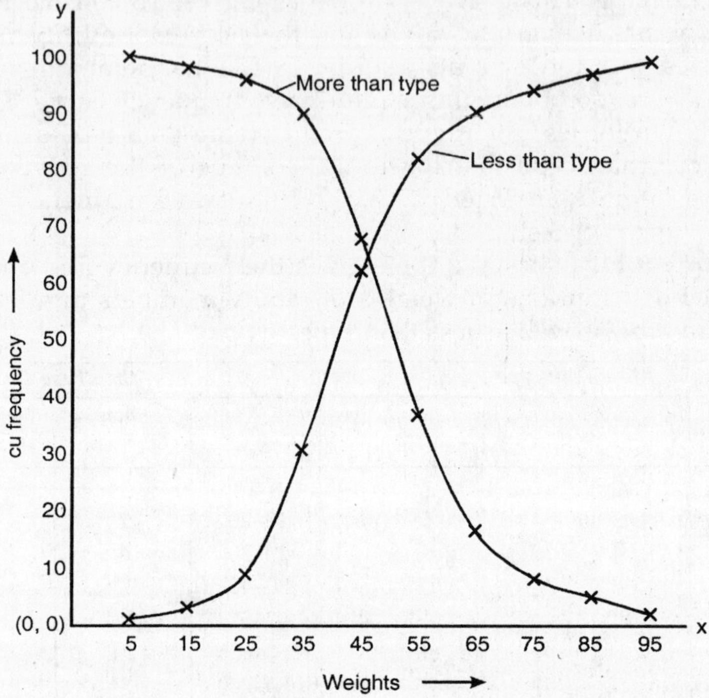

Fig. 3.12: Cumulative frequency or Ogive curves

FREQUENCY POLYGON

A frequency distribution can be represented by a **frequency polygon**. Obviously, a many sided closed figure is called a polygon. A frequency polygon can be constructed by two methods as discussed below.

1. **With the help of histograms:** Draw a histogram for a (grouped) continuous frequency distribution. Mark the mid points of the upper side of the rectangles erected on the class intervals. Join these mid points by straight lines in order of rectangles. The mid-points located at the first and last rectangles are joined with the mid-points of the extended class intervals on X-axis to the left of the first class interval and to the right of the last class interval respectively. The graph so obtained is a frequency polygon.

Example 3.12. Frequency polygon is constructed for the following grouped distribution of age.

Age (years)	*No. of persons*
10 – 20	4
20 – 30	11
30 – 40	15
40 – 50	18
50 – 60	12
60 – 70	10
70 – 80	3

Frequency polygon is drawn in the manner described in theory and shown below.

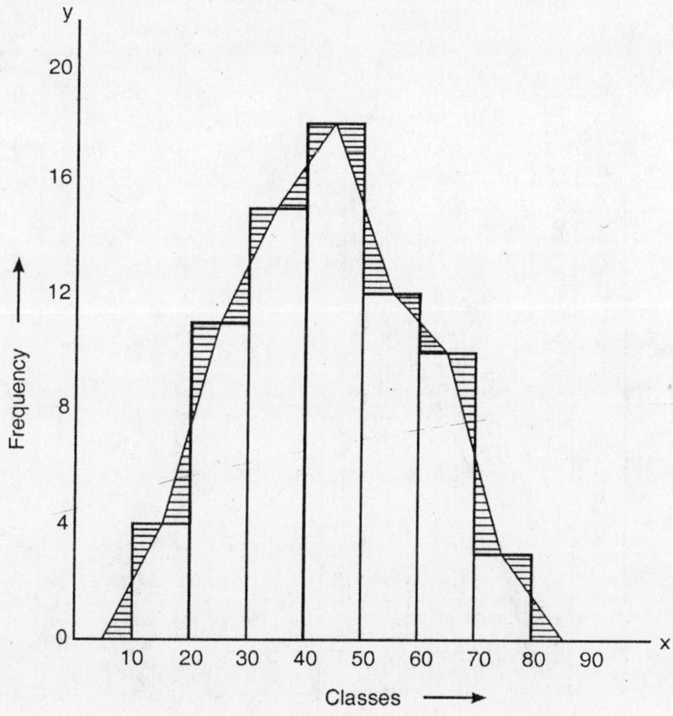

Fig. 3.13: Frequency polygon from histogram

The shaded area is shown in the figure for use hereafter. Frequency polygon is the eight sided closed diagram without rectangles and shaded areas in the graph 3.13.

BY PLOTTING THE POINTS

In this method, no histogram is constructed. Instead the mid-points of the class intervals and corresponding frequencies are plotted directly.

The plotted points are joined by line segments in order. The first and last points are joined to the mid-values of the extended class intervals on the x-axis. The figure so obtained is a frequency polygon.

Frequency Curve

A smoothened frequency polygon is called a frequency curve.

Example 3.13. The frequency distribution of the mid-values of class intervals of the example 3.12 is given below and frequency polygon is constructed.

Mid-values	*Frequency*
15	4
25	11
35	15
45	18
55	12
65	10
75	3

Frequency polygon is drawn and displayed below.

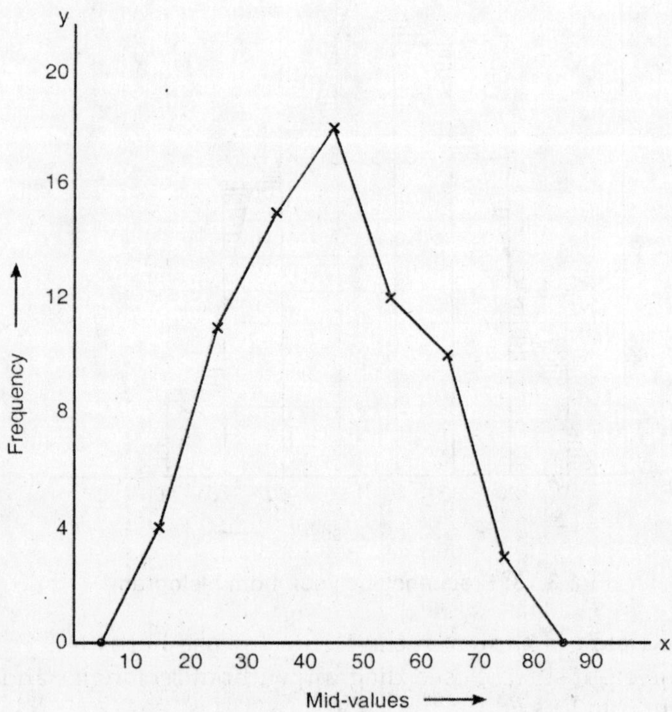

Fig. 3.14: Frequency polygon from mid-values

Frequency polygon in Fig. 3.14 is same as in Fig. 3.13.

PRACTICE QUESTIONS AND EXERCISES

1. Discus the role of diagrams in statistics.
2. What procedure will you adopt in constructing a graph.
3. Discuss the following adequately:

   a. Bar diagram b. Sub-divided bar diagram
   c. Ogive curve d. Histogram
   e. Pie chart

4. Data below give the production of rice in India from 1988 to 1992. Display the data by a bar diagram.

Years	1988	1989	1990	1991	1992
Production (Million Tonnes)	56.9	70.5	73.5	74.3	73.7

5. Following table gives the production of four crops (in Million Tonnes) in India for four years.

Food Grains	*Years*			
	1982-83	*1983-84*	*1984-85*	*1985-86*
	Production (Mn. Tonnes)			
Rice	47	66	58	64
Wheat	43	45	44	47
Pulses	12	13	12	13
Oilseeds	10	13	13	11

Construct a sub-divided bar diagram.

6. Following table gives the percentages of Boys and girls in five schools.

	Schools				
	A	B	C	D	E
	Percentage				
Boys :	67	55	70	45	50
Girls :	33	45	30	55	50

Prepare a percentage bar diagram.

7. Given the age and weight of six persons, draw a graph between age and weight.

Age (years)	*Weights (kg)*
5	15
7	18
10	22
14	35
16	42
19	50

8. Given the following frequency distribution, draw a cumulative frequency diagram (Ogive curve) for less than type distribution.

x :	7.5	9.5	12.5	16.5	20.5	25.5
f :	4	8	14	13	7	3

9. Following table gives the percentage of consumption of three types of fertilizers during the year 1986-87.

Type of fertilizer	*Percentage*
Nitrogenous	66
Phosphatic	24
Potassic	10

Draw a pie diagram.

10. The distribution of marks of students of a class in continuous group distribution is given below. Construct a histogram and a frequency polygon.

Groups of marks	*No. of students*
0 – 10	3
10 – 20	6
20 – 30	8
30 – 40	14
40 – 50	22
50 – 60	16
60 – 70	7
70 – 80	4

11. Population of India during 1976 to 1981 is as follows:

Years	*Population in Millions*
1976	612
1977	626
1978	640
1979	655
1980	670
1981	685

Display the data by a bar diagram.

12. Differentiate between a diagram and a graph.
13. What are the special features of a sub-divided bar diagram?
14. When should a percentage bar diagram be used?
15. What does a Frequency polygon represents?
16. Discuss a frequency polygon.
17. Total deaths due to various diseases in the years 1988 and 1989 are as follows:

Diseases	*1988*	*1989*
Asthm & Bronchitis	2097	1885
Heart attack	1261	1236
Pneumonia	1204	1190
T.B. of lungs	1222	1106
Cancer	654	685
Anemia	697	677
Others	865	721
Total	8000	7500

Prepare a sub-divided bar diagram to be displayed in public interest.

18. The table presents the pulse rate and systolic blood pressure of ten patients at rest.

Patient No.	*Pulse rate per minute*	*Blood pressure mm*
1.	70	127
2.	68	136
3.	74	139
4.	75	143
5.	73	136
6.	74	145
7.	69	136
8.	73	133
9.	76	140
10.	68	126

Draw a graph between blood pressure and pulse rate to show the relationship between them.

OBJECTIVE TYPE QUESTIONS

Select the best choice out of four choices for the given statement or question.

19. A diagram is an alternative display of:
    a. Tabulated data b. Comparitive statement of data
    c. Frequency distribution d. All of the above
20. Most suitable diagram for periodic display of data is:
    a. Pic-chart b. Sub-divided bar diagram
    c. Bar diagram d. A graph
21. Different expenditure under various heads on year basis can best be depicted by:
    a. Bar diagram b. Sub-divided bar diagram
    c. Histogram d. Frequency polygon
22. Consumption of electricity in different sectors can better be represented by:
    a. Pic-chart b. Bar diagram
    c. Component bar diagram d. All of the above
23. A frequency distribution of a variable can properly be shown by:
    a. Frequency polygon b. A simple graph
    c. Ogive curve d. None of the above
24. A cumulative frequency curve is called:
    a. Pic-chart b. Ogive curve
    c. Frequency curve d. Frequency polygon
25. Divided component bar chart is used for:
    a. Comparing various components of a variable.
    b. Comparing frequencies of variate values
    c. Showing the relation between variables
    d. None of the above

26. Diagrams are capable of providing:
    a. An exact idea of data
    b. An exact idea of minute differences
    c. Pictures for any number of variables
    d. None of the above
27. Grouped data are diagramatically presented by:
    a. Bar diagram b. Histogram
    c. Simple graph d. Pictogram
28. Most attractive technique of data presentation is:
    a. Diagramatic b. Tabular
    c. Textual d. All of the above
29. Most accurate way of data presentation is:
    a. Diagramatic b. Textual
    c. Tabular d. None of the above
30. Which of the following statements does not hold true in case of tabulation?
    a. Tabulation is the basis of statistical analysis.
    b. Tabulation in required to simplify data.
    c. To compare row data with column data.
    d. To understand better the salient features of data.

CHAPTER 4

Statistical Central Values

PREAMBLE

In statistics one is to deal with large number of values in general. To draw any conclusion about the units to which the values represent is not straight forward. For instance, a factory has 800 employees. If a person wants to give a statement about the salaries of all employes, it is not possible to remember the salary of each individual. Hence, it is considered fit to know a central value which represents the salary of all workers. Let the total monthly salary of 800 workers be Rs. 5,60 ,000. Thus, the average salary per worker is 5,60,000 ÷ 800, i.e. Rs 700 per month. So one can easily understand that most of the workers get around Rs 700 per month.

As another example, there is a need to report which class is better than the other. Students secure diferent marks in all the classes. So it is not possible to say as such which class is better than the other. But it seems appropriate to find average marks of each class. Suppose the average marks of three sections A, B, C of class IX in a school are 67, 72 and 54 respectively. From these values, one can easily conclude that section B is better than sections A and C. Also section A is better than C. This gives an idea that an average can represent the whole mass or population which makes possible to draw conclusions about them.

Three statements given by renowned statisticians are quoted below which throw light on the importance and utility of averages.

1. **R. A. Fisher:** The inherent inability of the human mind to grasp in its entirely a large body of numerical data, compels us to seek relatively few constants that will adequately describe the data.
2. **Moroney** (Facts from figures): The purpose of an average is to represent a group of individual values in a simple and concise manner so that the mind can get a quick understanding of general size of the individuals in the group.
3. **Croxton and cowden:** An average is a simple value within the range of the data that is used to represent all the values in the series since an average is somewhere within the range of the data, it is sometimes called a measure of central values.

USES OF STATISTICAL AVERAGES

1. **An average is a concised statement:** It represents a complicated group of observations in a simple manner. A large number of values are reduced to one value which can easily be remembered and in a broad sense it represents the whole mass.
2. **Easy for comparison:** In case of more than one series of items, they can not be compared as such. But if one finds the average of each series, the averages can easily be compared and conclusion can be drawn which series is better than the other. For example, it is easy to say that the average age of people in America is more than in India. One can not say so without statistical basis. But if one knows that average life of a person in America is 71 years while in India it is 62 years, then it is justified to say that Americans live longer in general than people in India.
3. **A basis for interpretation of data:** In a series of data, each item has its own measure which differs from each other. So on the basis of these values nothing can be stated. But on getting an average value, an interpretation can be given. For instance, the ages of five students of class VII are, 10, 11, 12, 14 and 18.
   No comment can be made on the basis of this data. Anyhow on getting an average age, i.e. $65 \div 5 = 13$ years, it can be inferred that on an average, 13 year old children study in class seventh.
4. **Basis for decision making:** An average can be a logical basis for taking decisions. For instance, the postal department can decide about opening a post office in a locality if the numbers of letters delivered per day on an average in that locality fulfils the minimum requirement.
   Stoppage of a train at a railway station depends on the average number of passengers boarding the train and getting down from it. Above examples clearly show that an average is a basis for making decision.
5. **Usefulness in industry:** An average like **mode** (discussed later) makes possible for a manufacturer to know which size of an item is most required.
   So on the basis of such an information he produces items of that size in greater number. It is known that the shoes of size 7 mostly fit to the people. Naturally a shoe manufacturer will produce shoes of No. 7 in larger number than other shoe sizes.
   As another example, a garment making factory manufactures clothes of average sizes so that they fit to most of the people.
6. **Another important measure of central values is median** (discussed ahead). It is a very useful measure because median can be found out in cases where measurements are not quantified such as health, intelligence, etc. It is frequently used in socialogical studies.

Properties of a good average

1. It must be rigidly defined. It means that an average is defined in such a way that anybody calculating it, gets the same value.
2. An average should be based on all observations. If one or more values are not involved in calculating it, then it will not be a good representative of the entire data.
3. It should be easily understandable.
4. Its calcuation must be simple.
5. It must be useable in further statistical formulae.

CENTRAL TENDENCY MEASURES FOR UNGROUPED DATA

This section covers the following central values, namely, i. Arithmetic mean or Average, ii. Geometric mean iii. Harmonic mean iv. Median, v. Quartiles, vi. Mode.

ARITHMETIC MEAN OR AVERAGE (AM)

It is a most popular type of average. When one talks of an average or mean, it means that he is concerned with arithmetic mean.

Definition:

Arithmetic mean of a finite number of values of individual items is a single value obtained by dividing the sum of values by the number of values.

Let the marks of five students be 42, 55, 38, 69 and 74. Here the sum of marks is 278 and number of students is 5. Thus, the average of marks is 278 ¸ 5, i.e. 55.6.

Formula for arithmetic mean is,

$$\text{A.M.} = \frac{\text{Sum of values}}{\text{Number of values}} \qquad (4.1)$$

If $X_1, X_2, ..., X_N$ are N values, then

$$\bar{X} = \frac{\Sigma_i X_i}{N} \qquad (4.1.1)$$

for $i = 1, 2, ..., N$.

Where,

Σ – Stands for summation
$\Sigma_i X_i$ – Sum of values
N – Number of values
$\bar{X}$ – Mean of values.

Example 4.1. The birth weight of eight babies in kilograms are, 2.4, 2.8, 3.2, 1.9, 2.7, 4.2, 3.8, 2.2.

The average birth weight of babies by the formula 4.1 is,

$$\bar{X} = \frac{2.4 + 2.8 + 3.2 + 1.9 + 2.7 + 4.2 + 3.8 + 2.2}{8}$$

$$= \frac{23.2}{8} = 2.9 \text{ kg.}$$

ARITHMETIC MEAN IN CASE OF FREQUENCY DISTRIBUTION

If the data are given or arranged in the form of frequency distribution, the average value of the character under study can be obtained as follows:

i. Multiply each value by its corresponding frequency.
ii. Calculate the sum of the cross products obtained in step i.
iii. Find the sum of all frequencies.
iv. Divide the sum of cross products by the total of frequencies. The value so obtained is the average (A.M.).

Following the above steps, the formula for arithmetic mean is as given below:

Values (X)	*Frequency* (*f*)	*Cross Product* (*f*X)
X_1	f_1	f_1X_1
X_2	f_2	f_2X_2
$\vdots$	$\vdots$	$\vdots$
X_K	f_K	f_KX_K
Total	$\Sigma_i f_i$	$\Sigma_i f_i X_i$

The arithmetic mean,

$$\overline{X} = \frac{\Sigma_i f_i X_i}{\Sigma_i f_i} \qquad (4.2)$$

for $i = 1, 2, K$.

Example 4.2. The frequency distribution of marks in a test (out of ten) in mathematics of class X is given below.

Marks gained (X)	*No. of students* (*f*)
2.0	2
3.5	4
4.5	7
5.5	8
6.0	4
7.5	2
8.0	1
9.5	2
	30

Average marks of the class by the formula (4.2) can be worked out in the following manner.

First calculate $\Sigma_i f_i X_i$, i.e.

$$\Sigma_i f_i X_i = 2.0 \times 2 + 3.5 \times 4 + 4.5 \times 7 + 5.5 \times 8 + 6.0 \times 4 + 7.5 \times 2 + 8.0 \times 1 + 9.5 \times 2$$
$$= 159.5$$

Again, $\Sigma_i f_i = 2 + 4 + 7 + 8 + 4 + 2 + 1 + 2$
$= 30$

Average marks of the class by the formula 4.2 are,

$$\bar{X} = \frac{159.5}{30}$$
$$= 5.32.$$

Example 4.3. Wages per month and the number of workers in a factory are tabulated below

Wages (Rs) (x)	*No. of workers* (f)
550	6
650	8
750	11
850	18
950	5
1100	3

On an average, the wages per worker can be calculated by the formula (4.2) as follows:

$$\Sigma_i f_i X_i = 550 \times 6 + 650 \times 8 + 750 \times 11 + 850 \times 18 + 950 \times 5 + 1100 \times 3$$
$$= 3300 + 5200 + 8250 + 15300 + 4750 + 3300$$
$$= 40100$$
$$\Sigma_i f_i = 6 + 8 + 11 + 18 + 5 + 3 = 51$$

Thus, $$\bar{X} = \frac{40100}{51} = 786.27 \text{ Rs.}$$

MEAN BY SHORT-CUT METHOD

Often the magnitude of data is large and it is inconvenient to find the average of the data as such. In this situation a short-cut method reduces the labour of calculating mean or average. In this method an appropriate constant value either from the data or any other value, say a, is chosen. Then this value a is subtracted from each value, i.e. the deviations of each value from a are found out maintaining their proper sign (– or +). Let the deviations be denoted by dx. The sum of all dx is worked out. The average is calculated by the formula,

$$\bar{X} = a + \frac{\Sigma dx}{n} \qquad (4.3)$$

where n is the number of observation.

In case of frequency distribution, all steps remain same except that each deviation is multiplied by its corresponding frequency 'f' and then added maintaining their sign. So in this case $\Sigma f dx$ is calculated. Now the formula is,

$$\bar{X} = a + \frac{\Sigma fdx}{n} \qquad (4.4)$$

where $$n = \Sigma f$$

If the class intervals are given instead of individual values, formula (4.4) is used in which X is the mid-value of each class-interval.

Example 4.4. Calculate the average of the income per month by short-cut method.

Income in Rs (x): 1560, 1490, 1610, 1580, 1640, 1470.

$$\text{Suppose } a = 1500$$

dx : 60, – 10, 110, 80, 140, – 30

$$\Sigma dx = 350, n = 6$$

$$\therefore \quad \bar{X} = 1500 + \frac{350}{6}$$

$$= 1500 + 58.33 = 1558.33$$

Example 4.5. For the data given in example (4.3), find the average wages by short-cut method.

Let $a = 800$

X	X – 800 = dx	f	fdx
550	– 250	6	– 1500
650	– 150	8	– 1200
750	– 50	11	– 550
850	50	18	900
950	150	5	750
1100	300	3	900
		51	– 700

By the formula (4.4) ,

$$\bar{X} = 800 - \frac{700}{51}$$

$$= 800 - 13.725$$

$$= 786.275$$

Average wages of workers by short method is same as in example 4.3.

Example 4.6. For the following frequency distributions with class intervals, calculate arithmetic mean by short-cut method. Here, a = 225.

Calculations

Class	*Frequency* (*f*)	*Mid-values* (X)	X – 225 (*dx*)	*f dx*
50 – 100	3	75	– 150	– 450
100 – 150	6	125	– 100	– 600
150 – 200	8	175	– 50	– 400
200 – 250	12	225	0	00
250 – 300	7	275	+ 50	350
300 – 350	5	325	+ 100	500
350 – 400	2	375	+ 150	300
Total	43			– 300

$$\Sigma f = 43 \text{ and } a = 225$$

By the formula (4.4),
$$\bar{X} = 225 - \frac{300}{43}$$

$$= 225 - 6.98 = 218.02.$$

GEOMETRIC MEAN (GM)

In most of the cases arithmetic mean is a desirable central value. But in cases where the observations are given in ratios, percentages or proportions, geometric mean is more appropriate than other means. The geometric mean of two observations X_1 and X_2 is $\sqrt{X_1 \cdot X_2}$, i.e. the square root of the product of two values. Similarly, the geometric mean of three values X_1, X_2 and X_3 is $\sqrt[3]{X_1 \cdot X_2 \cdot X_3}$, i.e. the cube root of the product of three values. In general, if there are N values $X_1, X_2, ..., X_N$, then the geometric mean of N values is

$$\text{GM} = \sqrt[N]{X_1 \cdot X_2 \cdots X_N} \tag{4.5}$$

From the formula (4.5), it is clear that the geometric mean is the Nth root of the product of N values. Nth root can easily by found out with the help of logarithm. These days scientific calculators have the facility of getting the Nth root directly. So, readers can make use of calculators.

Example 4.7. The percentage increase in production of milk in a milk bottling factory during the last four years was 19.2, 14.1, 6.9 and 7.8 percent.

The average percentage increase can be found out by calculating the geometric mean of these values. Thus,

$$\begin{aligned} \text{GM} &= \sqrt[4]{19.2 \times 14.1 \times 6.9 \times 7.8} \\ &= \sqrt[4]{14570.1504} \\ &= 10.987\% \end{aligned}$$

Here the value of GM is obtained by taking the square root of the square root.

N.B.:

1. If any one or more values are zero, geometric mean can not be calculated. The reason is obvious. The product of values will always be zero and hence the geometric mean will be zero.
2. If some observation (s) is/are negative, in that situation either the geometric mean will not be calculable or the value of geometric mean will be redundant in most of the cases.
3. The main property of geometric mean is that it give less weightage to the extreme values. Hence, the influence of very small and very large values is minimized. In other words, small values get more weightage and large values get less weightage.
4. Many times geometric mean is preferred over arithmetic mean if the differences between values are large in magnitude.

HARMONIC MEAN (HM)

Harmonic mean is suitable for the data pertaining to time, rates, speed, velocity, etc.

Definition:

The harmonic mean of a series of values is the reciprocal of the arithmetic mean of the reciprocals of the values.

If $X_1, X_2, \ldots, X_N$ are the N values, the formula for harmonic mean as per definition is,

$$HM = \frac{1}{\frac{1}{N}\left(\frac{1}{X_1}+\frac{1}{X_2}+\ldots+\frac{1}{X_N}\right)} \quad (4.6)$$

$$= \frac{N}{\frac{1}{X_1}+\frac{1}{X_2}+\ldots+\frac{1}{X_N}} \quad (4.6.1)$$

$$= \frac{N}{\Sigma_i \frac{1}{X_i}} \quad (4.6.2)$$

To calculate HM, first work out the inverse of each value and then find the sum of these reciprocals. Divide N, (the number of values) by the sum value of reciprocals. The value so obtained is the harmonic mean.

Example 4.8. A motorist drives five cars in a sequence at the speeds 45, 64, 70, 80 and 55 km. per hour. The average speed of cars can be obtained by calculating the harmonic mean by the formula (4.6.1).

$$HM = \frac{5}{\frac{1}{45}+\frac{1}{64}+\frac{1}{70}+\frac{1}{80}+\frac{1}{55}}$$

$$= \frac{5}{0.0222+0.0156+0.0143+0.0125+0.0182}$$

$$= \frac{5}{0.0828}$$

$$= 60.39 \text{ Kph.}$$

Nota bene

1. If any one value is zero, harmonic mean can not be calculated as its value will also become zero.
2. In the calculation of harmonic mean, smaller value gets more weightage. Hence, harmonic mean is suitable for highly variable series.

Relation between three Means

An inequality between arithmetic mean (AM), geometric mean (GM) and Harmonic mean (HM) always hold, i.e.

$$AM \geq GM \geq HM \quad (4.7)$$

$$AH = G^2 \quad (4.8)$$

The proof is avoided.

In the relation (4.8), M is silent.

MEDIAN

This is another frequently used measure of central values. It is positional average. Need for this measure arises when in a series of values, a few value(s) is/are either very large or small as compared to most of the other values. In this situation, mean does not give a value which is nearer to most of the values.

Further mean can not be calculated when lower limit of the first class interval or upper limit of the last class interval or both in a frequency distribution are not given. In other words, mean can not be obtained in case of open end intervals.

Example 4.9. In case of the following intervals of a frequency distributions, mean can not be calculated

Income per person per day	*Freq.*	*Income per person per day*	*Freq.*	*Income per person per day*	*Freq.*
< 50	5	0 – 50	5	< 50	5
50 – 100	12	50 – 100	12	50 – 100	12
100 – 150	17	100 – 150	17	100 – 150	17
150 – 200	13	150 – 200	13	150 – 200	13
200 – 250	8	200 – 250	8	200 – 250	8
250 – 300	4	> 250	4	> 250	4
Type (*a*)		Type (*b*)		Type (*c*)	

Definition:

Median is that value in an ordered series of observations which divides the series into two parts in such a manner that half of the values are exceeded by it and half of the values exceed it.

Locating the Median

Arrange the values in order (ascending or descending) and find the value which is exactly in the middle of the ordered series. This value is the median.

The idea that mean is not a good measure of central value in certain situations but median is more adequate measure will be explained by the following example.

Example 4.10. A factory has six workers and one executive officer. The salaries per month of workers are 3650, 2600, 5900, 4740, 6400, 7200, rupees whereas the executive officer gets Rs. 24000 per month.

The average salary of a person in the factory, say $\overline{S}$ is,

$$\overline{S} = \frac{1}{7}(3650 + 2600 + 5900 + 4740 + 6400 + 7200 + 24000)$$

$$= 7784.28 \text{ Rs.}$$

Now to find the median salary, arrange the salaries in ascending order as given below :

2600, 3650, 4740, 5900, 6400, 7200, 24000

The number of values is 7. So the middle value will be the 4th value, i.e. 5900. The median value is more nearer to salaries of six workers whereas the salaries are much different from the mean salary of Rs. 7784.28. Hence, in this case median is a superior measure of central value than mean. It means that an average is sensitive to sampling fluctuations whereas median is not.

General Case

Suppose X_1 , X_2, ..., X_N are N values for some variable X after arranging in ascending order. It means that X_1 is the smallest value of X, X_2 is the next higher value and so on upto X_N, the largest of X.

Now to find the median value, the middle value will depend whether N is odd or even number.

Case (i): When N is odd.

In this situation, the value located at $\frac{(N+1)\text{th}}{2}$ position will be the median. $\frac{(N-1)}{2}$ values will be less than or equal to this median value and $(N-1)/2$ will be greater than the median value.

Consider data of example 4.7. Number of values $N = 7$. Thus, $\frac{N+1}{2} = \frac{7+1}{2} = 4$. Therefore, 4th value is the median value which is 5900 Rs.

Case (ii): When N is even.

In this case there can not be a single value as middle value, i.e. there will always be two values of the ordered series as mid-values. For even N, $N/2$ th and $(N + 2)/2$ th values of the ordered series will be mid-values. The average of $N/2$th and $(N + 2)/2$th values will be the median value. It is further elucidated by the following numerical example.

Example 4.11. Let the values in a set of observations are 4, 3, 6, 3, 4, 7, 6, 5, 3, 4, 7, 3, 3. On arranging these values in ascending order, the observations are as 3, 3, 3, 3, 3, 4, 4, 4, 5, 6, 6, 7, 7. For this series, number of values is 13, i.e. $N = 13$.

The median shall be the $\frac{(13+1)}{2}$, i.e. seventh value in the series. Hence, median = 4. Writing the values repeatedly is a cumbersome job particularly when N is large . But this process is simplified when they are given in the form of frequency distribution. In the given set of data, the value 3 is repeated 5 times, 4 occurs thrice, 5 only once, 6 and 7 are repeated twice. Hence, for the given set of values, it is easy to make the following frequency distribution.

Values (x)	*Frequency* (f)	*Cumulative* ($c.f.$)
3	5	5
4	3	8
5	1	9
6	2	11
7	2	13

To find the median, do the following steps.

1. First find the cumulative frequencies and write them in the next column. Here, it is given in the third column.
2. Find $N/2$. In the given distribution $N = 13$ and thereby $N/2 = 6.5$.
3. In the column of cumulative frequencies, search minimum cumulative frequency which contains the value $N/2$. In the above distribution, the value 6.5 is contained in the minimum cumulative frequency 8.

   The variate value infront of this cumulative frequency is the median value. In this case, it is 4.

Nota bene: Readers should note that median by this approach is same as obtained directly.

Example 4.12. Consider a series of observations having eight values, say 4, 9, 6, 12, 5, 15, 19 and 22.

Letting these values be arranged in descending order, the series is 22, 19, 15, 12, 9, 6, 5, 4. Since $N = 8$ is an even number, median will be the average of $\frac{8}{2}$th and $\frac{(8+2)}{2}$th, i.e. 4th and 5th values of the series. In the above series, these values are 12 and 9. Hence, median denoted as M_d is,

$$M_d = \frac{12+9}{2} = 10.5.$$

Note: In case of frequency distribution, it makes no difference whether N is odd or even.

Example 4.13. Following is the frequency distribution of daily wages of 120 labourers of a factory.

Wages per day (Rs)	*No. of workers*	*Cu. Frequency*
60.00	4	4
62.50	4	8
65.00	14	22
67.50	28	50
70.00	40	90
75.00	24	114
90.00	6	120

Median wages of labourers can be worked out in the following manner.

To save space, cumulative frequencies are also displayed in the last column.

In this example $N = 120$ and so, $\frac{N}{2} = 60$. The frequency 60 is contained in the minimum cumulative frequency 90. The wages against 90 are Rs. 70.00 per day. Hence, Rs. 70.00 are the median wages.

MEDIAN FOR GROUPED DATA

It has already been mentioned that for a large number of values, data are preferably grouped and presented in the form of frequency distribution having an adequate number of class intervals. It is recalled that it is not necessary for median to have open end intervals. It can be found in both the situations, i.e. with open end interval(s) or for any grouped distribution. The method for determining median in case of continuous grouped data with equal class intervals is given below. Also it is assumed that the classes are arranged in ascending order.

Consider the following frequency distribution.

Class intervals	*Frequency*	*Cu. frequency*
$X_1 — X_2$	f_1	F_1
$X_2 — X_3$	f_2	F_2
$X_3 — X_4$	f_3	F_4
$\vdots$	$\vdots$	$\vdots$
$X_{i-1} — X_i$	f_{i-1}	F_{i-1}
$X_i — X_{i+1}$	f_i	F_i
$X_{i+1} — X_{i+2}$	f_{i+1}	F_{i+1}
$\vdots$	$\vdots$	$\vdots$
$X_K — X_{K+1}$	f_K	$F_K = N$

The last cumulative frequency is always equal to the sum of all frequencies, i.e. the total number of variate values 'N'.

Step 1. Find the cumulative frequencies.
They are displayed in the last column.

Step 2. Find $\frac{N}{2}$.

Step 3. Locate–the minimum cumulative frequency in which the value $\frac{N}{2}$ is contained. Let this value be F_i.

Step 4. The class infront of this minimum cumulative frequency is the median class. Here it is $X_i - X_{i+1}$.

As per definition, median is an unique value. So the question remains to locate the single value within this class interval which is median value. Median is obtained by the formula,

$$M_d = X_i + \frac{\frac{N}{2} - C}{f_i} \times I \qquad (4.9)$$

where,

X_i – lower limit of the median class.

C – Cumulative frequency just above F_i.
$I = X_{i+1} - X_i$, the class interval,

Example 4.14. Find the median for the grouped frequency distribution of wages per month.

Income groups (Rs)	*No. of workers (f)*	*Cu. frequency (F)*
1500 – 1600	6	6
1600 – 1700	8	14
1700 – 1800	11	25
1800 – 1900	18	43
1900 – 2000	5	48
2000 – 2100	3	51

Calculate values step by step.

$$\frac{N}{2} = \frac{51}{2} = 25.5$$

The value 25.5 lies in the minimum cumulative frequency 43. So 1800 – 1900 is the median class.

Further, $X_i = 1800, C = 25, f_i = 18$ and $I = 1900 - 1800 = 100.$

By the formula (4.9) the median,

$$M_d = 1800 + \frac{25.5 - 25}{18} \times 100$$

$$M_d = 1800 + \frac{50}{18}$$

$$= 1800 + 2.78 = 1802.78 \text{ Rs per month}$$

Remark: Unit of measurement should always be given with the median value.

QUARTILES

Quartiles are also the partitional averages. They are used in the same manner as the median.

Definition:

Three variate values which divide an ordered series into four equal parts are called quartiles.

These variate values are denoted by Q_1, Q_2 and Q_3. Q_1 is the value which have 25% values below it. Q_2 is the value such that 50% values are below it and 50% are above it. As a matter of fact Q_2 is same as median. Q_3 is the value which has 75% values below it and 25% above it. In a way, quartiles balance the number of values into four equal parts.

Methods of finding Quartiles

Let there be N values in a series arranged in order of magnitude and $(N + 1)$ is divisible by 4, then the quartiles are located as follows:

Q_1 is the value located at $\frac{N+1}{4}$ th position.

Q_2 is the value located at $\frac{N+1}{2}$th position.

Q_3 is the value located at $\frac{3(N+1)}{4}$ th position.

Example 4.15. Eleven values of a series are given below

11.2, 6.5, 3.7, 4.2, 5.6, 4.8, 9.6, 7.7, 12.9, 6.9, 5.5.

Values arranged in order are,

3.7, 4.2, 4.8, 5.5, 5.6, 6.5, 6.9, 7.7, 9.6, 11.2, 12.9

Here, $N = 11$, For the first quartile, $\frac{N+1}{4} = \frac{11+1}{4} = 3$,

Therefore, $Q_1 = 4.8$

Similarly for the second quartile, $\frac{N+1}{2} = \frac{11+1}{2} = 6$. Hence, $Q_2 = 6.5$

For the third quartile, $\frac{3(N+1)}{4} = 9$. Ninth value in the series is 9.6. Thus, $Q_3 = 9.6$.

Quartiles in Case of Frequency Distribution

The method is same as for median. Arrange the frequency distribution in order of magnitude of individual variate values. The corresponding frequencies are written accordingly. Find the cumulative frequencies and enter them in the next column. For Q_1, Q_2, Q_3, calculate, $\frac{N}{4}, \frac{N}{2}, \frac{3N}{4}$ and note in which minimum cumulative frequencies these values are contained in respectively. The respective variate values corresponding to these cumulative frequencies will be Q_1, Q_2 and Q_3. Method given over here is applied directly in the following example.

Example 4.16. The distribution of age of a group of persons is available as displayed below

Age (years) X	*No. of persons* (*f*)	*Cu. frequency* (*c.f.*)
5	12	12
15	25	37
25	27	64
35	15	79
45	19	98
55	13	111
65	10	121
75	9	130
85	1	131

Cumulative frequencies are calculated and entered in the third column.

For Q_1, Q_2 and Q_3, $\frac{N}{4} = \frac{131}{4} = 32.75$, for second quartile, $\frac{N}{2} = \frac{131}{2} = 65.5$ and

for the third quartile, $\frac{3N}{4} = 98.25$ respectively.

Frequency 32.75 lies in minimum cu. freq., 37. Hence, $Q_1 = 15$ yrs. Similarly 65.50 lie in 79 and thus, $Q_2 = 35$ yrs.

Also 98.25 is contained in 111. So $Q_3 = 55$ yrs.

Quartiles for Grouped Data

Just like median, quartiles can also be found out for a frequency distribution with equal class intervals arranged in ascending order by the formulae similar to median. Find $\frac{N}{4}, \frac{N}{2}$ and $\frac{3N}{4}$ for Q_1, Q_2 and Q_3 respectively. In the distribution as given for median with class intervals, locate the quartile classes for Q_1, Q_2, and Q_3 and find the values of Q_1, Q_2 and Q_3 by the following formulae.

$$Q_1 = l_{01} + \frac{\frac{N}{4} - C_1}{f_1} \times I \qquad (4.10)$$

$$Q_2 = l_{02} + \frac{\frac{N}{2} - C_2}{f_2} \times I \qquad (4.11)$$

$$Q_3 = l_{03} + \frac{\frac{N}{4} - C_3}{f_3} \times I \qquad (4.12)$$

where, l_{01}, l_{02}, l_{03} are the lower limits of the quartile classes Q_1, Q_2 and Q_3 respectively.

C_1, C_2, C_3 are the cumulative frequencies just above the cu. freq. of the respective quartile classes.

f_1, f_2 and f_3 are the frequencies of the corresponding quartile classes.

I is the class interval.

Note: The first quartile is also known as *lower quartile* and third quartile as *upper quartile*.

Example 4.17. The distribution of marks of 98 students of class-X is as give below

Class intervals of marks	*No. of students*	*Cu. frequency*
0 – 10	3	3
10 – 20	8	11
20 – 30	12	23
30 – 40	7	30
40 – 50	25	55
50 – 60	23	78
60 – 70	14	92
70 – 80	5	97
80 – 90	1	98

Three quartiles Q_1, Q_2, Q_3 can be calculated by the formulas (4.10), (4.11) and (4.12) respectively.

For Q_1,

$\frac{N}{4} = \frac{98}{4} = 24.5$. The value 24.5 lies in the minimum cumulative frequency 30. Therefore,

$$l_{01} = 30, C = 23, f_1 = 7 \text{ and } I = 40 - 30 = 10$$

By (4.10),

$$Q_1 = 30 + \frac{24.5 - 23}{7} \times 10$$

$$= 30 + \frac{15}{7} = 32.14 \text{ marks}$$

For Q_2, $\frac{N}{2} = \frac{98}{2} = 49$. This value lies in the min.

Cu. freq. 55. Therefore,

$$l_{02} = 40, C = 30, f_2 = 25 \text{ and I} = 10$$

By (4.11),

$$Q_2 = 40 + \frac{49 - 30}{25} \times 10$$

$$= 40 + \frac{190}{25}$$

$$= 47.60 \text{ marks.}$$

Similarly,

For Q_3, $\frac{3N}{4} = 79.5$. This value lies in cu. freq., 92.

Hence,

$$l_{03} = 60, C = 78, f_3 = 14 \text{ and } I = 10$$

By (4.12),

$$Q_3 = 60 + \frac{79.5 - 78}{14} \times 10$$

$$= 60 + \frac{15}{14} = 61.07 \text{ marks.}$$

MODE

It is another kind of statistical central value. The world 'mode' is taken from french language *La Mode*, a french word which means a thing in maximum fashion. A thing which is in maximum fashion has maximum sale. Hence, mode may be defined as,

"Mode is that value which occurs more frequently than any other value in a frequency distribution of variate values".

In other words, it can be said that most of the items concentrate at this value. For instance, largest number of men have their shoe size No. 7. It means, modal value is 7. Most prevalent shirt collar size is 34 cm. Hence, modal value for collar size is 34 cms.

In a frequency distribution, mode can be judged visually by seeing which variate value has maximum frequency. That value is the modal value.

Example 4.18. The income (rupees per month) of twelve families is, 3600, 12820, 8750, 5680, 12820, 8750, 4650, 5680, 8750, 8750, 12820, 8750.

Now prepare the frequency distribution with the help of tally marks.

Income (Rs/month)	*Tally*	*Frequency*
3600	|	1
4650	|	1
5680	||	2
8750	~~||||~~	5
12820	|||	3

Family income of Rs. 8750 has maximum frequency,, i.e. 5. Hence, Rs 8750 is the modal value.

Mode in case of grouped data

Consider the frequency distribution given in case of median for grouped data. Also supposing that f_i is the maximum frequency, mode can be calculated by the following formula.

$$M_0 = l_0 + \frac{f_i - f_{i-1}}{(f_i - f_{i-1}) + (f_i - f_{i+1})} \times I \tag{4.13}$$

$$= l_0 + \frac{f_i - f_{i-1}}{2f_i - f_{i-1} - f_{i+1})} \times I \tag{4.13.1}$$

Putting $f_i - f_{i-1} = \Delta_1$ and $f_i - f_{i+1} = \Delta_2$ [Δ-capital delta]

Also Δ_1 and Δ_2 will always be positive as f_i is maximum frequency. So the formula (4.13) can be written as,

$$M_0 = l_0 + \frac{\Delta_1}{\Delta_1 + \Delta_2} \times I \tag{4.13.2}$$

where,

l_0 — Lower limit of the modal class.
f_i — frequency of the modal class.
f_{i-1} — frequency just about f_i.
f_{i+1} — frequency just below f_i.
I — class interval equal to $(X_{i+1} - X_i)$.

Further it is once again to emphasize that the distribution should be written in ascending order as per magnitude of the variate values.

MERITS

1. Mode is not affected by extreme values or open end intervals.
2. It can be used in case of ranks also.
3. If two values in a frequency distribution have equal maximum frequencies, then the distribution will have two modal values. In this situation, the distribution is said to be *bimodal*.
1. It is hardly used for further, statistical formulae.

2. It can not be meaningfully determined when there are a few frequencies.
3. It becomes meaningless when each value occurs once or an equal number of times.

Example 4.19. Given below is a frequency distribution of age with class intervals.

Age groups (years) (*X*)	*Frequency* (*f*)
0 – 10	13
10 – 20	17
20 – 30	12
30 – 40	32
40 – 50	26
50 – 60	11
60 – 70	5

Mode for the given distribution can easily be found out by the formula (4.13.2).

32 is the maximum frequency. Therefore, the mode, M_0 lies in the class interval 30 – 40.

Therefore, $l_0 = 30, \Delta_1 = 32 - 12 = 20, \Delta_2 = 32 - 26 = 6$

and $I = 40 - 30 = 10.$

$$M_0 = 30 + \frac{20}{20+6} \times 10.$$

$$= 30 + \frac{200}{26}$$

$$= 37.69 \text{ years.}$$

PRACTICE QUESTIONS AND EXERCISES

1. Why measures of central values so important in statistics?
2. Define arithmetic mean and geometric mean.
3. What do understand by quartiles?
4. Discuss median and give situations in which it becomes essential to calculate median.
5. Define median and give the method of finding it in case of grouped data.
6. How can the median be located in case of individual data.
7. What are the requirements which a good average should possess?
8. Calculate arithmetic mean and median of the following data.
   96, 105, 87, 92, 78, 88, 95, 102.
9. Calculate median for the following frequency distribution of a variable *X*.

X:	1	2	3	4	5	6	7
f:	6	8	10	14	13	9	4

10. Given the grouped distribution of salaries per day of workers in a construction company, find the average salary per day, the modal salary and the three quartiles.

Salary (Rs/day)	*No. of Workers*
85–100	2
100–115	5
115–130	10
130–145	16
145–160	13
160–175	7
175–190	3

11. Find the geometric mean of the following values.
    18, 16, 22, 12
12. Reproduce the definitions of averages given by R.A. Fisher, Croxton and Cowden and Moroney.
13. What are various uses of averages?
14. Obtain the missing frequency f for the following frequency distribution when the value of median is 86.

Classes	*Frequency*
40–50	2
50–60	1
60–70	6
70–80	6
80–90	f
90–100	12
100–110	5

15. Which quartile is same as median?
16. Give the areas in which mode is preferable than other measures of central values.
17. What is the origin of the word mode?
18. How can you calculate arithmetic mean in case of frequency distribution of individual values?
19. What shall be the geometric mean of a set of values having an observation equal to zero?
20. When harmonic mean should preferably be used in comparison to any other central value?

OBJECTIVE TYPE QUESTIONS

Choose the most suitable one out of four alternatives for the given statement or question.

21. Calculation of a central value in a case of grouped data is usually based on the assumption that:

    a. Classes are continuous　　b. Each class has same class width
    c. There is no open end class　　d. All of the above

22. A large number of values can be condensed to a single figure by:
a. The mean of the value
b. The modal value
c. The second quartile
d. All of the above
23. Which of the following statement is not correct?
a. Arithmetic mean is rigidly defined.
b. Arithmetic mean cannot be used for further statistical formulae.
c. Arithmetic mean is more used than any other central value.
d. Arithmetic mean is very much affected by sampling fluctuations.
24. When the measurements are in ratio or proportion, then the most suitable central value is:
a. Arithmetic mean
b. Median
c. Geometic mean
d. Mode
25. If a value in a set of values is zero, then one can not calculate:
a. Arithmetic mean
b. Median
c. Harmonic mean
d. Mode
26. If the sum of positive and negative values in a data series is same, then the average value is:
a. One
b. Zero
c. Not calculable
d. Two
27. Which of the following relation between A.M., G.M. and H.M. holds?
a. A.M. = G.M. = H.M.
b. A.M. ≤ G.M ≤ H.M.
c. A.M. ≥ G.M. ≥ H.M.
d. A.M. ≥ G.M. ≤ H.M
28. Median is a value which divides an ordered series into:
a. Four equal parts
b. Three equal parts
c. Two equal parts
d. All of the above
29. Median of a frequency distribution is:
a. Unique
b. The maximum value
c. The maximum frequency
d. None of the above
30. The relation that holds between arithmetic mean (*M*), geometric mean (G) and harmonic mean (H) is:
a. $\sqrt{H.A} = G$
b. $\frac{A}{G^2} = \frac{1}{H}$
c. $A.H. = G$
d. (*a*) and (*b*) but not (*c*)
31. Median is always same as:
a. Mode
b. Second quartile
c. Third quartile
d. Half of the number of values
32. If two values in a frequency distribution have an equal maximum frequency, then the distribution is:
a. Unimodal
b. Without mode
c. Bimodal
d. Any of these
33. Third quartile divides the frequency distribution in the ratio:
a. 3 : 2
b. 2 : 1
c. 2 : 3
d. 3 : 1

34. If X and Y are two linearly related variables such that $-3X + 2Y = 7$. Given that the arithmetic mean of X is 9. What is the mean of Y?
    a. 20 b. – 20
    c. 17 d. – 10
35. If a variable X takes on the values 2, 3, 5, 8 with respective frequencies 3, 2, 5 and 8, then the arithmetic mean of X is:
    a. 18/4 b. 49/9
    c. 36/4 d. None of the above
36. The arithmetic mean of a set of values is 16 and harmonic mean is 9. The geometic mean for the same set of values is:
    a. 144 b. 12
    c. 12.5 d. 36
37. A modal value in a frequency distribution has:
    a. Maximum frequency b. Minimum frequency
    c. Middle frequency d. Zero frequency.
38. Which of the following measure of central tendency is not necessarily unique for a frequency distribution ?
    a. Mean b. Median
    c. Mode d. Third quartile
39. Which of the following statement is not true?
    a. No measure of central value is perfect.
    b. Median is the best measure of central value.
    c. Second quartile and median are same.
    d. Mean, Median and mode can have the same value for a specific frequency distribution.
40. If a data set contains some extreme values, then a preferable measure of central tendency is:
    a. Geometric mean b. Arithmetic mean
    c. Median d. Mode

CHAPTER 5

Measures of Dispersion

CONCEPT

In the last chapter, central values which represent a series of values were discussed adequately. Those values present a good deal of information but fail to reveal about their spread. Unless one knows whether the values are close to each other or far apart, the information remains incomplete. This fact is substantiated with the help of three series given below.

Series A :	8	8	8	8	8
Series B :	0	4	8	12	16
Series C :	1	3	8	10	18

In all the above series, mean is 8 and median is also 8. At the same time it is visually apparent that they are very much different. In series A, all values are equal, i.e. there is no variation. In series B, two values are less than 8 and two are greater than 8 that too on equal distances. Series C has values which are far apart and indicate lot of variability.

From the above discussion of three series it is evident that mean, median and mode are not enough to give full information about a series. In addition to it there is a need of some other measure which reveals about the spread amongst values. Hence, the measures which provide information about variation are discussed in this chapter.

Two statements about dispersion are quoted which may be taken as definitions of dispersion.

1. **Spiegel:** "The degree to which numerical data tend to spread about an average value is called the variation or dispersion of the data."
2. **John I Griffin:** "A measure of variation or dispersion describes the degree of scatter shown by the observations and is usually measured as an average deviation about some central value or by an order statistics."

Uses of Dispersion

1. Measures of dispersion indicate how exactly a central value represents a series of values. If the value of a dispersion is less, more reliable is the central value and vice-versa.

2. It enables one to compare two series in respect of their variability.
3. If a series has more variation, one can find ways to reduce it so that the results become more reliable.

Dispersion Measures

Six measures of dispersion are succinctly discussed namely—

i. Range
ii. Interquartile range
iii. Variance
iv. Standard deviation
v. Mean deviation
vi. Coefficient of variation.

Range

It is the simplest type of measure of dispersion and is widely used. This measure is given in two ways.

First find the lowest and highest value of a series.

Way I : Write, lowest value – highest value

Way II : It is also given as the difference between the highest value and lowest value. If we denote range by R, highest value by M, lowest value by L, then the range,

$$R = M - L \tag{5.1}$$

Rather than giving the difference, the range is better represeted in way I, i.e.

$$L–M \tag{5.2}$$

An absolute measure of range is **coefficient of range**. The formula for this is,

$$\text{coeff. of range} = \frac{M - L}{M + L} \tag{5.3}$$

Less is the value of coefficient of range, better it is. The value of coefficient of range lies between 0 and 1.

Example 5.1. Let the five observations be,

10, 14, 13, 19, 6

The range and coefficient of range can be found out as follows:

Range can be expressed as 6–19.

Here $M = 19, L = 6$

$R = 19 - 6 = 13$

$$\text{Coefficient of range} = \frac{19-6}{19+6} = \frac{13}{25} = 0.52$$

Example 5.2. Given the frequency distribution of individual values of X as,

X	*f*
3	2
8	5
12	6
17	8
19	7
23	4

The range of X can be found out as

$$R = 23 - 3 = 20$$

$$\text{Coefficient of range} = \frac{23-3}{23+3} = \frac{20}{26} = 0.769$$

Example 5.3. For the following frequency distribution of the age of students.

Age groups X (*years*)	*No. of students* (*f*)
5 — 10	16
10 — 15	19
15 — 20	23
20 — 25	17
25 — 30	5

The range and coefficient of range of age can be calculated as follows:
Here, $M = 30$, $L = 5$
Range is 5–30 years or $R = 30 - 5 = 25$ years. By the formula (5.3),

$$\text{coeff. of range} = \frac{30-5}{30+5} = \frac{25}{35} = 0.714$$

Remark: In open-end grouped frequency distribution, range can not be found out.

Uppers

1. Range is a crude measure of dispersion as it is based on only two extreme values.
2. It gives information about largest and smallest values within which all other values lie.
3. Range is routinely used to give an idea about weather conditions of a city in the form of maximum and minimum temperatures of a day.
4. Range is extremely used in statistical quality control of products as a measure of variation.

Lowers

1. Range is a crude measure of dispersion as it is based on only two extreme values.
2. Range does not provide any information about the values lying in between two extreme values.

3. Whatever changes may occur in between the two extreme values, range remains same.

Interquartile range (IQR)

This is a measure of partial range as it gives the range of 50 per cent middle values of an ordered series.

If Q_1 is the first quartile and Q_3 is the third quartile, then,

$$IQR = Q_3 - Q_1 \tag{5.4}$$

Quartile deviation or semi-interquartile range is given by,

$$QD = \frac{Q_3 - Q_1}{2} \tag{5.5}$$

Coefficient of quartile range is similar to coefficient of range and is obtained by the formula,

$$\text{Coeff. of } QR = \frac{Q_3 - Q_1}{Q_3 + Q_1} \tag{5.6}$$

A small value of coeff. of QR indicates less variation in the series. It has no unit.

Example 5.4. In example 4.14, $Q_1 = 32.14$ and $Q_3 = 61.07$. Then for these values of Q_1 and Q_3.

$$IQR = 61.07 - 32.14$$
$$= 28.93$$

Also,

$$QD = \frac{28.93}{2} = 14.465$$

$$\text{coeff. of range} = \frac{61.07 - 32.14}{61.07 + 32.14}$$
$$= \frac{28.93}{93.21}$$
$$= 0.310$$

VARIANCE

This is the backbone of statistics. In most of the studies variance is involved. The reliability of an average is adjudged on the basis of variance. Lesser the variance, more reliable is the mean.

Definition:

Variance of a series is the average of the sum of squares of deviations from its own mean.

Variance of Individual Series

If a series consists of single values, i.e. no frequency is given, then it can be calculated in the following manner. Variance is usually denoted by σ^2 (sigma - σ).

1. Let the N observations be $X_1, X_2, ..., X_N$.
2. Find the mean of values by the formula, $(\Sigma X)/N = \bar{X}$ (say)
3. Find the deviation of each observation from mean $\bar{X}$ such as $(X_1 - \bar{X}), (X_2 - \bar{X}), ..., (X_N - \bar{X})$.
4. Find the square of each deviation, i.e. $(X_1 - \bar{X})^2, (X_2 - \bar{X})^2, ..., (X_N - \bar{X})^2$
5. Add these squared values, i.e. find $\sum_i (X_i - \bar{X})^2$ for $i = 1, 2, ..., N$.
6. To obtain the value of variance, divide $\Sigma(X_i - \bar{X})^2$ by N. Thus, the formula for variance is,

$$\sigma^2 = \frac{1}{N}\Sigma(X_i - \bar{X})^2 \tag{5.7}$$

Sometimes taking deviation from mean and squaring deviations become cumbersome. Hence, the formula (5.7) can be written in another form (5.7.1) where there is no need of taking deviations from mean and squaring them. The two formulae are equivalent and yield same value of σ^2. It will be shown by numerical example as well.

$$\sigma^2 = \frac{1}{N}\left[\Sigma X_i^2 - \frac{(\Sigma X_i)^2}{N}\right] \tag{5.7.1}$$

(5.7.1) can also be written as,

or
$$\sigma^2 = \frac{1}{N}\left[\Sigma X_i^2 - N\bar{X}^2\right] \tag{5.7.2}$$

Example 5.5. Given the series of seven values,

11, 7, 6, 8, 5, 9, 10

the variance can be calculated following the steps (2) to (6).

Sum of values,

$$\Sigma X = 11 + 7 + 6 + 8 + 5 + 9 + 10 = 56$$

$$\bar{X} = \frac{56}{7} = 8 \text{ since N} = 7.$$

Deviations from mean are,

$11 - 8 = 3,\quad 7 - 8 = -1,\quad 6 - 8 = -2,\quad 8 - 8 = 0,\quad 5 - 8 = -3,\quad 9 - 8 = 1,$ $10 - 8 = 2.$

Sum of squares of deviations,

$$\sum_{i=1}^{7}(X_i - \bar{X})^2 = 3^2 + (-1)^2 + (-2)^2 + 0^2 + (-3)^2 + 1^2 + 2^2$$

$$= 9 + 1 + 4 + 0 + 9 + 1 + 4$$
$$= 28$$

$$\therefore \quad \sigma^2 = \frac{28}{7} = 4.0 \qquad \text{(By 5.7)}$$

To make use of (5.7.1), find the sum of square.

$$\Sigma X_i^2 = 11^2 + 7^2 + 6^2 + 8^2 + 5^2 + 9^2 + 10^2$$
$$= 121 + 49 + 36 + 64 + 25 + 81 + 100$$
$$= 476$$

Now,
$$\sigma^2 = \frac{1}{7}\left[476 - \frac{(56)^2}{7}\right]$$
$$= \frac{1}{7}[476 - 448]$$
$$= \frac{28}{7} = 4.0.$$

Thus, it is verified that the formulae (5.7) and (5.7.1) yield the same value of σ^2.

Variance in Case of Frequency Distribution

If data are given in the form of frequency distribution such as,

Values (X)	*Frequency* (f)
X_1	f_1
X_2	f_2
X_3	f_3
⋮	⋮
X_K	f_K

Variance can be determined in the same way as in case of individual values except that X-values and deviations from mean are multiplied by their corresponding frequencies. Also sum of frequencies, i.e. $\Sigma f_i = N$ for $i = 1, 2, 3, ..., K$

For the given distribution, the mean

$$\bar{X} = \frac{\sum f_i X_i}{\sum f_i}$$

Then find,

$$(X_1 - \bar{X}), (X_2 - \bar{X}), (X_3 - \bar{X}), ..., (X_K - \bar{X})$$

Square each deviation and multiply the squared deviation by the corresponding frequencies. Sum these quantities and divide it by $\Sigma f_i = N$. The resulting value will be the variance. Hence, obtain

$$(X_1 - \overline{X})^2, (X_2 - \overline{X})^2, (X_3 - \overline{X})^2, ..., (X_K - \overline{X})2$$

and $f_1(X_1 - \overline{X})^2, f_2(X_2 - \overline{X})^2, f_3(X_3 - \overline{X})^2, ..., f_K(X_K - \overline{X})^2$

$$\text{Sum} = f_1(X_1 - \overline{X})^2 + f_2(X_2 - \overline{X})^2 + f_3(X_3 - \overline{X})^2 + ... + f_K(X_K - \overline{X})^2$$

$$= \Sigma f_i (X_i - \overline{X})^2$$

Variance,
$$\sigma^2 = \frac{\Sigma f_i (X_i - \overline{X})^2}{\Sigma f_i} \tag{5.8}$$

Formula (5.8) can be written in another form where the complexity of taking the deviations from mean can be avoided. The alternative formula is,

$$\sigma^2 = \frac{1}{N}\left[\Sigma f_i X_i^2 - \frac{(\Sigma f_i X_i)^2}{N}\right] \tag{5.8.1}$$

$$= \frac{1}{N}\left[\Sigma f_i X_i^2 - N\overline{X}^2\right] \tag{5.8.2}$$

It is convenient to use formula (5.8.1) or (5.8.2) when mean is not a whole number.

Nota bene: In case of grouped data, mid-value of each class (group is taken as a variate value and rest of the procedure remains same as for ungrouped frequency distribution.

Example 5.6. The frequency distribution of a Variable X is given below:

Values X :	5,	7,	9,	12,	6,	3
Frequency f :	2,	3,	5,	4,	1,	2

To calculate the variance, prepare the following table.

i. X	*ii.* f	*iii.* fX	*iv.* X^2	*v.* fX^2	*vi.* $(X - \overline{X})$	*vii.* $(X - \overline{X})^2$	*viii.* $f(X - \overline{X})^2$
5	2	10	25	50	– 3	9	18
7	3	21	49	147	– 1	1	3
9	5	45	81	405	1	1	5
12	4	48	144	576	4	16	64
6	1	6	36	36	– 2	4	4
3	2	6	9	18	– 5	25	50
Total	**17**	**136**		**1232**			**144**

$$\overline{X} = \frac{136}{17} = 8$$

For the variance by the formula (5.8), use totals of columns (ii) and (viii). Thus,

$$\sigma^2 = \frac{144}{17} = 8.47$$

To use alternative formula (5.8.1), utilize the totals of cols. (ii), (iii) and (v)

Hence,

$$\sigma^2 = \frac{1}{17}\left[1232 - \frac{(136)^2}{17}\right]$$

$$= \frac{1}{17}[1232 - 1088]$$

$$= \frac{144}{17}$$

$$= 8.47$$

It is noteworthy that the unit of variance is the square of the unit of measurement of the variable *X*. For instance, if height is measured in cms, the unit of variance will be cm^2. Again if unit of weight is kg, then the unit of variance shall be kg^2.

Standard Deviation (SD)

Definition:

Standard deviation is the positive square root of the variance. It is denoted by σ. Therefore,

$$SD = \sigma = +\sqrt{\sigma^2} \tag{5.9}$$

By definition, it is clear that to find out standard deviation, one has to work out the variance. Directly formula can be given as,

$$\sigma = \sqrt{\frac{1}{N}\sum(X_i - \bar{X})^2} \tag{5.10}$$

Keeping in view the formula (5.10), standard deviation can also be defined as,

"Standard deviation is the root mean square deviation about the mean."

Its unit is same as the unit of measurement of the variable. Standard deviation is considered as the best measure of dispersion and is a most used measure.

Merits

1. Standard deviation is based on all observations.
2. Square of deviations are always taken from mean. In this situation sum of squares of the deviations is minimum.
3. The unit of standard deviation is same as that of variate values.

Demerits

1. It has unit of measurement. Hence, two series having different units of measurement can not be compared for their variability. For instance, if one series is measured in cms and the other in gms, then the variation in the two series can not be compared through standard deviation.

Example 5.7. Variance for the data given in example 5.5 is 4.0.

Standard deviation for the same data can be obtained by the formula (5.9). Thus,

$$\sigma = \sqrt{4.0} = 2.0$$

Example 5.8. For the frequency distribution given in example 5.6, the value of $\Sigma f_i (X_i - \bar{X})^2$ is 144. Hence, the standard deviation by the formula (5.10) will be,

$$\sigma = \sqrt{\frac{144}{17}}$$

$$= \sqrt{8.47} = 2.91$$

Mean Deviation (MD)

Mean deviation is also called average deviation (AD)

Definition:

Mean deviation is the average of the absolute deviations of each value taken from arithmetic mean or median.

In absolute deviations, the signs (plus or minus) of the deviations are disregarded (ignored).

Formula for mean deviation for individual series $X_1, X_2, X_3, ..., X_N$ is,

$$MD = \frac{1}{N}\sum|X_i - A| \qquad (5.11)$$

for $i = 1, 2, ..., N$.

A may be mean or median.

Also for a frequency distribution as given in case of variance, the formula for mean deviation is,

$$MD = \frac{1}{N}\sum f_i\,|X_i - A| \qquad (5.12)$$

Mean deviation is minimum when A is taken to be median.

Nota bene: For a frequency distribution with class intervals, mid-value of each class is taken as X_i and MD is calculated in the same way as in (5.12)

The greatest objection to this measure is that all signs of deviation are ignored without any algebraic justification.

Relation between MD, QD and SD

An empirical relation between MD about mean, QD and SD is as follows.

$$4\ SD = 5\ MD = 6\ QD \qquad (5.13)$$

Relation between R and SD

Empirical relation between R and SD is,

$$R = 6\ SD \qquad (5.14)$$

Example 5.9. Birth weights of seven children are as given below.

Birth weights (kg) X : 2.3, 1.8, 3.2, 2.7, 2.5, 3.0, 2.7

Mean deviation about mean and also about median can be worked out as follows:

i. Mean deviation about mean.

$$\text{Mean, } \bar{X} = \frac{2.3 + 1.8 + 3.2 + 2.7 + 2.5 + 3.0 + 2.7}{7}$$

$$= \frac{18.2}{7} = 2.6$$

$$\text{MD} = \frac{1}{7}[|2.3 - 2.6| + |1.8 - 2.6| + |3.2 - 2.6| + |2.7 - 2.6| + |2.5 - 2.6| + |3.0 - 2.6| + |2.7 - 2.6|]$$

$$= \frac{1}{7}[0.3 + 0.8 + 0.6 + 0.1 + 0.1 + 0.4 + 0.1]$$

$$= \frac{2.4}{7} = 0.34 \text{ kg}$$

ii. Mean deviation about median.

For median, arrange the data in ascending order.

1.8, 2.3, 2.5, 2.7, 2.7, 3.0, 3.2

4th value is 2.7. Therefore, median = 2.7.

$$\text{MD} = \frac{1}{7}[|1.8 - 2.7| + |2.3 - 2.7| + |2.5 - 2.7| + |2.7 - 2.7| + |2.7 - 2.7| + |3.0 - 2.7| + |3.2 - 2.7|]$$

$$= \frac{1}{7}[0.9 + 0.4 + 0.2 + 0 + 0 + 0.3 + 0.5]$$

$$= \frac{2.3}{7} = 0.33 \text{ kg}$$

Remark: Above example substantiates that MD about median is less than MD about mean.

Example 5.10. For the frequency distribution given in example 5.6, mean deviation about median and mean can be claculated in the manner given below.

First write the frequency distribution in ascending order and then proceed for further calculations

X	*f*	cu.fr.	*f*X
3	2	2	6
5	2	4	10
6	1	5	6
7	3	8	21
9	5	13	45
12	4	17	48
	17		136

For median, $\frac{N}{2} = \frac{17}{2} = 8.5$, which is contained in the minimum cumulative frequency 13.

Hence, $M_d = 9$

Also, $\bar{X} = \frac{136}{17} = 8.0.$

Mean deviation about median is,

$$\begin{aligned} MD &= \frac{1}{17} [2\ |3 - 9| + 2\ |5 - 9| + 1\ |6 - 9| \\ &\qquad + 3\ |7 - 9| + 5\ |9 - 9| + 4\ |12 - 9|] \\ &= \frac{1}{17} [12 + 8 + 3 + 6 + 0 + 12] \\ &= \frac{41}{17} = 2.412 \end{aligned}$$

Mean deviation about mean,

$$\begin{aligned} MD_{\bar{X}} &= \frac{1}{17} [2\ |3 - 8| + 2\ |5 - 8| + 1\ |6 - 8| \\ &\qquad + 3\ |7 - 8| + 5\ |9 - 8| + 4\ |12 - 8|] \\ &= \frac{1}{17} [10 + 6 + 2 + 3 + 5 + 16] \\ &= \frac{42}{17} = 2.4706 \end{aligned}$$

Note: Example 5.10 further verify that the mean deviation about median is minimum.

COEFFICIENT OF VARIATION (CV)

This is an unitless measure of dispersion. It is given in percentage. Hence, any two series can be compared for variability by comparing their coefficients of variation. Lesser the value of CV, more consistent is the series.

Formula for coefficient of variation is,

$$CV = \frac{\text{Standard deviation}}{\text{Mean}} \times 100 \tag{5.15}$$

Notationally,

$$CV = \frac{\sigma}{\bar{X}} \times 100 \text{ per cent} \tag{5.15.1}$$

Note: For sample, use sample standard deviation s instead of σ.

Example 5.11. Coefficient of variation for the series given in example 5.5 can easily be obtained by utilizing the values of variance and mean already worked out. Obviously,

$$\sigma^2 = 4.0 \text{ and } \bar{X} = 8.0. \text{ Thus, } \sigma = \sqrt{4.0} = 2.0.$$

$$CV = \frac{2.0}{8.0} \times 100$$

$$= \frac{200}{8} = 25.0 \text{ per cent.}$$

Example 5.12. Coefficient of variation of the variable X for the frequency distribution given in example 5.6 is easily calculable by making use of the values $\sigma^2 = 8.47$ and $\bar{X} = 8.0$.

Therefore,

$$CV = \frac{\sqrt{8.47}}{8} \times 100$$

$$= \frac{2.91}{8} \times 100$$

$$= 36.38 \text{ per cent}$$

SHAPES OF FREQUENCY DISTRIBUTION CURVES

Symmetric Curve

As discussed earlier, a frequency polygon represents a frequency distribution of continuous type. Frequency polygon takes the shape of a smooth curve when the points are smoothly joined by free hand. If the rectangles on both the sides of the highest rectangle are equal in number and have same heights, then the smoothened curve obtained by joining mid-points of the tops of the rectangles will be a *symmetric curve* as shown in Fig. 5.1.

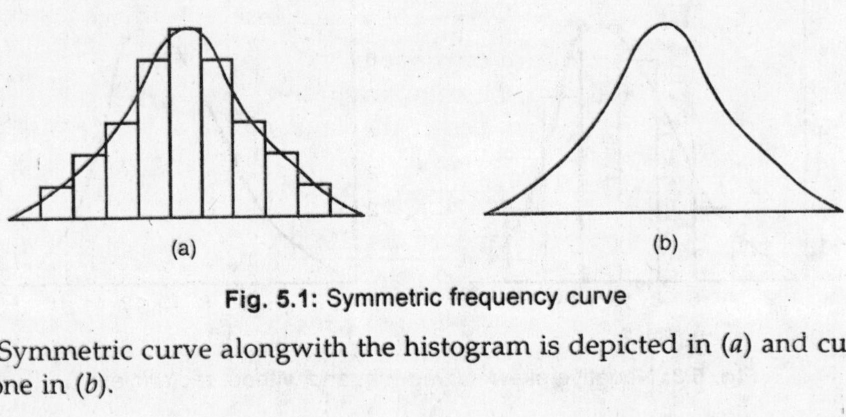

Fig. 5.1: Symmetric frequency curve

Symmetric curve alongwith the histogram is depicted in (*a*) and curve alone in (*b*).

Skew Curve

When a curve is not symmetrical about its mean, it is called a skew curve. This statement implies that the tail of a curve is elongated to either right side or to left side. If the tail of a curve is elongated to the right side, then it is called a *positive skew curve.* Positive skew curves with and without histogram are shown in Fig. 5.2. In Fig. 5.2(a), there are a few rectangles to the left of highest rectangle and more to its right side. Positive skew curve alone is displayed in Fig. 5.2(b).

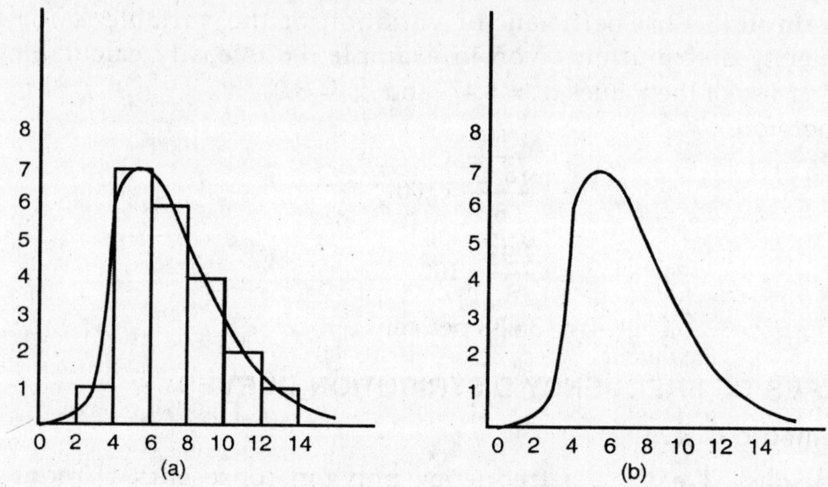

Fig. 5.2: Positive skew curves

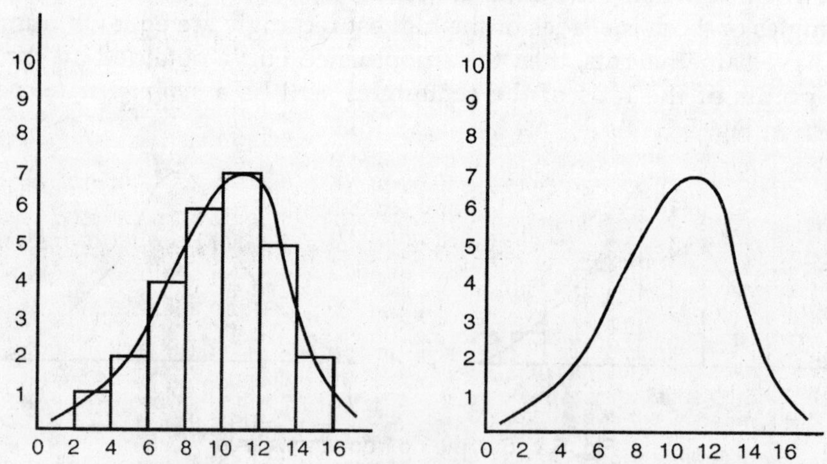

Fig. 5.3: Negative skew curves with and without rectangles

If the tail of a frequency curve is elongated to left side of the highest point, then it is called a *negative skew curve.* Shape of the negative skew curves with and without histogram are shown in figure 5.3. There are hardly one or two tails to the right of highest rectangle of the histogram in (a) whereas a large number of rectangles of decreasing heights occur to the left. Negative skew curve is shown in (b).

Determination of skewness through formulas

Whether a distribution is symmetrical, positive or negative skew can better be ascertained with the help of various formulae. Skewness is measured in terms of coefficient of skewness denoted by *J*.

A formula for *J* is,

$$J = \frac{\text{Mean} - \text{Mode}}{\text{S.D.}} \tag{5.16}$$

For any frequency distribution, it is simple to calculate value of *J* by (5.16). This value of *J* is interpreted according to the following norms.

(i) If $J = 0$, the curve is symmetrical.

(ii) If $J < 0$, the curve is negative skew.

(iii) If $J > 0$, the curve is positive skew.

The degree of skewness depends on the value of *J*. Greater is the value of *J*, more is skewness.

Another formula for *J* given by Professor A.L. Bowley is in terms of quartiles.

Formula is,

$$J = \frac{Q_3 + Q_1 - 2Q_2}{Q_3 - Q_1} \tag{5.17}$$

Recall that Q_1, Q_2 and Q_3 stand for first, second and third quartiles respectively.

Any formula can be used depending on the convenience of calculations.

Example 5.13. For a frequency distribution

Mean = 43.17, Mode = 53.50

and Standard deviation = 17.57

Coefficient of skewness for the given distribution can be calculated by the formula (5.16). Thus,

$$J = \frac{43.17 - 53.50}{17.57}$$

$$= \frac{10.33}{17.57} = -0.588$$

Value of *J* is negative and of medium magnitude. Hence, it is easy to conclude that the curve is moderately skew towards left tail.

Example 5.14. It is known that for a frequency distribution, three quartiles are :

$Q_1 = 174.90$, $Q_2 = 246.50$ and $Q_3 = 369.75$

Value of J in this case can be obtained by the formula (5.17). Thus,

$$J = \frac{174.90 + 369.75 - 2 \times 246.50}{369.75 - 174.90}$$

$$= \frac{544.65 - 493.00}{194.85}$$

$$= \frac{51.65}{194.85} = 0.265$$

Since J has a small positive value, it is inferred that the curve is slightly positive skew.

Kurtic Curve

Another important property of a curve given by Karl Pearson is with regard to its *peakedness*. If a frequency curve is properly peaked, then it is called a normal curve. Pearson called it a *mesokurtic curve*. If the top of a curve is flat as compared to a normal curve, then it is called a *platykurtic curve*. Again, in case the top of the curve is more peaked than normal curve, then it is known as a *leptokurtic curve*.

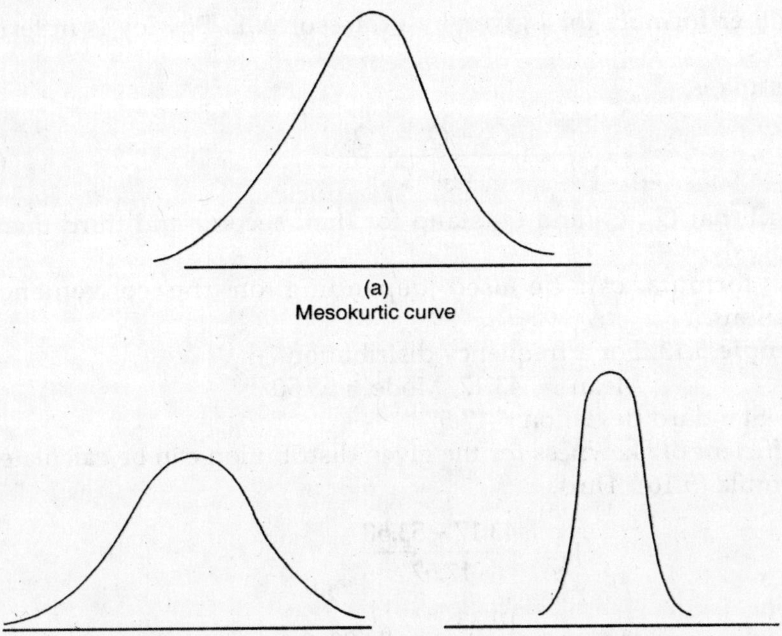

(a)
Mesokurtic curve

(b)
Platykurtic curve

(c)
Leptokurtic curve

Fig. 5.4: Kurtic curves

Abnormality in peakedness of frequency distribution curve is termed as **Kurtosis.** Three types of Kurtic curves are shown in Fig. 5.4; (a), (b) and (c).

Extent of Kurtosis can also be measured mathematically through formula. But it has been kept out of the scope of this book. Anyhow, coefficient of Kurtosis is denoted by β_2.

If $\beta_2 = 3$, the curve is properly peaked, i.e. mesokurtic.
If $\beta_2 < 3$, the curve is flat, i.e. platykurtic.
If $\beta_2 > 3$, the curve is highly peaked, i.e. leptokurtic.

PRACTICE QUESTIONS AND EXERCISES

1. Name different measures of dispersion.
2. What is interquartile range and quartile deviation?
3. Throw light on the need of measures of dispersion.
4. Discuss range and its merits and demerits.
5. Why standard deviation is considered to be the best measure of disperision?
6. Can a frequency distribution curve be skew as well as kurtic? Justify your answer.
7. How will you know about the skewness of a frequency curve?
8. What is the advantage of coefficient of variation over other measures of dispersion?
9. For the following series of values,
   10, 3, 7, 9, 8, 6, 5, 2, 4
   Find (i) standard deviation, (ii) coefficient of variation, (iii) range, (iv) Mean deviation about median.
10. For the following grouped data,

Classes	*Frequency*
2–4	4
4–6	8
6–8	16
8–10	28
10–12	13
12–14	10
14–16	6
16–18	4
18–20	2

    Find (i) Interquartile deviation, (ii) coefficient of skewness, (iii) variance, (iv) Mean deviation about mean.

11. Given the following frequency distribution,

x:	2.0,	6.0,	3.5,	6.5,	10.0
f:	3,	5,	8,	4,	2

    Find (i) Range, (ii) Standard deviation, (iii) coefficient of skewness and interpret it.

12. Calculate the coefficient of variation of series *A* and *B*. Find out which of the two series is more variable.

A:	12	18	27	33	19	11
B:	19	21	28	23	15	14

13. Discuss standard deviation in case of grouped data and its main characteristics.
14. Find the range and coefficient of range for the following observations.
15, 20, 32, 31, 26, 7, 10, 5
15. Given the following grouped data.

0 — 10	6
10 — 20	4
20 — 30	10
30 — 40	8
40 — 50	2
50 — 60	7
60 — 70	3

Find (i) Interquartile range, (ii) Mean deviation about median, (iii) standard deviation.

16. The mean μ and variance σ^2 of 6 observation are 8 and 7 respectively. If four observations are 7, 6, 12 and 9, then find the remaining two observations.

OBJECTIVE TYPE QUESTIONS

Select the correct option out of given ones for each statement or question.

17. The measures of dispersion characterize about:
a. Spread of values b. Scatleredness of observations
c. Distance of values from each other d. All of these.
18. Which measure of dispersion is maximally used in statistical formulae?
a. Range b. Standard deviation
c. Mean deviation. d. Quartile deviation.
19. A measure of dispersion is useful in revealing about:
a. The degree of scatter of values
b. How well a central value represents a series of values
c. Comparative variablity of two series
d. All the above.
20. Range is mostly used in describing:
a. Every day temperature fluctuations
b. Salary structure
b. Price structure of an electronic watch
d. All of these.
21. The relation between interquartile range (I.Q.R.) and quartile deviation (Q. D.) is:
a. IQR = 2 QD b. 2 IQR = QD
c. IQR = QD d. None of the above

22. Variance is defined as:
    a. An average of the square of deviations taken from medium.
    b. An average of the square of deviations taken from mean
    c. An average of the deviations taken from mean
    d. All of these
23. Variance of a series of observations is minimum when:
    a. The observation are in arithmetic progression
    b. The sum of values is zer
    c. All values are same
    d. The sum of deviations from mean is zero
24. Formula for calculating variance with usual notations is:
    a. $\frac{1}{N}\left[\sum_{i=1}^{N} x_i^2 - N\bar{x}^2\right]$ b. $\frac{1}{N}\sum_{i=1}^{N}(x_i - \bar{x})^2$
    c. $\frac{1}{N}\sum_{i=1}^{N} x_i^2 - \frac{\left(\sum_{i=1}^{N} x_i\right)^2}{N}$ d. All the above
25. Variance can never be:
    a. Negative b. Zero
    c. One d. Positive
26. Relation between variance and standard deviation (SD) is:
    a. Square of variance is SD
    b. Square root of variance is SD
    c. positive under-root of variance is SD
    d. Variance is same as SD
27. The best measure of dispersion is:
    a. Variance b. Mean deviation
    c. Quartile deviation d. Standard deviation
28. Mean deviation is minimum when the deviations are taken from:
    a. Mean b. Mode
    c. Median d. None of the above
29. The range of a variable X is 3. What would be the range of a variable y where $y = -2x + 20$?
    a. 6 b. 14
    c. 26 d. 18
30. Bulginess of a frequency distribution curve indicates towards its:
    a. Peackedness b. Kurtosis
    c. Both (*a*) and (*b*) d. Only (*a*) but not (*b*)
31. If a frequency distribution curve is either more peaked or flat than a normal curve, then it is called:
    a. Kurtic curve b. Mesokurtic curve
    c. Normal curve d. Leptokurtic curve

32. If the tails of a frequency distribution curve are asymmetric, then it is called:
    a. Kurtic curve
    b. Skew curve
    c. Normal curve
    d. None of the above
33. The value of measure of skewness is – 3.2, than the curve is:
    a. Symmetrical
    b. Normal
    c. Flat
    d. Highly negatively skew
34. There are two series A and B. If series A has coefficient of variation (CV) 7.8 and series B has CV, 8.7. Which of the following statement is correct?
    a. Series A is more variable than series B
    b. Series A and B are at par form variability point of view
    c. Series A is more consistent than series B
    d. Series A is not comparable with series B
35. If each value in a series of data is reduced by 12, then the coefficient of variation:
    a. Increases
    b. Decreases
    c. Remains unaltered
    d. Reduces by 12 percent
36. If the range of a series of 10 observations is 60, then standard deviation is:
    a. 6
    b. 10
    c. 50
    d. 15
37. If the mean deviation of a series of values is 12, then the quartile deviation is:
    a. 15
    b. 12
    c. 10
    d. 14.4
38. If the quartile deviation of a set of values is 24, then the standard deviation of values is:
    a. 16
    b. 36
    c. 20
    d. 6
39. Check the correctness of the statement, 'relative measures of dispersion makes different sets of data comparable.'
    a. False
    b. True
    c. Partially true
    d. Makes no sense
40. If three quartiles of a variable series are 15, 25 and 30, then the coefficient of quartile deviation is:
    a. 3
    b. $\frac{1}{4}$
    c. $\frac{1}{3}$
    d. $\frac{1}{11}$
41. If all values in a data set are same, then the value of any measure of dispersion is:
    a. One
    b. Same as any single value
    c. Zero
    d. Equal to the number of values.

CHAPTER 6

Empirical Probability

INTRODUCTION

Every one talks in probable terms. Generally the statements given by a person have an element of doubt. For example, some person asks a student whether he will get first position in the class, he may say, let us hope so. In the statement of the student, there is no certainity whether to stand first or not. On a particular day, a person going out of the house has to decide whether he should carry an umbrella or not to protect from rain. So he has to think of the chance whether there will be rain or not. But more problems arise in the games of chance. Person betting on cards would always be interested to know what are the chances of getting winning cards. So in daily life, one has an element of doubt in most of the affairs and wants to know mathematically, what are the chances of occurrence?

REPEATED EXPERIMENTS

In tossing a coin again and again, one gets either a head or a tail each time. In this way there is a sequences of heads and tails in repeated tossings. In the game of ludo, a die is thrown every time. Number of spots from 1 to 6 turn up on the upper face. Such experiments are known as repeated experiments (trials).

HISTORICAL BACKGROUND

The credit of origin of probability theory goes to the gamblers of seventeenth century. They put up their problems related to chance of betting situations to mathematicians. A gambler Chevalier De Mere put a number of problems to his mathematician friend Blaise Pascal in 1654. Fermat also initially contributed to the theory of probability. Mainly the probability theory developed in nineteenth century and this credit goes to the mathematician P. Laplace, Gauss, De Moivre, A.A. Markov. A.N. Kolmogorov, J. Bernoulli, Euler, D' Almbert, etc. In twentieth century Karl Pearson, R.A. Fisher, E.S. Pearson, J. Neyman, etc. contributed a lot of theory which enhanced the use of probability theory in various disciplines.

EVENT

From the above discussion it is clear that whenever one talks of probability, an event is associated with it. So one may ask what is probable? The answer is a particular event.

In the context of probability theory, an event can be defined as:

"An event is a happening or occurrence which can be numerically enumerated or listed".

For instance, a coin is tossed twice and noted each time whether it is a head or a tail upside. Let a head be denoted by **H** and a tail by **T**. Only four outcomes are possible as described below.

a. In the first tossing there is a head **(H)** and in the second tossing also there is a head **(H)**, i.e. **HH**.
b. In the first tossing there is a head **H** and in the second tossing there is a tail **(T)**, i.e. **HT**.
c. In the first tossing there is a tail **(T)** and in the second tossing there is a head **(H)**, i.e. **TH**
d. Lastly in the first tossing there is a tail **(T)** and in the second tossing also there is a tail **(T)**, i.e. **TT**. In this way all possible outcomes in tossings of a coin twice are:

HH, HT, TH, TT

In this experiment, a number of events can be described as follows:

Event I: That the coin shows head both the times. It consists of one point, **HH**.

Event II: That the coin turns up with one head and one tail. This event contains two points **HT** and **TH**.

Event III: That the coin has at least one head up. This event consists of three points, **HH, HT, TH**.

Similarly many other events can be considered. Consider another example. In the game of ludo a die is thrown which has six faces marked with spots 1, 2, 3, 4, 5 and 6 on each face below.

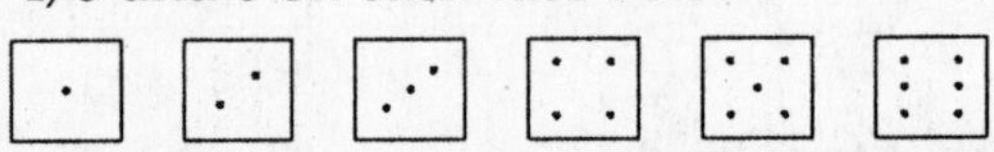

There faces are mutually exclusive in the sense that no two or more faces can turn up simultaneously. If a die is rolled once various events may be given as follows:

Event I: The die turns up with 5 spots. This event will have only one point i.e., 5.

Event II: The die turns up with spots more than three. The points favourable to this event 4, 5 and 6.

Event III: The upper face of a die has spots less than three. This event will have only two points, i.e. 1 and 2.

Similarly many other events can be framed.

Games of cards are very popular all over the world. A pack has 52 cards. There are four cards of same value, i.e., 4 Aces, 4 King, 4 Queen, 4 Jacks, 4 Tens, and so on upto 4 Two's. The pack has 13 cards of each suit namely, spade, heart, diamond and club. Heart and diamond cards are of red colour whereas spade and club are of black colour.

Large number of events can be constructed in the game of cards. A few are exemplified over here. Suppose a card is drawn randomly from the pack.

Event I: The card drawn is an ace. It means that this can have 4 cards, i.e., the ace of any of the four suits.

Event II: The cards drawn is a club. There are 13 cards of club suit. So this contains 13 cards.

Event III: The card drawn is an ace of spade. There is only one spade ace in the pack. So this event has only one card.

From the above examples it is clear that from the totality of elements (all possible outcomes), an event consists of some elements (outcomes) which are favourable to an event.

Simple and Composite Event

An event is called **simple** if it corresponds to a single element (outcome) and otherwise it is known as **composite** or **compound event**.

In the game of cards, event-III is a simple event whereas events I & II are composite or compound events.

Mutually Exclusive Events

Two or more events are said to be mutually exclusive if the happening of one precludes the happening of others in the same experiment.

For example, in tossing of a coin the events of getting either a head or a tail are mutually exclusive because if head turns up, tail can not come and vice-versa. So they are mutually exclusive. Similarly, in rolling of a die, turning up of faces with spots 1, 2, 3, 4, 5 and 6 leads to mutually exclusive events because no two faces can turn up simultaneously.

Independent Events

In case of consecutive experiments, two or more events are said to be **independent** if the happening of one event in no way affects the occurrence of the other events otherwise they are called **dependent**.

For example, in tossing of a coin two or more times, the result in second or subsequent tossing is in no way affected by the result of the previous tossing. Hence, the event of turning up head in one trial is independent of the result of the previous trial.

Again, if a card is drawn from a pack and its face value is noted. At the time of second, there are only 51 cards left over in the pack. So the second draw is affected by the previous draw. Thus, the events related to first and second draw are dependent. But if first drawn card is replaced to the pack before the second draw, the events in the first and second draw become independent.

EMPIRICAL PROBABILITY

In case of repeated trials (experiments), one observes the number of trials that are favourable to an event out of total number of trials conducted. Probability solely based an experimental results or surveys is known as empirical probability. Formula for empirical probability of an event 'E' can be gives as,

$$P(E) = \frac{\text{Number of trails which yieleded results favourable to an event E}}{\text{Total number of trials}} \quad (6.1)$$

In case of surveys or enumeration studies, the probability of an event 'E' is given by the formula,

$$P(E) = \frac{\text{Number of units favourable to an event E}}{\text{Total number of units surveyed or enumerated}} \quad (6.1.1)$$

Definition:

If a trial is repeated a number of times under homogeneous and identical conditions, then the ratio of the number of times 'm' the event E *happens to the total number of trials 'n' conducted is called the probability of the even* E. *When* n *is indefinitely large but finite, then the empirical probability of* E *becomes apposite.*

$$P(E) = \frac{m}{n} \quad (6.2)$$

PROPERTIES OF PROBABILITY

1. Probability of an event is never negative.
2. The value of probability of an event 'E' varies from 0 to 1, i.e., $0 \leq P(E) \leq 1$.
3. If two events A and B are independent, then the probability of their product event AB, i.e., $(A \cap B)$ is equal to the product of their individual probabilities.
4. If two events A and B are mutually exclusive, then the probability of their product AB is zero.

   In empirical probability, the result of each trial is considered independently. Following examples will clearly reveal the method of calculation.

Example 6.1. An experiment was conducted by tossing a fair coin 12 times. It was noted each time whether the coin falls with head or tail upside. The results are as tabulated on next page.

No. of trials	*No. of heads*	*No. of tails*
12	4	8

Empirical probability of getting a head say E_1, is

$$P(E_1) = \frac{4}{12} = \frac{1}{3}$$

Again the probability of getting a tail, say E_2, is

$$P(E_2) = \frac{8}{12} = \frac{2}{3}$$

Let the trial be conducted further for 15 times. The results of obtaining heads and tails in 15 tossings are as tabulated below:

No. of trials	*No. of heads*	*No. of tails*
15	11	4

In this trial the probabilities of E_1 and E_2 comes out to be,

$$P(E_1) = \frac{11}{15} \quad \text{and} \quad P(E_2) = \frac{4}{15}$$

From these trials it is easy to infer that empirical probability is fluctuating fast and may not be justifying our conceptual probability. It is well known that the probability of a head or a tail in tossing a fair coin in $\frac{1}{2}$. But this value is not evinced usually in small number of trials as is seen in case of above two trials. But nearness to this value $\frac{1}{2}$ increases as the number of trials increases. Now consider the two trials jointly. In that case, the results are as given below.

No. of trials	*No. of heads*	*No. of tails*
12 + 15 = 27	4 + 11 = 15	8 + 4 = 12

From the combined results.

$$P(E_1) = \frac{15}{27} \quad \text{and} \quad P(E_2) = \frac{12}{27}$$

Empirical probabilities are nearing to $\frac{1}{2}$. Thus, one can conclude that in the long run of trials, it is expected that empirical probability approaches to theoretical probability of an event.

Example 6.2. A general insurance company conducted the survey of 1000 pilots of whom 450 had an experience of flying aeroplanes less than 5 years, 360 had an experience of 5 to 10 years and 190 were with a flying experience of more than 10 years. Number of accidents faced by the pilots of various experience groups were as tabulated on next page.

Pilots' flying experience	*No. of accidents during last one year*						*Total*
	0	*1*	*2*	*3*	*4*	*5*	
Less than 5 years	270	55	44	62	12	7	**450**
5 to 10 years	195	60	39	31	29	6	**360**
More than 10 years	145	21	15	4	3	2	**190**
Total	**610**	**136**	**98**	**97**	**44**	**15**	**1000**

i. Probability of exactly four accidents in a year, E_1, faced by a randomly selected pilot having an experience of less than 5 years is,

$$P(E_1) = \frac{12}{1000} = 0.012$$

ii. Probability of committing more than one accident, E_2, by a randomly chosen pilot having flying experience of 5 to 10 years can be calculated as follows:
No. of pilots having more than one, i.e., 2, 3, 4 and 5 accidents = 39 + 31 + 29 + 6 = 105
Total no. of pilots = 1000

$$\therefore \quad P(E_2) = \frac{105}{1000} = 0.105$$

iii. Probability of committing no accident by a pilot, E_3, can be obtained as, number of pilots who met no accident = 270 + 195 + 145 = 610. Probability of no accident by a pilot.

$$P(E_3) = \frac{610}{1000} = 0.610$$

iv. Probability of one or less accident E_4, by a randomly selected pilot can be calculated as, No. of pilots facing one or zero accident
= 610 + 136 = 746

$$\therefore \quad P(E_4) = \frac{746}{1000} = 0.746$$

Note: In the same manner probability of any other event can be worked out.

Example 6.3. Two coins were tossed simultaneously 300 times. Number of times two heads, one head and one tail, both the tails turned up were as follows:

Two heads (*HH*) = 80
One head & one tails (*HT*) = 175
Both the tails (*TT*) = 45

i. Probability of getting both the heads in a single tossing of two coins can be calculated by the formula (6.1).

No. of trials favourable to $HH = 80$
Total no. of trials = 300

$$\therefore \qquad P(HH) = \frac{80}{300} = \frac{4}{15}$$

ii. Similarly, the probability of obtaining only one head (or only one tail, or one head and one tail) in a tossing of two coins is,

$$P(TH) = \frac{175}{300} = \frac{7}{12}$$

iii. Probability of getting both the tails in tossing two coins once is,

$$P(TT) = \frac{45}{300} = \frac{3}{20}$$

Check: On tossing two coins simultaneously, the possible outcomes are *HH*, *TH*, *TT*. So the sum of probabilities of these outcomes should be unity. To verify,

$$P(HH \text{ or } HT \text{ or } TT) = \frac{4}{15} + \frac{7}{12} + \frac{3}{20}$$

$$= \frac{16 + 35 + 9}{60} = \frac{60}{60} = 1$$

Example 6.4. Three students of a class were asked to throw a fair die 120 times and record the number of spots that turned up in each throw. Number of times the students obtained the spots 1, 2, 3, 4, 5 and 6 on the upper face are tabulated below.

No. of spots	*Student - I*		*Student - II*		*Student - III*	
	Frequency	*Probability*	*Frequency*	*Probability*	*Frequency*	*Probability*
1	16	$\frac{16}{120} = 0.133$	15	$\frac{15}{120} = 0.125$	25	$\frac{25}{120} = 0.208$
2	25	$\frac{25}{120} = 0.208$	19	$\frac{19}{120} = 0.158$	20	$\frac{20}{120} = 0.167$
3	14	$\frac{14}{120} = 0.117$	16	$\frac{16}{120} = 0.133$	30	$\frac{30}{120} = 0.250$
4	20	$\frac{20}{120} = 0.167$	30	$\frac{30}{120} = 0.250$	15	$\frac{15}{120} = 0.125$
5	15	$\frac{15}{120} = 0.125$	25	$\frac{25}{120} = 0.208$	24	$\frac{24}{120} = 0.200$
6	30	$\frac{30}{120} = 0.250$	15	$\frac{15}{120} = 0.125$	6	$\frac{6}{120} = 0.050$

In case of tossing a fair die, theoretically the probability of obtaining either of 1, 2, 3, 4, 5 or 6 spots on the upper face is $\frac{1}{6}$, i.e., 0.167. But an inspection of the above table reveals that the probabilities of spots in case of individual students are quite different from 0.167. Now pool the frequencies of various spots for I and II student and again for all the three students. Then calculate the respective probabilities as depicted in the following table.

No. of spots	*Pooled results of I and II students*		*Pooled results of all the three students*	
	Frequency	*Probability*	*Frequency*	*Probability*
1	31	$\frac{31}{240} = 0.129$	56	$\frac{56}{360} = 0.155$
2	44	$\frac{44}{240} = 0.183$	64	$\frac{64}{360} = 0.178$
3	30	$\frac{30}{240} = 0.125$	60	$\frac{60}{360} = 0.167$
4	50	$\frac{50}{240} = 0.208$	65	$\frac{65}{360} = 0.180$
5	40	$\frac{40}{240} = 0.167$	64	$\frac{64}{360} = 0.178$
6	45	$\frac{45}{240} = 0.188$	51	$\frac{51}{360} = 0.142$

On pooling the frequencies of students I and II and calculating the probabilities of 1, 2, 3, ...6 sports individually, it is noticed that they are approaching to 0.167, i.e., $\frac{1}{6}$. Further on pooling the frequencies for 1, 2, 3, ...6 spots obtained by the three students and calculating the respective probabilities, it is apparent that they are very near to 0.167. It means that for verification of theoretical probabilities, one should conduct a large number of trials.

Example 6.5. Table below give the distribution of monthly wages of 1000 employees of a company.

Monthly wages (Rs)	*No. of wage earners*
2000 – 2500	8
2500 – 3000	109
3000 – 3500	428
3500 – 4000	290
4000 – 4500	104
4500 – 5000	38
5000 – 5500	13
5500 – 6000	10

Footnote: Lower class limit are included in the classes.

An individual is selected at random from among the above wage earners.

N.B.: When one specks of random selection of fixed number of units (sample of fixed size) from a target population of units, the word random implies that each unit has same chance of selection in the sample. Also the word random signifies that all possible samples have the same chance of occurrence.

The probability that this employee is getting.

(i) Over Rs 5000 (E_1), (ii) between 3000 – 3500 per month (E_2), (iii) either between 4000 to 4500 or 5500 to 6000 (E_3), can be found by the formula (6.1.2) in the following manner.

Total number of wage earners = 1000

i. No. of wage earners having income over

$$\text{Rs } 5000 = 13 + 10 = 23$$

Hence, the probability of an individual getting over Rs 5000 is

$$P(E_1) = \frac{23}{1000} = 0.023$$

ii. Employees earning below Rs 3500 = 428 + 109 + 8 = 545. Probability of a selected individual of getting wages below Rs 3500 is,

$$P(E_2) = \frac{545}{1000} = 0.545$$

iii. Number of persons drawing wages between (4000 – 5000) and (5500 – 6000) = (104 + 38) + 10 = 152 Hence, the required probability of the event 'E_3' is

$$P(E_3) = \frac{152}{1000} = 0.152$$

Example 6.6. A fair die is thrown 600 times and the number of times the spots 1, 2, 3, 4, 5 and 6 turning up are tabulated below:

No. of spots	1	2	3	4	5	6
No. of times the spots turned up	93	96	108	102	106	95

(i) Probability of turning up only 1 spots (E_1) is

$$P(E_1) = \frac{93}{6000} = 0.155$$

(ii) Probability of getting 3 spots or less say, E_2 can be obtained in the following manner

Frequency favourable to E_2 = 93 + 96 + 108 = 297

Total frequency = 600

$$\therefore \quad P(E_2) = \frac{297}{600} = 0.495$$

(iii) Probability of the event to obtain 4 or more spots, say E_3 can be calculated as,

Frequency favourable to E_3 = 102 + 106 + 95 = 303

Thus, $P(E_3) = \frac{303}{600} = 0.505$

Note : On throwing a die, a player will get either the spots 1, 2, 3 or 4, 5 and 6. So the sum of probabilities obtained in (ii) and (iii) is 1.

(iv) Probability of the event that a player will get either 1 or 6, say E_4, can be worked out as given below.

Frequency favourable to E_4= 93 + 95 = 188

Therefore, $P(E_4) = \frac{188}{600} = 0.313$

Example 6.7. In a city on an average 2500 persons go to office by their own cars every day. Average number of deaths due to car accidents on seven days of a week is as follows:

Days	Mon	Tue	Wed	Thur	Fri	Sat	Sun
No. of deaths	12	9	7	11	13	8	7

(i) Probability that a person going out with his own car on Monday will die of car accident say E_1, is

$$P(E_1) = \frac{12}{2500} = 0.0048$$

(ii) Probability that a person going out in his car on Thursday and Friday will die because of car accident, Say E_2, is

$$P(E_2) = \frac{11}{2500} + \frac{13}{2500} = \frac{24}{2500} = 0.0096$$

Example 6.8. Pass percentage in mathematics of class X students taught by a teacher during last nine years is tabulated below:

Years	1996	1997	1998	1999	2000	2001	2002	2003	2004
Pass percentage	56.9	62.5	70.0	55.5	61.0	85.3	81.4	73.2	76.6

Based on the above information, find the probability that the teacher will give the result next year better than 70%.

Total number of years having the record = 9

No. of years in which the pass percentage of students is better than 70% = 4

Hence, the required probability = $\frac{4}{9}$

Check that the probability of the result being 70 percent or less next year = $\frac{5}{9}$.

Example 6.9. Monthwise distribution of births of students of IX class in a school in tabulated below.

Months	Jan	Feb	Mar	Apr	May	Jun	July	Aug	Sept	Oct	Nov	Dec
No. of students	86	74	55	61	76	38	46	57	68	72	92	75

Total number of students = 800

i. A student is selected at random. What is the probability that he had borned in the month of April.
No. of students who borned in April = 61

Hence, the required probability = $\dfrac{61}{800} = 0.076$

ii. Probability that a student picked up randomly was borned before July, can be calculated as follows:
No. of students who borned before July

$$= 86 + 74 + 55 + 61 + 76 + 38 = 390$$

Thus, the required probability = $\dfrac{390}{800} = 0.4875$

iii. Similarly the probability that a student chosen randomly was borned in Dec. or Jan.

$$= \frac{86+75}{800} = \frac{161}{800} = 0.201$$

Example 6.10. A survey was conducted in a colony regarding distribution of number of children in the families. The distribution of houses according to the number of children per family was found to be as follows:

No. of children	0	1	2	3	4	5
No. of families	56	78	184	146	64	32

Total number of families = 560

A family is selected at random.

(i) The probability that this family has two children (E_1) can be obtained in the following manner.
No. of families with two children = 184
Hence, by the formula (6.2),

$$P(E_1) = \frac{184}{560} = 0.328$$

(ii) Probability of the event, E_2, that a randomly chosen family has not more than 3 children can be found as follow:
No. of houses having 0, 1, 2, 3, children

$$= 56 + 78 + 184 + 146 = 464$$

$$\text{Thus, } P(E_2) = \frac{464}{560} = 0.828$$

(iii) Now the probability of the event E_3, that a randomly chosen family has four or more children can be calculated as given below. No. of families which have 4 or more children = 64 + 32

$$\text{Hence,} \quad P(E_3) = \frac{96}{560} = 0.171$$

Example 6.11. In a book the distribution of errors on various pages was found to be as follows:

No. of errors	0	1	2	3	4	5	6
No. of pages	270	138	155	86	76	38	27

A page is opened randomly.

(i) The probability of the event E_1, that this page contains no error can be obtained in the following manner.

No. of pages which have no error = 270

Total no of pages = 790

$$\text{Hence, } P(E_1) = \frac{270}{790} = 0.342$$

(ii) Probability of randomly selected page having more than 3 errors can be calculated as follows:

No. of pages having 4, 5 or 6 errors = 76 + 38 + 27 = 141

$$\text{Hence, the required probability} = \frac{141}{790} = 0.178$$

(iii) Probability of a page with 2 or less errors can be worked out as given below:

No. of pages which have two or less errors = 270 + 138 + 155 = 563

$$\text{Probability of a page having two or less errors} = \frac{563}{790} = 0.712$$

Example 6.12. The forecast by the meteorological department of a rainy day in 120 days was correct on 85 days.

(i) The probability of correct forecast that today it will rain

$$= \frac{85}{120} = 0.708$$

(ii) Probability of wrong forecast of raining on a day

$$= \frac{120 - 85}{120} = \frac{35}{120} = 0.292$$

Note: Obviously the forecast of raining on a day will either be correct or wrong. Hence, the sum of probabilities obtained in (i) and (ii) is 1.0 as the two events are exhaustive.

CONCLUDING REMARK

Empirical probability is based on the result of trials. Hence, the probability of the same event varies from trial to trial. This makes no sense. This probability is conceptually very week. Therefore, in the theory of probability it stands no where. This is being considered simply to give a vague idea of the ratio of favourable outcomes to an event out of total outcomes. For beginners, it is easy to understand. Hence, it is preliminary covered. Anyhow, when the number trials '*n*' under identical condition becomes very large assuming *n* to be finite, the probability becomes conceptually correct.

PRACTICE QUESTIONS AND EXERCISES

1. Write a short note on the origin of probability.
2. What do you understand by repeated trials?
3. Define an event and give five examples of events.
4. Differentiate between simple and composite events.
5. Define mutually exclusive events and explain them through practical examples.
6. When do you call the two events to be independent? Give two examples of independent events.
7. Give an example when two events are dependent.
8. Eight hundred families having 3 children were surveyed. The distribution of families with 0, 1, 2 and 3 boys was as follows:

No. of boys	0	1	2	3
No. of families	56	268	307	169

   Calculate the probability of a randomly chosen family having (i) 3 boys (ii) no boy (iii) one boy (iv) 2 boys. Also show that the sum of four probabilities is equal to unity.

9. An opinion survey was conducted and a question was canvassed among 1200 secondary students seeking their opinion about introduction of statistics from class IX to XII. 970 students answered in affirmative and 180 were against it and 50 students gave no opinion.

   Find the probability that the opinion of a randomly chosen student is (i) against introducing statistics, (ii) in favour of introducing statistics, (iii) having no opinion. Also verify your answer.

10. Frequency of trains arriving on time or late at Delhi railway station on an average each day is as given below.

Train arriving late (hours):	0	1	2	3	4	5
Frequency:	112	75	68	34	24	7

   A man is to depart from Delhi by train on a particular day. What is the probability that (i) his train will be late by one hour? (ii) his train will be late by not more than 2 hours? (iii) his train will be late by 3 hours or more?

11. A pen producing company supplies pens in boxes containing 50 pens. The experience tells that in a box there are 5 pens whose nib is defective,

7 pens are leaking and 3 pens have defective ink filling system. What is the probability that a pen taken out of box at random (i) has defective nib? (ii) has no defect? (iii) is defective?

12. A tea company supplies bags in one kilogram packages. But a lot of 15 packages weighted as follows:

Weight in kg.

1.050, 1.020, 0.960, 0.980, 0.850, 1.006, 0.970, 0.980, 0.950, 0.990, 0.995, 1.030, 0.976, 0.987, 1.010

A bag is sold to a customer. What is the probability that (i) this bag contains tea less by 20 grams or more? (ii) the bag is overweight (iii) the bag differs from 1 kg. weight by 10 grams? (iv) the bag contains tea leaves less than 1 kg.

13. The distribution of wages (Rs per week) of labourers of a factory is given below:

Wages :	700 – 800	800 – 900	900 – 1000	1000 – 1100	1100 – 1200	1200 – 1300	1300 – 1400	1400 – 1500
No. of labourers :	14	19	35	30	28	17	9	8

A labourer is picked up at random. Find the chance that (i) he gets Rs 950 per week, (ii) his salary is Rs 900 or less per week, (iii) his wages are Rs 1200 or more per week, (iv) he is one of the highest wage earner.

14. In a locality, the distribution of persons according to blood groups is as follows:

Blood group :	O	A	B	AB
No. of person :	160	78	92	65

A person is called by a hospital to donate his blood. What is the probability that

i. his blood group is AB?
ii. his blood group is either O or B?
iii. his blood group is A?

15. The frequency of accidents per week in a city of pedestrians, cyclists, motor cyclists and four wheeler vehicle drivers, is as tabulated below

Type of persons :	Pedestrians	Cyclists	Motor cyclists	Four wheeler vehicle drivers
No. of person :	18	22	118	52

A person is called by a hospital to donate his blood. What is the probability that (i) the injured person is a pedestrian? (ii) he is neither a pedestrian nor a motor cyclist? (iii) he is a motor cyclist?

16. Three fair coins were tossed simultaneously 180 times. The frequencies of getting 3, 2, 1 and no heads are displayed below:

HHH	**HHT**	**HTT**	**TTT**
25	66	74	15

Three coins are tossed once again, (i) what is the probability of getting all the three tails? (ii) find the probability of at least two heads (iii) Find the probability of obtaining either all heads or all tails (iv) Find the probability of not getting all heads and all tails.

17. A fair die is thrown 90 times. Number of times the spots 1 to 6 appeared on the upper face are delineated below:

No of spots	:	1	2	3	4	5	6
Frequency of spots	:	18	12	16	17	13	14

A fair die is thrown once again. (i) what is the chance that 3 spots will appear upside? (ii) Find the probability of getting 5 or 6 spots? (iii) what chance is there of falling the die with 4 or less spots? (iv) what is the probability that the member of spots turning up on the die is an even number?

18. A lot of 30 TV sets contains 5 defective sets. A TV set is supplied to a customer from this lot. Calculate the probability of this set to be (i) non-defective (ii) defective.

19. A box contains 20 switches of which 14 are non defective. Four switches have two defects and two switches have three defects. A switch is taken out of the box and sold to a customer. What is the probability that this switch has (i) two defects? (ii) no defects (iii) three defects?

20. In a tea party 50 cups of tea were prepared. Out of 50 cups, tea in 10 cups was prepared without sugar. Somehow the cups of tea with sugar and without sugar mixed up. A cup was served to a diabetic patient. What is the probability that tea in this cup is (i) with sugar? (ii) without sugar?

OBJECTIVE TYPE QUESTIONS

Solve the given problems and choose one correct option

21. A survey was conducted in 300 houses of a locality. A question was asked whether they purchased a big screen LC television (LCTV) and also a DVD. Their responses LC television (LCTV) and also a DVD. Their responses were as tabulated below.

	Purchased DVD		
Purchased LCTV	*Yes*	*No*	*Total*
Yes	136	64	200
No	28	72	100
Total	164	136	300

The probability that a randomly selected house purchased a LCTV is:

a. 4/5 b. 41/75
c. 2/3 d. 17/25

22. If a fair coin is tossed only once, then the two events, appearance of a head or a tail are:

a. Mutually exclusive b. Exhaustive
c. Equally likely d. All of the above

23. If A and B are two events such that $P(AB) = P(A)\ P(B)$, then the events A and B are:

a. Mutually exclusive b. Mutually independent
c. Complementary d. None of the above

24. Observe that forecast for raining on days 1, 2, 3, 4, 7 and 10 were true out of 10 consecutive days. Based on this information, we may say that the probability for a correct forecast is:
    a. 2/5 b. 1/2
    c. 1/10 d. 3/5
25. *A* and *B* play 10 games of chess of which *A* won 5 games, *B* won 3 games and 2 games ended in a draw. The probability of *B* winning a game in future is:
    a. 1/2 b. 3/10
    c. 1/5 d. 1
26. The probability '*P*' of an event '*E*' can lie within the range,
    a. $-1 \leq P \leq 1$ b. $-1 \leq P \leq 0$
    c. $0 \leq P \leq 1$ d. $0 \leq P \leq \infty$
27. If *A* and *B* are two mutually exclusive and exhaustive events, then *P*(*A*) + *P*(*B*) is equal to
    a. 1 b. 0
    c. 1/2 d. 1/4
28. Empirical probability due to Von Mixes is subject to the condition,
    a. Number of trials must be infinite
    b. Number of trials is very large but finite
    c. Number of trials favourable to an event *E* are not exactly countable
    d. None of the above
29. A fair die is rolled 28 times. Number of times spots 1 to 6 appeared upside are:

Spots	:	1	2	3	4	5	6
No. of times	:	3	4	6	8	2	5

    The probability that the die shows 4 spots in the next throw is:
    a. 4/5 b. 1/4
    c. 2/7 d. 6/7
30. Which of the following four pairs of events *A* and *B* are mutually exclusive?
    a. A : Mr X is a college student ; B: he studies
    b. A : Mr X lives in Mumbai ; B: he is an IT man
    c. A : Mr X is a graduate ; B : he is listed an illiterate
    d. A : Mr X is an Indian ; B : he is an American national

CHAPTER 7

Classical Probability

INTRODUCTORY COMMENT

In the previous section probability of events was confined to frequencies observed by way of trials or survey conducted for some phenomena leading to events out of total number of trials conducted or the number of units belonging to a certain class out of total units surveyed or enumerated. But the scope of theory of probability widened in financial management, armed forces, political areas, theory of games, etc. Therefore, instead of confining to probability based on counts or frequencies in trials or surveys, probability theory was conceptualised and was applied to various disciplines like economics, biology, insurance, decision theory, etc.

CLASSICAL PROBABILITY

In this section, probability will be calculated in those situations, experiments or phenomenon in which a particular outcome is not predictable but it is possible to enumerate all possible outcomes. Notable development of probability took place in sixteenth century. Major credit of this development goes to B. Pascal, J. Bernoulli, De-Moivre, P.S. Laplace, etc. Most commonly used definition of probability is due to Laplace. It is also named after him as *Laplacian definition of probability*. This definition of probability is also known as *classical, Mathematical* or *a priori probability.*

Laplacian definition of probability: Suppose in a trial[1], there are n equally likely[2], mutually exclusive[3] and exhaustive outcomes. Out of n outcomes, m are favourable to an event E, then the probability of E can be calculated by the formula,

$$P(E) = \frac{\text{Number of outcomes favourable to E}}{\text{Total number of outcomes}} \tag{7.1}$$

$$= \frac{m}{n} = p \text{ (say)} \tag{7.1.1}$$

Obviously, the number of outcomes not favourable to E are $(n - m)$. Hence, the probability of not happening E, say the event E′ is,

$$P(E') = \frac{n-m}{n} = 1 - \frac{m}{n} \quad (\because 7.2)$$

$$= 1 - p = q \text{ (say)} \quad (\because 7.2.1)$$

Also $$p + q = 1 \quad (\because 7.3)$$

Nota bene: 1. Trial is a random experiment.

2. Equally likely means that each possible outcome of a trial has same chance to occur.

3. Mutually exclusive means that no two or more outcomes can occur simultaneously in the same trial.

Properties

1. Probability ranges from 0 to 1, i.e. $0 \leq p \leq 1$
2. Probability can never be negative, i.e. $P(E) \geq 0$
3. Probability of an impossible event is zero, i.e. $P(E) = 0$ and of a certain event is 1, i.e. $P(E) = 1$. For example, if a die is rolled, then the event E that the die will show up the number of spots from 1 to 6 is a certain event and hence $P(E) = 1$. Again the die will show up the face with 7 spots is an impossible event and $P(E) = 0$.
4. If an event is dichotomous, i.e. it has only two options like success and failure, pass and fail, etc., then the sum of probabilities of success and failure is unity.

Note: Above properties of probability will help the students to ensure the answer of a question.

Limitations

1. If various outcomes of a trial are not equally likely, probability by Laplace's formula can not be calculated. For example, the chance of a student to pass in a test is not 50%, then the outcomes pass and fail are not equally likely.
2. If the number of all possible outcomes is either unknown or infinite, formula (7.1) fails to calculate probability.

Following examples will elucidate the method of calculation of probabilities by Laplace's approach.

Example 7.1. From a well shuffled pack of playing cards, a card is drawn at random.

i. The probability of the event E_1, that the card drawn is of black colour, can be calculated from the formula (7.1).
Total number of cards in a pack = 52
Number of black cards in a pack = 26

Hence, $P(E_1) = \frac{26}{52} = \frac{1}{2}$

ii. The probability of the event, that the card drawn is a queen (E_2) can be worked out in the following manner.
In a pack of cards, number of queens = 4.

$$P(E_2) = \frac{4}{52} = \frac{1}{13}$$

iii. The probability of the card drawn to be a king of spades (E_3) is obtainable as follows: there is only one spade king in a pack

therefore, $P(E_3) = \frac{1}{52}$

iv. The event that the card drawn be a diamond (E_4), has the chance,

$$P(E_4) = \frac{13}{52} = \frac{1}{4}$$

Since the number of diamond cards in a pack = 13

Example 7.2. A fair die is rolled once, the event E_1, that there appears less than 7 dots, is a certain event. Because six faces of a die have dots 1 to 6 which are less than 7. Hence, the number of outcomes favourable to E_1 is 6.

Total number of possible outcome is also 6.

$$\text{Thus, } P(E_1) = \frac{6}{6} = 1$$

Again the probability of a die showing up 3 dots is $\frac{1}{6}$. Since only one face is marked with 3 dots out of total six faces. Also the probability of not getting 3 dots is $\frac{5}{6}$. Because any of the five faces may appear except the face marked with 3 dots. Since a die can show up 3 dots or other than 3 dots, there are mutually exclusive and exhaustive events. Hence, the sum of probabilities of these two events say E and E' is 1, i.e.

$$P(E) + P(E') = \frac{1}{6} + \frac{5}{6} = \frac{1}{6} = 1.$$

Example 7.3. Two fair coins are tossed simultaneously.

i. The probability that both the coins will fall with head upside, HH, can be obtained conceptually as given below.
In tossing two coins at a time, all possible outcomes are : HH, HT, TH, TT
Therefore, total no. of outcomes = 4
One outcome favourable to the given event is HH. Hence,

$$\text{P(both heads)} = \frac{1}{4}$$

ii. To find the probability of at least one head, favourable outcomes are HH, HT, TH.

∴ No. of favourable outcomes = 3

Thus, P (at least one head) = $\frac{3}{4}$

iii. For finding the probability of no head, only favourable outcome is TT.

No. of favourable outcome = 1

∴ P(no head) = $\frac{1}{4}$

iv. For probability of only one head (one tail), the outcomes favourable to this event are HT, TH. So the no. of favourable outcomes = 2

$$P(\text{one } H) = \frac{2}{4} = \frac{1}{2}$$

Check that the probability of one head and one tail will also be $\frac{1}{2}$.

Note: Same situation arises if a coin is tossed twice as given in example 7.3.

Example 7.4. Consider the situation when two fair dice are rolled simultaneously. Then there will be 36 combinations of spots on two dice as listed below.

1, 1	1, 2	1, 3	1, 4	1, 5	1, 6
2, 1	2, 2	2, 3	2, 4	2, 5	2, 6
3, 1	3, 2	3, 3	3, 4	3, 5	3, 6
4, 1	4, 2	4, 3	4, 4	4, 5	4, 6
5, 1	5, 2	5, 3	5, 4	5, 5	5, 6
6, 1	6, 2	6, 3	6, 4	6, 5	6, 6

A large number of events can be created out of this trial. But a few are considered here and the method of calculating their probabilities is explained.

In this trial total number of pairs of spots = 36.

i. E_1: The event that both dice show the same number of spots has six pairs which satisfy this condition, namely (1,1), (2, 2), (3, 3), (4, 4), (5, 5), (6, 6).

Hence, $$P(E_1) = \frac{6}{36} = \frac{1}{6}$$

ii. E_2: Pair of dice show up the number of spots whose sum is an even number. Obviously it is easy to note that half of the pairs have their sum which is an even number and other half pairs have their sum as odd number.

In this way, no. of pairs in favour of E_2 = 18.

$$\therefore \quad P(E_2) = \frac{18}{36} = \frac{1}{2}$$

Note: Same will be the probability of obtaining the odd sum of pair of spots.

iii. E_3 : Sum of spots on the two dice is equal to 8. Pairs which satisfy the condition of E_3 are (2, 6), (3, 5), (4, 4), (5, 3), (6, 2).
No. of pairs which are favourable to $E_3 = 5$

$$\therefore \quad P(E_3) = \frac{5}{36}$$

iv. E_4 = Pair of dice show up the faces with number of spots whose sum is 10 or less. All pairs have their sum 10 or less except the pairs (5, 6), (6, 5) and (6, 6).
Hence, the number of pairs which satisfy $E_4 = 33$

$$\therefore \quad P(E_4) = \frac{33}{36} = \frac{11}{12}$$

v. E_5 : Sum of spots on the pair of dice is divisible by 3.
Pairs of spots whose sum is divisible by 3 are,

(1, 2), (1, 5), (2, 1), (2, 4), (3, 3), (3, 6)
(4, 2), (5, 1), (4, 5), (5, 4), (6, 3), (6, 6)

No. of pairs which fulfil the condition of $E_5 = 12$.

$$\therefore \quad P(E_5) = \frac{12}{36} = \frac{1}{3}$$

Example 7.5. A bag contains 3 white and 4 red balls. The bag is shaked and a ball is drawn from it. The probability of the event (E_1), that the ball drawn is of white colour can be found as follows:

Total no. of ways in which a ball can be drawn = 7

There are three white balls. So the number of ways in which a white ball can be drawn = 3

$$\therefore \quad P(E_1) = \frac{3}{7}$$

(i) In the same manner, probability of a ball drawn to be red (E_2) is,

$$P(E_2) = \frac{4}{7}$$

Note: This is to point out that a ball drawn will either be white or red. Hence, the sum of $P(E_1)$ and $P(E_2)$ is unity

Example 7.6. There are three groups of children whose compositions are:

Group I: 1 boy and 3 girls
Group II: 2 boys and 2 girls
Group III: 3 boys and 1 girl

One child is selected randomly from each group. Probability of the event that the group of three selected children comprises of 2 boys and 1 girl, can be calculated in the following manner.

Possibilities of selection of 2 boys and 1 girl from three groups are:

a. one boy each from Groups II and III and one girl from group I.
b. one boy each from group I and III and one girl from group II.
c. one boy each from group I and II and one girl from group III.

The occurrences within (a), (b) and (c) are independent.

$$\therefore \quad \text{Probability of the event (a)} = \frac{2}{4}\times\frac{3}{4}\times\frac{3}{4}=\frac{18}{64}=\frac{9}{32}$$

$$\text{'' '' '' '' (b)} = \frac{1}{4}\times\frac{3}{4}\times\frac{2}{4}=\frac{6}{64}=\frac{3}{32}$$

$$\text{'' '' '' '' (c)} = \frac{1}{4}\times\frac{2}{4}\times\frac{1}{4}=\frac{2}{64}=\frac{1}{32}$$

Since the events (a), (b) and (c) are mutually exclusive, the required probability is the sum of P(a), P(b) and P(c).

$$\therefore \quad \text{The required probability} = \frac{9}{32}+\frac{3}{32}+\frac{1}{32}=\frac{13}{32}$$

Note: It is to remember that in case of independent events, their probabilities are multiplied whereas in case of mutually exclusive events, their probabilities are added.

Example 7.7. Three persons X, Y, Z travel by car from Jaipur to Delhi on the same day. Odds in favour of their reaching Delhi safe are 3 : 4 ; 4 : 5 ; 5 : 9 respectively.

Probability that they all reach Delhi safe can be calculated as follows:

$$\text{Probability of X reaching safe} = \frac{3}{7}$$

$$\text{'' '' Y '' ''} = \frac{4}{9}$$

$$\text{'' '' Z '' ''} = \frac{5}{14}$$

All the above three events are independent. Hence, the probability of their reaching safe $= \frac{3}{7}\times\frac{4}{9}\times\frac{5}{14}=\frac{10}{147}$

Remark:

1. Odds in favour of an event $E = \dfrac{\text{No. of favourable outcomes to } E}{\text{No. of unfabourable outcomes to } E}$

2. Odds against an event $E = \dfrac{\text{No. of unfavourable outcomes to } E}{\text{No. of fabourable outcomes to } E}$

Example 7.8. In a shooting competition, an Indian can hit the bull's eye 7 times in 15 shots, an American 6 times in 13 shots and a Chinese 4 times in 9 shots. A shooter from each country shoots the target once. The probability that the target will be hit by two shooters can be worked as follows:

For the given event there are three possibilities.

a. Indian and American hit the target and Chinese misses it.
b. Indian and Chinese hit the target and American misses it.
c. American and Chinese hit the target and Indian misses it.

Probability of hitting by an Indian $= \frac{7}{15}$ and of missing $= 1-\frac{7}{15}=\frac{8}{15}$

" " " " American $= \frac{6}{13}$ " " " $= 1-\frac{6}{13}=\frac{7}{13}$

" " " " Chinese $= \frac{4}{9}$ " " " $= 1-\frac{4}{9}=\frac{5}{9}$

Hitting by a shooter is independent of the other.

$$\therefore \quad P(a) = \frac{7}{15}\times\frac{6}{13}\times\frac{5}{9}=\frac{210}{1755}$$

$$P(b) = \frac{7}{15}\times\frac{4}{9}\times\frac{7}{13}=\frac{196}{1755}$$

$$P(c) = \frac{6}{13}\times\frac{4}{9}\times\frac{8}{15}=\frac{192}{1755}$$

Probability of the given event will be sum of the probabilities of the events (a), (b) and (c) as the three events are mutually exclusive.

Thus, required probability $= \frac{210}{1755}+\frac{196}{1755}+\frac{192}{1755}=\frac{598}{1755}$

Example 7.9. An urn *A* contains 4 white and 5 black balls. Another urn B contains 3 white and 6 black balls. One ball is taken out from each urn. Probability of the events.

i. E_1 : both the balls are white.
ii. E_2: both the balls are black.
iii. E_3: one ball is white and one is black.

Can be worked out in the following manner.

Probability of drawing from urn A, a white ball $= \frac{4}{4+5}=\frac{4}{9}$

" " " " " " a black ball $= \frac{5}{4+5}=\frac{5}{9}$

" " " " " B a white ball $= \frac{3}{3+6}=\frac{3}{9}=\frac{1}{3}$

" " " " " " a black ball $= \frac{6}{3+6}=\frac{6}{9}=\frac{2}{3}$

$$P(E_1) = \frac{4}{9} \times \frac{1}{3} = \frac{4}{27}$$

$$P(E_2) = \frac{5}{9} \times \frac{2}{3} = \frac{10}{27}$$

$P(E_3) = P$ (White ball from A) × P (Black ball from B)
+ P (Black ball from A) × P (White ball from B)

$$= \frac{4}{9} \times \frac{2}{3} + \frac{5}{9} \times \frac{1}{3} = \frac{8+5}{27} = \frac{13}{27}$$

Note: Events E_1, E_2 and E_3 are mutually exclusive and exhaustive. Hence, it is easy to verify that $P(E_1) + P(E_2) + P(E_3) = 1$.

Example 7.10. A fair die is thrown twice. Probability of the event, that at first time the die will show up two or less dots and second time 5 or more dots, can be calculated as explained below.

In two throws, total no. of pairs of dots = 36

In the first throw the dots can be 1, 2 and in second throw 5, 6 for the event to happen. So in two throws, pairs of dots that can appear are (1, 5), (1, 6), (2, 5) and (2, 6). Thus, no. of pairs favourable to the given event = 4

Hence, the required probability $= \frac{4}{36} = \frac{1}{9}$.

Example 7.11. The probability of the event, that a randomly chosen leap year has 53 Sundays, can be obtained as follows: A leap year has 366 days. On dividing by 7, one finds that there are 52 complete weeks and any other two days of the week. A weak has 7 days named as, Sun., Mon., Tue., Wed., Thu., Fri. and Sat.

The left out two days will always be two consecutive days. Hence, the possible pairs of two consecutive days are :

1. Sun and Mon 2. Mon and Tue 3. Tue and Wed
4. Wed and Thu 5. Thu and Fri 6. Fri and Sat 7. Sat and Sun.

So the total no. of pairs of consecutive days = 7

If one is a Sunday, then two possibility remain there, i.e. Sunday followed by Monday and Saturday followed by Sunday, i.e. pairs 1 and 7. Thus, no. of pairs favouring for 53rd Sunday is 2.

∴ The probability of 53 Sundays in a leap year $= \frac{2}{7}$

PRACTICE QUESTIONS AND EXERCISES

1. Discuss briefly the areas in which probability is applied.
2. Give in brief the background of the theory of probability.
3. Give mathematical definition of probability.
4. What will happen if the number of all possible outcomes is infinite?

5. What is the range of probability?
6. Give an example of a certain and an impossible events.
7. Give an example when the results of a trial are not equally likely.
8. What do you understand by equally likely, exhaustive and mutually exclusive events?
9. What do you understand by an unbiased and fair die or a coin?
10. If there are four mutually exclusive and exhaustive events, what shall be the sum of probabilities of all these events?
11. Can the probability of an event be negative? Justify your answer.
12. There are two families *A* and *B*. Family *A* has two boys and one girl, family B has one boy and two girls. A child is selected from each family randomly. What is the probability that (i) both are boys? (ii) both are girls? (iii) one is a boy and other a girl?
13. A fair die is rolled once. What is the probability that the die will show up (i) more than 3 dots, (ii) 4 or less dots?, (iii) the die will turn up with either 1 or 6 dots.
14. A fair coin is tossed thrice. Find the probability of obtaining the sequence of head (H) and tail (T) (i) having at least two tails, (ii) having no tail, (iii) having only one head, (iv) having 2 heads and one tail.

    [Hint: All possible sequences of heads (H) and tails (T) are: HHH HHT HTH HTT THH THT TTH TTT]
15. A bag contains 5 red and 4 black balls and another bag contains 3 red and 5 black balls. A ball is drawn from each bag after shaking them. What is the probability that (i) both balls are black? (ii) both balls are red? (iii) one ball is black and other ball is red?
16. A bag contain 7 blue and 3 yellow balls. A ball is drawn in succession four times with replacement. What is the probability of getting blue and yellow balls and vice-versa alternatively?
17. If a student secures 60% marks, he gets first division and from 50 to 59 marks, he get second division. On securing less than 50% marks, he fails. The odds against first division are 3 to 5 and against second division 4 to 5. Find the odds against his failure.
18. A bag contains 4 red and 7 white balls. Two ball are drawn from the bag in order. What is the probability that a white and a red ball will be drawn when the first ball drawn is not replaced?
19. Odds against a person of 40 years of age to survive till the age of 70 years are 8 to 7 and that of a person of 50 years of age to survive till the age of 80 years are 5 to 7. What is the probability that at least one of them will survive 30 years from now.
20. An unbiased coin is tossed three times. Find the probability of the event that the coin shows up at least one tail in three tosses.
21. From a well shuffled pack of 52 playing cards, one card is drawn and noted its colour. The first card is replaced and again a card is drawn from the same pack of cards. What is the probability that one is of red colour and the other is of back colour?
22. What is the probability that a normal year (non leap year) has 53 Sundays?

OBJECTIVE TYPE QUESTIONS

Select the best answer out of given alternatives for the questions hereunder.

23. Classical probability approach becomes inapplicable if:
    a. All outcomes of a trial are not equally likely
    b. Total number of outcomes is uncountable
    c. An event is not clearly defined
    d. All of the above
24. If A and B are two independent event, then the probability of their joint event $P(AB)$ is:
    a. $P(AB) = P(A) + P(B)$ b. $P(AB) = P(A).\ P(B)$
    c. $P(AB) = 0$ d. $P(AB) = 1$
25. If A and B are mutually exclusive and exhaustive events, then the probability of the event $(A + B)$ is,
    a. $P(A + B) = P(A)\ .\ P(B)$ b. $P(A + B) = P(A) + P(AB)$
    c. $P(A + B) = 1$ d. $P(A + B) = 0$
26. If an event A denotes that a person serves a factory and event B denotes that he is an unemployed person, then the probability of the joint event is:
    a. $P(A \cap B) = 0$ b. $P(A \cap B) = 1$
    c. $P(A \cup B) = 0$ d. $P(A \cup B) = 1$
27. Probability of getting one head, when two fair coins are tossed simultaneously, is:
    a. 1.0 b. 0.25
    c. 0.50 d. 0.75
28. If an unbiased die is rolled once, the odds in favour of getting the face up with points which are a multiple of 2 is:
    a. 2 : 1 b. 1 : 1
    c. 1 : 3 d. 3 :1
29. A family has two children of whom one is a boy. What is the probability that other child is also a boy?
    a. 3/4 b. 1/3
    c. 1/2 d. none of the above
30. If A, B and C are three mutually exclusive and exhaustive events such that $2P(A) = 3P(B) = P(C)$, then $P(A)$ is equal to:
    a. 2/3 b. 1/2
    c. 1/3 d. 3/11
31. Marks of nine students are 42, 56, 62, 73, 58, 39, 66, 36 and 81. If a student is selected randomly, than what is the probability that his marks shall be more than the average marks of students?
    a. 4/9 b. 3/9
    c. 5/9 d. 7/9
32. From a well shuffled pack of cards, a card is drawn. What is the probability that it will be a queen?
    a. 1/52 b. 4/13
    c. 1/13 d. 1/4

CHAPTER 8

Statistical and Axiomatic Probability

GENERAL DISCUSSION

In the earlier two chapters, the chance of occurrence of an event was mathematically valued based on a finite number of trials. Mathematical approach to probability is credited to Laplace (1812) whose definition was based on the outcomes of a conceptual experiment e.g., tossing of fair coin(s), rolling of die or dice, etc. The probability based on a finite number of trials might be called physical or statistical probability. The credit of propounding statistical probability goes to Von Mises who emphasised on a large number of trials. This aspect is clearly reflected in the definition given by Von Mises.

DEFINITION

If an experiment can be repeated a large number of times under essentially identical conditions, the limiting value of the ratio of the number of times an event E happens to the total number of trials which increases indefinitely, is called the probability of the event E. If the event E occurs m times out of n trials, then the probability of E is given as,

$$P(E) = \lim_{n \to \infty} \frac{m}{n} \tag{8.1}$$

Actually it is a limiting case when n tends to a very large value. This makes the probability of E stable, i.e. it will not vary appreciably from trial to trial. But this definition has its own weaknesses.

A.N. Kolmogorov (1933) axiomatized the probability in his original work, 'Foundations of the theory of probability'. This extension led to measure theoretic approach. In view of this new approach, one to one correspondence was developed between events and sets. So some terms of set theory like sample space, subset or sub-space, Borel set, etc., are used and defined in this section. Different relations used for events are defined ahead in terms of sets and depicted through Venn diagrams.

Combinatorics is another important part of mathematics, which helps to calculate probability on finite sample spaces. In direct words, use of permutations and combinations makes simple to enumerate the number of arrangements or selections under sampling or experimentation with and without replacement. The readers will find themselves in a comfortable situation after learning about these terms and their uses given ahead in the calculation of probability of events.

RANDOM EXPERIMENT

An experiment is called random experiment if it possesses the following properties.

i. The experiment can be repeated any number of times under identical conditions.
ii. All possible outcomes can be enumerated prior to experimentation.
iii. It is not possible to predict the outcome or result of a particular experiment at any stage.

For instance, on tossing a fair coin it is certain that there will either be head (H) or tail (T). But one can never know whether it will fall with head or tail in a particular tossing.

In throwing of a fair die, it is sure that the die will show up a number from 1, 2, 3, 4, 5, 6. But no one never knows which of these number will be shown up.

SAMPLE SPACE AND EVENTS

The result of a particular trial in a random experiment is called an outcome and it represents an **elementary** or **simple event**. In set theory an outcome corresponds to only one sample point or an element. The totality of all possible sample points or elements is called **sample space**. It is denoted by Ω. It is not necessary that a trial is performed. But it is to be understood that each conceivable outcome of a conceptual experiment is a sample point and the totality of all such points is **sample space**. A sample space is said to be finite if the number of elements in Ω is finite otherwise infinite.

EVENT

The set of one or more sample points which possess the qualities of the described event constitutes an **event** for which the probability is to be calculated. In terms of sets, any event is a specified subset of Ω.

For instance, in tossing a coin twice, the possible sample points are : HH, HT, TH, TT. $\therefore \Omega$: {HH, HT, TH, TT}.

An events E_1, there is one head and one tail in two tosses of a coin, has two sample points HT, TH.

$\therefore \quad E_1$: {HT, TH}.

In rolling of a fair die, Ω: {1, 2, 3, 4, 5, 6}.

The event E_2 that the die show up an even number consists of the number of spots 2, 4, 6. $\therefore$ E_2 : {2, 4, 6}

So in this experiment $n(\Omega) = 6$ and $n(E_2) = 3$. Sample space of odd numbers is 1, 3, 5, 7, 9, ... This is an example of **infinite sample space** as it contains an uncountable odd integers.

A coin is continued to toss till a head (H) turns up. In this trial, the sample space will conceptually be of the type : H, TH, TTH, TTTH, ... This is also an infinite sample space.

Simple Event

An event having only one element of the sample space of a trial is called a **simple** or **elementary event.** In tossing a coin twice, each individual element HH, HT, TH, TT of Ω is a simple event.

Compound Event

An event which has more than one element of the sample space is called **compound event.** It is also called **joint event.** In rolling a die, each outcome of dots 1, 2, 3, 4, 5 and 6 is an elementary event. But the turning up of an even number of dots is a compound event as it consists of three elements 2, 4, 6.

Complementary Event

If A is an event in Ω, then the event consisting of all those points not contained in A is called a **complementary event** or **negation of A** and will be denoted by $\bar{A}$ in this book. For example, in tossing a coin twice, if A consists of the points HT and TH, then $\bar{A}$ has points HH and TT. It can be represented by the Venn diagram as follows.

Note: In all the Venn diagram Ω will be shown by a square and events by circles.

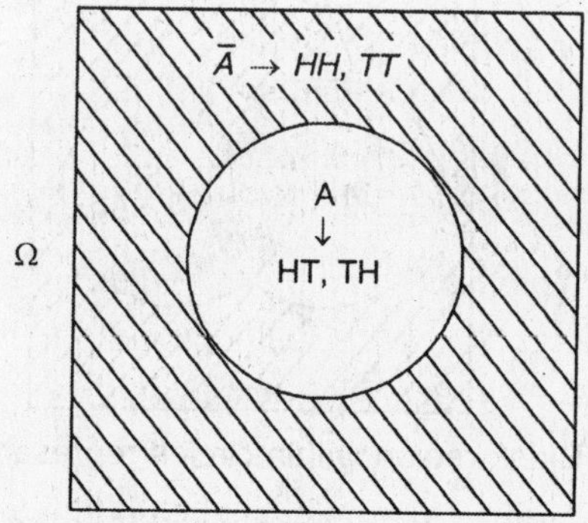

Fig. 8.1: Complementary event $\bar{A}$ is the shaded region

Impossible Event

A subset of Ω which contains no element of Ω, i.e. it is an empty set ϕ, which also represents an event, is known as an **impossible event**.

RELATIONS BETWEEN EVENTS

Different types of events are defined in terms of sets and are depicted through Venn diagrams.

Mutually exclusive events

Two event A and B are said to be mutually exclusive if there is no common point between A and B, i.e.

$A \cap B = \phi$. It implies that $P(AB) = 0$ and $P(A \cup B) = P(A) + P(B)$

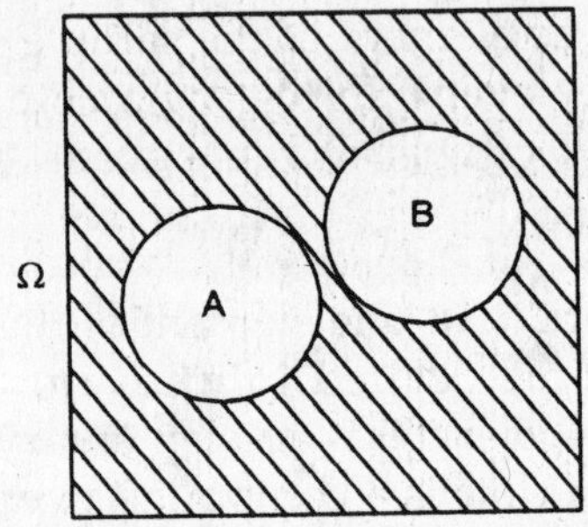

Fig. 8.2: Mutually exclusive events A and B are shown by blank circles

Events A and B are also called **disjoint events.**

Union of Events

Union of two events A and B (A ∪ B) represents an event which ensures the occurrence of either A or B or both. Entire area inside bold boundary represents A ∪ B.

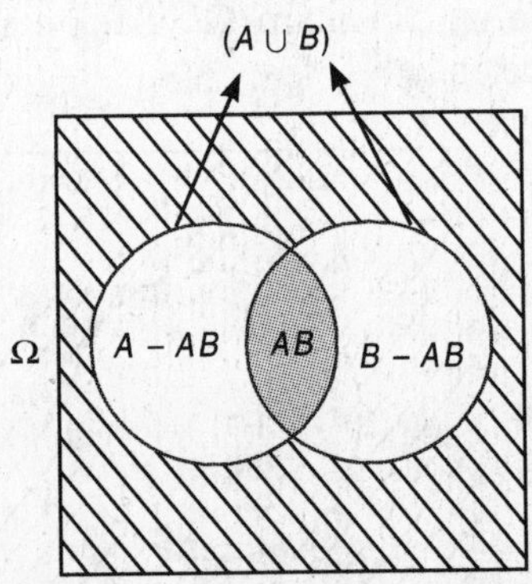

Fig. 8.3: Blank region within circles represents $A \cup B$

The event $A \cup B$ contains the elements of A plus elements of B minus the elements common to A and B.

Intersection of Two Events

Intersection of two events A and B is denoted by $A \cap B$ or simply AB. It is an event of those elements which are common to A and B. Refer to Venn diagram 8.3., the light shaded area inside circles represents $A \cap B$ or AB.

Independent Events

Two events A and B are said to be statistically independent if $P(A \cap B) = P(A) \cdot P(B)$. Its converse is also true, i.e. if two events are statistically independent, then $P(A) \cdot P(B) = P(AB)$.

AXIOMATIC PROBABILITY

Before discussing axiomatic probability it seems pertinent to discuss two more terms of the set theory as follows.

σ-FIELD

A non-empty class of subsets of Ω which is closed under the formation of countable unions and complement and also contains ϕ is known as σ-field.

BOREL SET

A σ-field generated by the class of all bounded semi closed intervals $(a,b]$ will be denoted by B. The sets B are called **Borel sets.**

Without entangling into the complexities of set theory, axiomatic definition of probability propounded by A.N. Kolmogorov in 1933 is given herewith. His theory introduces probability as a number associated with an event. The advantage of the axiomatic approach is that it covers all situations irrespective of whether the possible outcomes are equally likely, exhaustive, mutually exclusive, dependent and independent or not.

DEFINITION

Let Ω be the sample space and B be the Borel set of the class of events over σ-field and P be a real valued function defined on Ω. Then P is called a probability measure and $P(E)$, the probability of an event E if it satisfies the following conditions.

i. $0 \leq P(E) \leq 1$ for every E belonging to B.

ii. $P(\Omega) = 1$

iii. For every set of disjoint events $E_1, E_2, E_3, \ldots$
$P(E_1 \cup E_2 \cup E_3 \cup \ldots) = P(E_1) + P(E_2) + P(E_3) + \ldots$

ALGEBRA OF SETS

Following properties of sets will help the readers to solve numerical problems on probability.

i. $A \cup B = B \cup A$

ii. $A \cap B = B \cap A$

iii. $A \cup (B \cup C) = (A \cup B) \cup C$

$\cup \rightarrow$ Union

$\cap \rightarrow$ Intersection

iv. $A \cap (B \cup C) = (A \cap B) \cup (A \cap C)$

v. $A \cup (B \cap C) = (A \cup B) \cap (A \cup C)$

vi. $A - B = A \cap \bar{B} = (A \cup B) - B$

vii. $\overline{A \cup B} = \bar{A} \cap \bar{B}$

viii. $\overline{A \cap B} = \bar{A} \cup \bar{B}$ (De Morgan Laws)

ORDERED AND UNORDERED SELECTIONS

Consider a population of n objects marked as $a_1, a_2, ..., a_n$. From these n objects, r objects are selected randomly. The selection of r objects out of n can be made in two ways. Firstly an object is selected and replaced back. under this process, the number of objects remain n at the time of each draw. This process is known as **selection** or **sampling with replacement**. In case of sampling with replacement an object may be selected more than once. Also the sample size r may be greater than n. Therefore, the number of all possible samples with replacement is n^r.

Again consider the case when an object selected once is not replaced. In this situation, at first draw there are n units, at the time of second draw there remain $(n - 1)$ units, at third draw $(n - 2)$ units, ..., at r^{th} draw $(n - r + 1)$ units. This process of selection or sampling is known as **selection without replacement.** Hence, the number of ways in which r objects can be selected from n objects when the order of selection is considered are,

$$n(n-1)(n-2) \ldots\ldots (n-r+1) = nP_r \text{ or } (n)_r \tag{8.2}$$

Notation nP_r or $(n)_r$ are called the permutations of r objects out of n objects. nP_r is also the number of all possible sample without replacement. In this situation r can not be greater than n. If $r > n$, then $nP_r = 0$

If the order in which the objects are selected is ignored, then the selection of r objects out of n is called the combination and the number of combinations is denoted by nC_r or $\binom{n}{r}$.

It is obvious that r objects can be arranged in $r(r-1)(r-2) \ldots. 3.2.1$ ways. Hence, the number of ways in which r objects out of n can be arranged or selected when ordering does not matter are,

$$nC_r = \frac{n(n-1)(n-2)\ldots.(n-r+1)}{r(r-1)(r-2)\ldots.3.2.1} \tag{8.3}$$

We know factorial n is denoted as $\lfloor n$ or n!, where

$$\lfloor n = n(n-1)(n-2) \ldots. 3.2.1 \tag{8.4}$$

$$\therefore \quad nC_r = \frac{nP_r}{\lfloor r} \tag{8.5}$$

$$= \frac{n(n-1)(n-2)....(n-r+1)(n-r)(n-r-1)....3.2.1}{\lfloor r \cdot (n-r)(n-r-1)....3.21}$$

$$= \frac{\lfloor n}{\lfloor r \lfloor n-r} \tag{8.6}$$

Also $\qquad nC_r = nC_{n-r}$ (8.7)

For example, $9C_7 = 9\,C_{9-7} = 9\,C_2$

To make the ideas more clear, consider 3 objects x, y and z. A sample of two objects is drawn from x, y and z without replacement. The possible samples are xy, xz, yz, yx, zx, zy, i.e. in all six samples. By the formula of permutations as well, the number of samples,

$$3P_2 = 3\,(3-2+1) = 3 \times 2 = 6$$

Now if the order of selection does not matter, xy and yx is same, $xz \equiv zx$ and $yz \equiv zy$. Total number of possible samples is 3.

By the formula (8.6).

$$3C_2 = \frac{\lfloor 3}{\lfloor 2 \lfloor 3-2} = \frac{\lfloor 3}{\lfloor 2 \lfloor 1} = \frac{3.2.1}{2.1.1} = 3$$

Note that, $\lfloor 1 = 1, \lfloor 0 = 1, nC_0 = 1, nC_n = 1, nC_1 = n$ verify that $4P_2 = 12$, $4C_2 = 6$.

Now some examples are solved so as to explicate the application of probability theory covered hitherto. Use of permutations, combinations and concepts of set theory will profusely be made without further clarification.

Example 8.1. A bag contains 4 white and 5 black balls. Two ball are drawn from the bag at random.

i. Probability of getting 2 white balls in a single draw from the bag can be calculated as follows:

   2 white balls out of 4 white balls in the bag can be drawn in $4C_2$ ways.

   Total number of balls in the bag = 4 + 5 = 9

   Total number of ways in which 2 balls from the bag can be drawn $= 9C_2$

   $$\therefore \qquad \text{The required probability} = \frac{4C_2}{9C_2} = \frac{4.3}{9.8} = \frac{1}{6}$$

ii. Similarly the probability of getting both black balls

   $$= \frac{5C_2}{9C_2} = \frac{5.4}{9.8} = \frac{5}{18}$$

iii. Probability of obtaining 1 white and 1 black balls in a single draw is calculable as, 1 white ball out of 4 white balls can be drawn in $4C_1$ ways.

1 black ball out of 5 black balls can be drawn in $5C_1$ ways. Number of ways in which a white and a black ball can be drawn

$$= 4C_1 \times 5C_1$$

$$\therefore \quad \text{The required probability} = \frac{4C_2 \times 5C_1}{9C_2} = \frac{4 \times 5}{\frac{9.8}{2.1}} = \frac{5}{9}$$

Example 8.2. A Class consists of 9 boys and 7 girls. Four students from this class are to be selected randomly to represent their class in a debate competition. Probability that this group consists of (i) 3 boys and 1 girl, (ii) 2 boys and 2 girls, (iii) 1 boy and 3 girls, can be found out in the manner given below.

Total no. of students $= 9 + 7 + 16$

Total number of ways in which 4 students can be selected from the class $= 16C_4 = \dfrac{16 \times 15 \times 14 \times 13}{4 \times 3 \times 2 \times 1} = 1820$

i. Number of ways in which 3 boys and 1 girl can be selected from the class $= 9C_3 \times 7C_1$

$$\therefore \quad P\text{ (3 boys and 1 girl)} = \frac{9C_3 \times 7C_1}{1820} = \frac{9 \times 8 \times 7 \times 7}{3 \times 2 \times 1 \times 1820}$$

$$= \frac{588}{1820} = \frac{21}{65}$$

ii. No. of ways in which 2 boys and 2 girls can be chosen $= 9C_2 \times 7C_2$

$$\therefore \quad P\text{ (2 boys and 2 girls)} = \frac{9C_2 \times 7C_2}{1820}$$

$$= \frac{9 \times 8 \times 7 \times 6}{2 \times 1 \times 2 \times 1 \times 1820}$$

$$= \frac{756}{1820} = \frac{189}{455}$$

iii. No. of way in which 1 boy and 3 girl can be selected $= 9C_1 \times 7C_3$

$$\therefore \quad P\text{(1 boy and 3 girls)} = \frac{9C_1 \times 7C_3}{1820}$$

$$= \frac{9 \times 7 \times 6 \times 5}{1820 \times 3 \times 2 \times 1} = \frac{9}{52}$$

Example 8.3. Amit has taken 3 tickets randomly from a pack of 10 lottery tickets in which 3 are winning tickets and 7 are blanks. Somna has taken one ticket from a pack of 5 lottery tickets in which 2 are winning and 3 blank tickets. Amongst Amit and Somna who has a better chance of winning a prize. Out of 10 tickets, Amit can select 3 tickets in $10C_3$ ways. Amit will not win a prize if all the 3 tickets are blank. So 3 tickets out of 7 blanks can be selected in $7C_3$ ways.

$$\text{Prob. of Amit not winning a prize} = \frac{7C_3}{10C_3} = \frac{7.6.5}{10.9.8} = \frac{7}{24}$$

$$\text{Amit's prob of winning a prize} = 1 - \frac{7}{24}$$

$$= \frac{17}{24} = 0.708$$

Out of 5 tickets, somna can select 1 tickets in $5C_1$ ways. Somna will not win a prize if her ticket is blank.

So 1 blank ticket out of 3 blanks can be selected in $3C_1$ ways

$$\text{Somna's probability of not winning a prize} = \frac{3C_1}{5C_1} = \frac{3}{5}$$

$$\text{So probability of winning a prize by somna} = 1 - \frac{3}{5} = \frac{2}{5} = 0.40$$

Since the probability of winning a prize by Amit is more than that of Somna, Amit has greater chance of winning a prize.

Example 8.4. Three houses of the same category were advertized for allotment in a locality. Three persons applied for allotting a house giving their choice. What is the probability that (i) all 3 persons gave choice for the same house? (ii) each of them gave choice for a different house? (iii) two of them applied for the same house and the third person for one of the other two houses?

i. 3 persons can apply for any of the three houses. Hence, total number of ways in which they can apply = $3^3 = 27$.
   Since there are three houses, all the three persons can apply for the same house in $3C_1$ ways, i.e. 3 ways.

   $$\text{Hence, the required probability} = \frac{3}{27} = \frac{1}{9}$$

ii. Number of ways in which 3 persons can apply for 3 different houses is $3P_3$ as the ordering does not matter. Hence, number of favourable ways = $3P_3 = 3.2.\ (3 - 3 + 1) = 3.2.1 = 6$

   $$\therefore \quad \text{The required probability} = \frac{6}{27} = \frac{2}{9}$$

iii. There are only three possible ways in which 3 persons can apply for three houses as given in parts (*i*), (*ii*), and (*iii*). Hence, the sum of the probabilities of parts (*i*), (*ii*) and (*iii*) must be unity.

   $$\therefore \quad p\,(i) + p\,(ii) + p\,(iii) = 1$$

or $$p\,(iii) = 1 - P\,(i) - P\,(ii)$$
$$= 1 - \frac{1}{9} - \frac{2}{9} = \frac{6}{9} = \frac{2}{3}$$

Example 8.5. Two cards are drawn from a well shuffled pack of playing cards. Calculate the probability of the events, (i) there is one card of black suits and the other of red suits, (ii) both the cards are aces, (iii) both the cards are hearts.

No. of ways in which two cards can be drawn from a pack of 52 cards $= 52C_2$

i. There are 26 cards of black colour and 26 cards of red colour. One card of each colour from suits of 26 cards can be drawn in $26C_1 \times 26\,C_1$ ways.

$$\therefore P\,(\text{one black and one red card}) = \frac{26\,C_1 \times 26\,C_1}{52\,C_2}$$
$$= \frac{26 \times 26 \times 2 \times 1}{52 \times 51}$$
$$= \frac{26}{51}$$

ii. There 4 aces in a pack of 52 cards. Two aces out of 4 aces can be drawn in $4C_2$ ways.

$$\therefore \quad P\,(\text{both the aces}) = \frac{4\,C_2}{52\,C_2} = \frac{4 \times 3}{52 \times 51} = \frac{1}{221}$$

iii. There are 13 cards of heart suit. 2 cards out of 13 hearts can be selected in $13\,C_2$ ways.

$$\therefore P\,(\text{both the hearts}) = \frac{13\,C_2}{52\,C_2} = \frac{13 \times 12}{52 \times 51} = \frac{1}{17}$$

Example 8.6. Out of 25 employees of a company, 5 are engineers. Three employees are selected at random for granting leave. What is the probability that (*a*) all the three are engineers? (*b*) none of them is an engineer? (*c*) at least one of them is an engineer?

Number of ways in which three employees out of 25 can be selected = $25C_3$.

a. 3 engineers out of 5 can be selected in $5C_3$ ways.

$$P\,(\text{selecting all 3 engineers}) = \frac{5C_3}{25\,C_3}$$
$$= \frac{5.4.3}{25.24.23} = \frac{1}{230}$$

b. There are 20 employees other than engineers. Therefore 3 employee out of 20 can be selected in $20\,C_3$ ways.

$$P \text{ (selecting 3 non engineering employees)} = \frac{20\,C_3}{25\,C_3}$$

$$= \frac{20.19.18}{25.24.23} = \frac{57}{115}$$

c. Probability of selecting at least one engineer

$$= 1 - \text{P (selection of no engineer)}$$

$$= 1 - \frac{20\,C_3 \times 5\,C_0}{25\,C_3}$$

$$= 1 - \frac{57}{115} \times 1 = \frac{58}{115}$$

Example 8.7. From a batch of five salesmen A, B, C, D and E, three are to be sent to a trade fair. The chance of the salesman A to be selected for the trade fair can be worked out as follows:

Total no of ways in which 3 salesmen out of 5 can be selected = $5C_3$.

If *A* is supposed to be selected, then there remains to select 2 salesmen from B, C, D and E.

2 Salesmen out of there four can be selected in $4C_2$ ways.

$$\therefore \quad P \text{ (A to be selected)} = \frac{4\,C_2}{5\,C_3}$$

$$= \frac{4.3/2.1}{5.4.3/3.2.1} = \frac{3}{5}$$

Example 8.8. An urn contains 8 gold and 6 silver coins of the same shape and size. Four coins are drawn in succession. Find the probability of drawing 4 gold coins in first draw and 4 silver coins in second draw under the condition that

i. the coin are replaced before the second draw.

ii. the coins are not replaced before the second draw.

i. Total no. of coins = 8 + 6 = 14

Four gold coins in the first draw can be obtained 8 C_4 ways.

Total no. of ways of drawing four coins from the urn having 14 coins = 14 C_4.

$$\therefore \quad P(A)\text{: Prob of 4 gold coins in first draw} = \frac{8\,C_4}{14\,C_4}$$

Again 4 silver coins in second draw can be obtained in 6 C_4 ways.

$$P(B)\text{ : Prob of 4 silver coins in second draw} = \frac{6\,C_4}{14\,C_4}$$

First and second draw are independent. Hence,

the join probability of A and B; $P(AB) = P(A) \cdot P(B)$

$$\therefore \quad P(AB) = \frac{8C_4}{14C_4} \times \frac{6C_4}{14C_4}$$

$$= \frac{8.7.6.5}{14.13.12.11} \times \frac{6.5.4.3}{14.13.12.11}$$

$$= \frac{10}{143} \times \frac{15}{1001} = \frac{150}{143143}$$

ii. $P(A)$: In the first draw, prob. of drawing 4 gold coins $= \dfrac{8C_4}{14C_4}$.

When second draw is made from the urn without replacement, there remain 4 gold and 6 silver coins in the urn.

Total no. of ways in which 4 coins can be obtained in second draw = $10C_4$

4 silver coins out of 6 silver coins can be drawn in $6C_4$ ways.

$P(B_1)$: Prob. of 4 silver coins in second draw without replacement

$$= \frac{6C_4}{10C_4}$$

Again, the joint probability $P(AB_1) = P(A) \cdot P(B_1)$

$$= \frac{8C_4}{14C_4} \times \frac{6C_4}{10C_4}$$

$$= \frac{10}{143} \times \frac{6.5 \cdot 4.3}{10.9 \cdot 8.7}$$

$$= \frac{5}{1001}$$

Example 8.9. A bag contains 8 red, 5 yellow and 3 white balls. A ball is drawn from the bag at random. Find the probability of obtaining (i) a red ball, (ii) a yellow ball, (iii) a white ball, (iv) a red or a white ball, (v) a yellow or a white.

Total no. of balls in the bag = 8 + 5 + 3 = 16

One ball from the bag can be drawn in $16C_1 = 16$ ways

i. No. of ways in which a red ball can be drawn = $8C_1 = 8$

$$\therefore \quad P(\text{a red ball}) = \frac{8}{16} = \frac{1}{2}$$

ii. Similarly $P(\text{a yellow ball}) = \dfrac{5}{16}$

iii. Similarly P (a white ball) $= \dfrac{3}{16}$

Note: A ball drawn will either be red, yellow or white. So the sum of probabilities obtained in i., ii. and iii. is unity.

iv. If the ball drawn is either red or white, these two events are mutually exclusive since if the ball is red, it can not be white and vice versa. Hence, the probabilities of drawing a red ball or a white ball will be added.

$$P \text{ (a red or white ball)} = \frac{8}{16} + \frac{3}{16} = \frac{11}{16}$$

v. Similarly, P (a yellow or a white ball) $= \dfrac{5}{16} + \dfrac{3}{16} = \dfrac{8}{16} = \dfrac{1}{2}$

Example 8.10. Two cards are drawn from a deck of 52 cards and thrown away. A card is drawn randomly from the remaining 50 cards. What is the probability that this card is an ace.

The problem can be solved in the following manner.

Let us consider different eventualities.

a. Two cards thrown are aces.

b. None of the two thrown cards is an ace.

c. Out of two thrown cards, one is an ace and second is any other card except ace.

Above three situations are mutually exclusive Hence, first find the probabilities under situations. (*a*), (*b*) and (*c*) and then add them to find the probability of the given event.

a. P (Two thrown cards to be aces) $= \dfrac{4C_2}{52\,C_2}$

P (An ace from left out 50 cards) $= \dfrac{2\,C_1}{50\,C_1}$

These two events are independent.

Hence $$P\,(a) = \frac{4\,C_2}{52\,C_2} \times \frac{2\,C_1}{50\,C_1} = \frac{1}{5525}$$

b. When none of the two thrown cards is an ace, it means that two thrown cards will be drawn from the remaining 48 cards excluding four aces

$\therefore P$ (Two cards excluding aces) $= \dfrac{48\,C_2}{52\,C_2}$

Remaining 50 cards contain all the four aces.

$\therefore$ P (An ace from 50 cards left) $= \dfrac{4\,C_1}{50\,C_1}$

$\therefore$ P (Ace in situation b) $= \dfrac{48\,C_2}{52\,C_2} \times \dfrac{4\,C_1}{50\,C_1}$

$= \dfrac{376}{5525}$

c. When 1 card is an ace and 1 card is any other card excluding ace out of two thrown cards,

P (one ace and one other card) $= \dfrac{4\,C_1 \times 48\,C_1}{52\,C_2}$

Remaining 50 cards contain 3 aces and 47 other cards.

$\therefore$ P (An ace from remaining 50 cards) $= \dfrac{3\,C_1}{50\,C_1}$

P (An ace under situation c) $= \dfrac{4\,C_1 \times 48\,C_1}{52\,C_2} \times \dfrac{3\,C_1}{50\,C_1}$

$= \dfrac{48}{5525}$

Thus, the required probability $= \dfrac{1}{5525} + \dfrac{376}{5525} + \dfrac{48}{5525}$

$= \dfrac{425}{5525} = \dfrac{1}{13}$

Example 8.11: A die is thrown twice. What is the probability that (*i*) the sum of spots in two throws will be a multiple of 5? (*ii*) the sum of spots will be 5 or less than 5? (*iii*) both the time the die will show up the same number of spots and their sum is divisible by 3.

In two throws of a die, the sample space will have 6 × 6 = 36 sample points as displayed below:

	1,1	1, 2	1,3	1, 4	1, 5	1, 6
	2,1	2, 2	2,3	2, 4	2, 5	2, 6
Ω =	3,1	3, 2	3,3	3, 4	3, 5	3, 6
	4,1	4, 2	4,3	4, 4	4, 5	4, 6
	5,1	5, 2	5,3	5, 4	5, 5	5, 6
	6,1	6, 2	6,3	6, 4	6, 5	6, 6

i. suppose the sum of spots which are multiple of 5 is denoted by the event A.

Pairs of spots whose sum is 5 or 10 will be the subset of Ω satisfying the event A. There can not be a number 15 or more as the maximum sum of spots can be 12.

$\therefore$ Subset for A = (1, 4), (2, 3), (3, 2), (4, 1), (4, 6), (5, 5), (6, 4).

Hence, No. of elements favourable to $A = 7$

$$\therefore \quad P(A) = \frac{7}{36}$$

ii. Let the event that the sum of spots is 5 or less than 5 be represented by B.

Pairs of spots which satisfying B are:

(1, 1), (1, 2), (1, 3), (1, 4), (2, 1), (2, 2), (2, 3), (3, 1), (3, 2), (4, 1)

So no. of sample points favourable to event B = 10

$$\therefore \quad P(B) = \frac{10}{36} = \frac{5}{18}$$

iii. Let the event that pairs of spot are of same numbers and divisible by 3 be denoted by C.

Pairs of same number of spots are:

(1, 1), (2, 2) (3, 3), (4, 4), (5, 5) and (6, 6). Out of these 6 pairs only two pairs (3, 3) and (6, 6) satisfy the condition of divisibility by 3.

So the number of sample points favourable to $C = 2$

$$\therefore \quad P(C) = \frac{2}{36} = \frac{1}{18}$$

Example 8.12. A coin is tossed thrice. Find the probability of obtaining (i) at least one tail and one head. (ii) two or more tails. (iii) at least one tail.

On tossing a coin three times, sample space of heads (H) and tails (T) will have the following sample points.

HHH, HHT, HTH, HTT, THH, THT, TTH, TTT

i. A: The sample points which have at least one tail and one head are:

HHT, HTH, HTT, THH, THT, TTH

$$\text{so,} \quad n(A) = 6$$

$$\therefore \quad P(\text{ at least one tail and one head}) = \frac{6}{8} = \frac{3}{4}$$

ii. B: The sample points which have two or more tails are : HTT, THT, TTH, TTT

$$\therefore \quad n(B) = 4$$

$$P(\text{two or more tails}) = \frac{4}{8} = \frac{1}{2}$$

iii. C : All the elements in the sample space except HHH have one or more tails.

$$\therefore \quad n(c) = 7$$

$$P(\text{at least on tail}) = \frac{7}{8}$$

Example 8.13. A card is drawn from a pinochle deck. What is the probability of obtaining a king?

A pinochle deck of cards consists of 2 aces, 2 kings, 2 queens, 2 jacks, 2 tens, 2 nines of each suit and no other lower face value card.

Hence, there are only 48 cards in a pinochle deck.

There are 8 kings in a pinochle deck:

1 card from the deck of 48 cards can be drawn in $48\ C_1$ ways.

1 king out of 8 kings can be drawn in $8C_1$ ways

Hence, $$P\ (\text{An ace}) = \frac{8\ C_1}{48\ C_1} = \frac{8}{48} = \frac{1}{6}$$

Example 8.14. A box contains 4 chits bearing odd numbers 1, 3, 5, 7 and another box contains 4 chits bearing even numbers 2, 4, 6 and 8. A chit is drawn randomly from each box. Find the probability of an event A that the sum of numbers on the selected chits will be nine.

Sample space will consists of all possible pairs of numbers marked on the chits in the two boxes.

$$\Omega : (1, 2),\ (1, 4),\ (1, 6),\ (1, 8),\ (3, 2),\ (3, 4),\ (3, 6),\ (3, 8)$$
$$(5, 2),\ (5, 4),\ (5, 6),\ (5, 8),\ (7, 2),\ (7, 4),\ (7, 6),\ (7, 8)$$

$$\therefore \quad n\ (\Omega) = 16$$

Pairs of number satisfy the condition of the events 'A' are: (1, 8), (3,6), (5, 4), (7, 2)

Hence $$n\ (A) = 4$$

$$\therefore \quad P\ (A) = \frac{n\ (A)}{n\ (\Omega)} = \frac{1}{16} = \frac{1}{4}$$

PRACTICE QUESTIONS AND EXERCISES

1. Define sample space and give its two examples. Can a sample space be infinite? Justify your answer through proper examples.
2. Establish an equivalence between sets and events
3. What are the characteristics of a random experiment?
4. Differentiate between simple and compound events.
5. What do you understand by complementary event? Is a null set ϕ, a complementary event of Ω?
6. Define the following events and display them through Venn diagram.
   a. Mutually exclusive events.
   b. Intersection of two events.
   c. Union of two events.
7. Give the statistical definition of probability. In what way it is better than classical definition of probability?
8. Define the terms σ-field and Borel set.
9. Which definition of probability was given by A.N. Kolmogorov? In What sense this is considered to be the most exact definition of probability?

10. What are the De-Morgan's laws on sets?
11. Find the value of the following:

i $4\,C_3$ ii $6\,C_4$ iii $6\,P_3$ iv. $5\,C_0$ v $5\,C_1$

vi. $8\,C_8$. vii. $\underline{|6}$ viii. $5\,P_2$ ix. $10\,C_4$ x. $\frac{15\,C_3}{10\,C_2}$

xi $\underline{|0}$ xii. $\underline{|1}$ xiii. $20\,C_{18}$ xiv. $\frac{10\,C_1}{8\,C_0}$ xv. $\frac{52\,C_0}{52\,C_1}$

12. Give the relationship between nP_r and nC_r.
13. A cell producing company calls a cell good (G) if it has no defect and defective (D) if it has any defect. Three cells are drawn from the lot consecutively. Write the sample space of this experiment.
14. Write the sample space of integers divisible by 5.
15. Write the sample space of outcomes of a trial in which three fair coins are tossed simultaneously
16. Different probabilities were assigned to each element of a sample space of a trial by five experimenters.
Find out which of the experimenters have assigned faulty probabilities.

Experimenters	*Sample points*				
	e_1	e_2	e_3	e_4	e_5
A	$\frac{1}{5}$	$\frac{1}{5}$	$\frac{1}{5}$	$\frac{1}{5}$	$\frac{1}{5}$
B	$\frac{1}{5}$	$\frac{2}{5}$	$\frac{3}{5}$	$\frac{4}{5}$	$\frac{5}{5}$
C	.1	.2	.3	.4	.5
D	.1	.3	.1	.4	.1
E	.3	.2	– .3	.2	.6

17. A fair coin and a die are thrown together. Write down the sample space of the trial.
18. From the word STATISTICS, a letter is selected at random. Find the probability that (*a*) it is a vowel. (*b*) it is a consonant.
19. A book is sent to three reviewers A, B, C independently. The odds that the book will favourably be reviewed by A, B, C are 5 to 2, 4 to 3 and 6 to 1 respectively. What is the probability that the book will have a favourable report by the majority of reviewers.
20. Three students from a class are picked at random. What is the probability that-
    a. All the three were born on the same day?
    b. All were born on Sunday?
    c. Two of them were born on Monday and one on Wednesday?
    d. None was born on Monday?

21. A bag contains 7 red, 3 white and 5 blue balls. Three balls are drawn from the bag after shaking it. Calculate the probability that
    a. All three balls are red.
    b. 2 balls are red and 1 is white
    c. At least one ball is white.
    d. One ball of each colour comes out.
    e. The balls are drawn consecutively in the order red, white and blue and are not replaced.
22. Find the probability of obtaining two Jacks from a pinochle deck when two cards are drawn at random. Also find the probability of obtaining a card with face value 8.
23. Obtain the probability of securing 5 from two fair dice thrown simultaneously using the concept of sets.
24. A box contains chits numbered as 1, 2, 3, 4, and another box contains chits bearing numbers 2, 4, 5, 7, 8, 9. A chit is drawn randomly from each box. Find the probability that the chits will show the numbers 2 and 4. Solve the problem making use of sample space and subsets.
25. A fair die is thrown thrice. What is the probability of obtaining
    a. 3 sixes
    b. 4, 5 and 6 spots
    c. A total 12 of spots
    d. A total greater than 5 spots
26. In a bag there are 3 red and 2 white balls. Find the probability of drawing first ball red, the second ball white, the third red and so on; when the balls are drawn one at a time.
27. Cards from a well shuffled deck are distributed equally among four players. What is the probability that one players will have all the four aces.
28. A bag contains 12 balls of which 3 are red. If 5 ball are drawn together, determine the probability that all three balls are red among the five balls.
29. If A, B and C are three mutually exclusive and exhaustive events. If $\frac{1}{3}P(C)=\frac{1}{2}P(A)=P(B)$, then find $P(B)$,
30. A number is chosen at random from numbers ranging 1 to 50. What is the probability that the number chosen is a multiple of 3.

OBJECTIVE TYPE QUESTIONS

Pick the correct one alternative out of the given four answers for every question.

31. The concept of axiomatic probability was propounded by:
    a. Van-Mises
    b. Laplace
    c. A.N. Kolmogorov
    d. Karl Pearson
32. Statistical probability of an event emphasizes on:
    a. Large number of trials
    b. Small number of trials
    c. Adequate number of trials
    d. Infinite number of trials

33. A random experiment implies that-
    a. The experiment is repeatable any number of times
    b. Total outcomes can be predetermined
    c. An individual outcome cannot be predicted
    d. All of the above
34. A sample space is:
    a. The totality of all sample points
    b. The collection of simple events
    c. The number of trials conducted
    d. All of the above
35. An event can be delineated as:
    a. A set of sample points having specified characteristics
    b. A subset of sample space as per specifications
    c. Both (*a*) and (*b*)
    d. Neither (*a*) nor (b).
36. In rolling a die, an event A consists of the points 1, 4 and 5. The complementary event $\overline{A}$ has the points:
    a. 2, 4, 6
    b. 1, 3, 5
    c. 2, 3, 6
    d. 4, 5, 6
37. If A and B are two disjoint events defined over Ω such that $P(A) = \frac{2}{7}$ and $P(B) = \frac{6}{7}$, then probability $P(A \cup B)$ is:
    a. $\frac{8}{7}$
    b. $\frac{4}{7}$
    c. $\frac{12}{49}$
    d. Not calculable as given probabilities are impossible
38. If A and B are independent events such that $P(A) = \frac{1}{13}$ and $P(B) = \frac{1}{4}$, then $P(A \cap B)$ is:
    a. $\frac{5}{52}$
    b. $\frac{1}{52}$
    c. $\frac{9}{52}$
    d. $\frac{17}{52}$
39. If for any two independent events *A* and *B*, $P(A) = \frac{1}{3}$ and $P(B) = \frac{2}{3}$, then $P(\overline{A \cup B})$ is:
    a. 1
    b. $\frac{1}{3}$
    c. $\frac{2}{9}$
    d. $\frac{2}{3}$
40. If the number of favourable cases to an event *A* is 2 out of 12 cases, then $P(A)$ is equal to:
    a. $\frac{1}{2}$
    b. $\frac{1}{6}$
    c. $\frac{1}{12}$
    d. 1

41. In a throw of two fair dice simultaneously, the probability of getting a sum of five spots on the two dice is:

a. $\frac{1}{9}$ b. $\frac{1}{6}$

c. $\frac{5}{36}$ d. None of these

42. If two event cannot occur simultaneously in a trial, then they are called:

a. Mutually independent b. Mutually exclusive

c. Compound event d. All of the above

43. The probability that exactly one tail appears in tossing a pair of fair coins is:

a. $\frac{1}{4}$ b. $\frac{2}{4}$

c. $\frac{3}{4}$ d. $\frac{4}{4}$

44. The probability of an event cannot exceed:

a. 0 b. $\frac{1}{2}$

c. 1 d. $\frac{1}{4}$

45. If there are three exhaustive events A, B, and C defined over the sample space Ω such that $P(A) = \frac{1}{5}$ and $P(C) = \frac{1}{3}$, then $P(B)$ is:

a. $\frac{8}{15}$ b. $\frac{1}{15}$

c. $\frac{2}{15}$ d. $\frac{7}{15}$

46. A card is drawn from each of the two packs of cards. What is the probability that at least one card is an Ace?

a. $\frac{1}{169}$ b. $\frac{24}{169}$

c. $\frac{25}{169}$ d. None of the above

47. Two letters are randomly chosen from the word STATISTICS. What is the probability that they are vovels?

a. $\frac{3}{10}$ b. $\frac{1}{3}$

c. $\frac{1}{30}$ d. $\frac{1}{45}$

48. If A and B are two events such that $P(A) = P(B)$, then we can infer that:

a. *A* and *B* are mutually exclusive events

b. *A* and *B* may be different events

c. A and B are necessarily same events

d. A and B are independent events.

49. An urn contains 16 balls of which 10 are white and 6 are black. One ball is drawn and its colour is noted. The ball is returned to the urn and again a ball is drawn from the urn. What is the probability that both the balls are of different colours?

a. $\frac{15}{64}$ b. $\frac{49}{64}$

c. 1 d. $\frac{5}{32}$

50. If A and B are any two events, then which of the following relation is correct?

a. $P(A - B) = P(B - A)$ b. $P(A - B) = P(A) - P(B)$

c. $P(A - B) = P(A) - P(AB)$ d. None of the three

CHAPTER 9

Advanced Probability

UTILITY

The purpose of this chapter is to extend knowledge of probability theory by studying some theorems on probability. Some more advances in probability like conditional probability, Bayes' probability will also be covered in this section. It should be kept in mind that whatsoever is given in previous three chapters will be used freely under the tacit assumption that readers have thoroughly studied the same. Addition and multiplication theorems will provide simple methods of calculating probability for a large number of problems. Bayes' theorem is an unique approach to calculate posteriori probability.

ADDITIVE LAW OF PROBABILITY

If A and B are two events, both subsets of the sample space Ω, and are non-mutually exclusive, then the probability of $A \cup B$, *i.e.* the probability of occurrence of either A or B or both is given by the following rule.

$$P(A \cup B) = P(A) + P(B) - P(A \cap B) \qquad (9.1)$$

Set $A \cup B$ can be represented by the Venn diagram as follows:

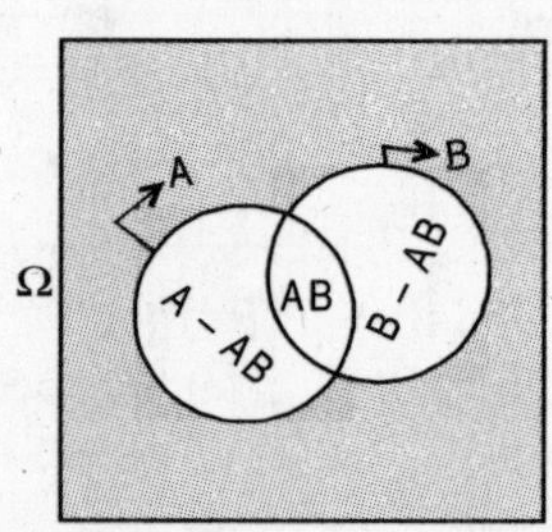

Fig. 9.1: Union of two non-disjoint sets

Sets $(A \cup B)$ is shown by the blank portion inside the circles. This portion consists of three disjoint set $(A - AB)$, AB and $(B - AB)$. Hence,

$$A \cup B = (A - AB) + AB + (B - AB)$$
$$P(A \cup B) = P(A - AB) + P(AB) + P(B - AB)$$

$$P(A \cup B) = P(A) - P(AB) + P(AB) + P(B) - P(AB)$$
$$P(A \cup B) = P(A) + P(B) - P(A \cap B)$$

Special Case : If A and B are mutually exclusive (disjoint), then $AB = \phi$ (null set). $\therefore P(AB) = 0$

Hence, $$P(A \cup B) = P(A) + P(B) \tag{9.2}$$

EXTENSION OF ADDITIVE LAW OF PROBABILITY

Additive law of probability can be extended to any number of events (subsets in Ω). But is confined to three events at present. If A, B and C are three non-disjoint events, then the probability of their union is given as,

$$P(A \cup B \cup C) = P(A) + P(B) + P(C) - P(AB) - P(AC) - P(BC) + P(ABC) \tag{9.3}$$

MULTIPLICATIVE LAW OF PROBABILITY

If A and B are two independent events, then the probability of the event of occurrence of A and B together, i.e. of intersection of A and B is given by the formula,

$$P(A \cap B) = P(A) \cdot P(B) \tag{9.4}$$

Similarly for three independent events A, B and C, probability of their intersection is given as,

$$P(A \cap B \cap C) = P(A) \cdot P(B) \cdot P(C) \tag{9.5}$$

Special Case

If $A \cap B = \phi$, then $P(A \cap B) = P(\phi) = 0$. Formulae (9.4) and (9.5) hold only if $P(A) > 0$, $P(B) > 0$ and $P(C) > 0$.

Also $P(AB) \leq P(A)$, $P(AB) \leq P(B)$, etc.

CONDITIONAL PROBABILITY

If A and B are any two events in sample space Ω, then the probability of an event A given that the event B has already occurred, denoted as $P(A \mid B)$, is given as,

$$P(A \mid B) = \frac{P(A \cap B)}{P(B)} \tag{9.6}$$

or $$P(A \cap B) = P(B)\, P(A \mid B) \tag{9.6.1}$$

Subject to the condition $P(B) > 0$. If $P(B) = 0$, the conditional probability is left undefined.

Equivalence

In terms of elements or sample points of sets, the conditional probability of A given B is

$$P(A \mid B) = \frac{n(A \cap B)/n}{n(B)/n} \tag{9.7}$$

$$= \frac{n(A \cap B)}{n(B)} \text{ provided } n(B) > 0 \qquad (9.7.1)$$

Similarly $$P(B \mid A) = \frac{n(A \cap B)/n}{n(A)/n} = \frac{n(A \cap B)}{n(A)} \qquad (9.8)$$

provided $n(A) > 0$

Nota bene: $P(A \mid A) = P(B \mid B) = 1$ only if $P(A) \neq 0$, $P(B) \neq 0$

Again if A and B are independent, then

$$P(A \mid B) = P(A) \text{ and } P(B \mid A) = P(B)$$

$$P(A \cap B) = P(A \mid B) \cdot P(B) = P(A) \cdot P(B) \qquad (9.9)$$

$$P(A \cap B) = P(B \mid A) \cdot P(A) = P(B) \cdot P(A) \qquad (9.10)$$

Relation (9.9) and (9.10) are also known as multiplication theorems (laws) of probability .

Axioms

Some self evident propositions are given below which shall enhance the knowledge and help to solve a variety of problems.

1. If A and B are independent events such that $P(A) > 0$ and $P(B) > 0$, then $P(A \cap B) = P(A) \times P(B)$. This is possible only when A and B are not mutually exclusive. Hence, two independent events, both of which exist, can not be mutually exclusive.

2. $$P(\Omega \mid B) = \frac{P(\Omega \cap B)}{P(B)} = \frac{P(B)}{P(B)} = 1$$

3. $$P(\bar{A} \cap \bar{B}) = P(\overline{A \cup B}) = 1 - P(A \cup B)$$

   If A and B are independent, then $P(A \cap B) = P(A) \cdot P(B)$

   $$\therefore \quad P(\bar{A} \cap \bar{B}) = [1 - P(A)]\,[1 - P(B)]$$

   $$= P(\bar{A})\, P(\bar{B})$$

   It means that if A and B are independent events, then their complementary event $\bar{A}$ and $\bar{B}$ are also independent.

4. If A and B are independent events and $\bar{A}$, $\bar{B}$ are their respective complements, then the following relations hold.

   $$P(\bar{A} \mid \bar{B}) + P(A \mid \bar{B}) = 1 \qquad (*)$$

   $$P(A \mid \bar{B}) = \frac{(A \cap \bar{B})}{P(\bar{B})} = \frac{P(A)\, P(\bar{B})}{P(\bar{B})} = P(A) \qquad (**)$$

   $$P(\bar{A} \mid \bar{B}) + P(A) = 1$$

   or $$P(\bar{A} \mid \bar{B}) = 1 - P(A) = P(\bar{A}) \qquad (***)$$

5. If A and B are two events and $P(B) \neq 1$, then

   $$P(\bar{A} \mid \bar{B}) = \frac{P(A) - P(A \mid B)}{1 - P(B)} \qquad (****)$$

Following examples will further elucidate the applications of additive and multicative laws of probability along with conditional probability in real life problems.

Example 9.1. A card is drawn from a well shuffled deck. The probability of the card drawn to be an ace or a spade can be calculated as given below.

There are 52 cards in the deck.

One card from the deck can be drawn in $52C_1$ ways. There are 4 aces. Hence, an event *A*, to draw an ace, can occur in $4C_1$ ways.

$$\therefore \qquad P(A) = \frac{4C_1}{52C_1} = \frac{4}{52} = \frac{1}{13}$$

Similarly there are 13 spades in a deck and event *B*, an spade out of 13 spade cards can be drawn in $13C_1$ ways.

$$\therefore \qquad P(B) = \frac{13C_1}{52C_1} = \frac{13}{52} = \frac{1}{4}$$

In 13 spade cards, there is only one ace. Hence, $(A \cap B)$ has only one card (element), i.e. ace of spade.

$$\therefore \qquad P(A \cap B) = \frac{1}{52}$$

Event an ace or a spade is $(A \cup B)$

By (9.1), $$P(A \cup B) = P(A) + P(B) - P(A \cap B)$$

$$= \frac{1}{13} + \frac{1}{4} - \frac{1}{52} = \frac{4+13-1}{52} = \frac{16}{52} = \frac{4}{13}$$

Example 9.2. A contractor applies for two contracts *A* and *B*. Contractor's chance of getting the contract *A* is $\frac{3}{7}$ and that of *B* is $\frac{2}{5}$. The chance that the contractor will get both the contracts is $\frac{1}{6}$. What is chance that the contractor will get at least one contract?

In this problem, the required probability is that of $(A \cup B)$.

Given that $$P(A) = \frac{3}{7}, P(B) = \frac{2}{3} \text{ and } P(A \cup B) = \frac{1}{6}$$

We know, $$P(A \cup B) = P(A) + P(B) - P(A \cap B)$$

$$= \frac{3}{7} + \frac{2}{5} - \frac{1}{6} = \frac{90+84-35}{210} = \frac{139}{210}$$

Example 9.3. A pair of fair dice is rolled. What is the probability that the sum of spots in the two dice is neither 7 nor 11?

Total number of pairs on the dice = $6^2 = 36$

Let *A* and *B* denote the events of getting the sums equal to 7 and 11 respectively.

Elements of A : (1, 6), (2, 5), (3, 4), (4, 3), (5, 2), (6, 1)

No. of element in $A = 6$ $\quad \therefore P(A) = \frac{6}{36} = \frac{1}{6}$

Pairs whose sum is 11 are the elements of B.
Elements of B : (5, 6), (6, 5)

No. of elements in $B = 2$. Hence, $P(B) = \frac{2}{36} = \frac{1}{18}$

Event that the sum is neither 7 nor 11 is equivalent to $(\bar{A} \cap \bar{B})$.

There is no element in common between A and B.
Thus, $A \cap B = 0$.

$$\text{By Axion (3), } P(\bar{A} \cap \bar{B}) = 1 - (A \cup B)$$
$$= 1 - P(A) - P(B)$$
$$= 1 - \frac{1}{6} - \frac{1}{18} = \frac{14}{18} = \frac{7}{9}$$

Example 9.4. A fair coin is tossed thrice. Find the probability of obtaining head all the three times.

$$\text{Probability of head} = \frac{1}{2}$$

Since the tossing of a coin are independent,

P (*Head* all the three times) $= \frac{1}{2} \cdot \frac{1}{2} \cdot \frac{1}{2} = \frac{1}{8}$.

Example 9.5. The probability that a problem of statistics will be solved by a student X is $\frac{1}{3}$ and a student Y is $\frac{2}{3}$. What is the chance that the problem will be solved?

The problem will be solved if it is solved either by X and Y or both.

Let the event that will be solved by X is denoted by A, and by Y is denoted by B.

The required probability is to find $(A \cup B)$.

The phenomenon of finding the solution of the problem by X is independent of solving the problem by Y.

$$\therefore \quad P(A \cap B) = P(A) \cdot P(B)$$
$$P(A \cup B) = P(A) + P(B) - P(A) \cdot P(B)$$

$$\text{Given that } P(A) = \frac{1}{3},\ P(B) = \frac{2}{3}$$

$$P(A \cup B) = \frac{1}{3} + \frac{2}{3} - \frac{2}{9} = \frac{7}{9}$$

Example 9.6. In cricket world cup 2007, India has to play 3 matches against three countries to enter into super 8. Probability of Indian team winning a match against any country is $\frac{1}{3}$. What is the probability that (i) Indian team will lose all the three matches? (ii) Indian team will win at least one match?

Indian team wins a match is denoted by the event A.

Indian team lose a match is denoted by $\bar{A}$.

Given that $P(A) = \frac{1}{3}$,

$$\therefore \qquad P(\bar{A}) = 1 - \frac{1}{3} = \frac{2}{3}$$

Winning or losing a match against a country is independent of winning or losing or match against any other country.

i. $\therefore$ P (*losing* all the three matches) $= \frac{2}{3} \times \frac{2}{3} \times \frac{2}{3} = \frac{8}{27}$

ii. India's win of at least one match amounts to winning 1, 2, or all 3 matches, i.e. not losing all the matches.

   P (at least winning one match)

$$= 1 - P \text{ (losing all three matches)}$$

$$= 1 - \frac{8}{27} = \frac{19}{27}$$

Example 9.7. Given that $P(A) = \frac{1}{5}$, $P(B) = \frac{2}{3}$, and $P(A \cup B) = \frac{4}{5}$. Find $P(A \mid B)$ and $P(B \mid A)$.

First obtain $P(A \cap B)$ by the additive law, i.e.

$$P(A \cap B) = P(A) + P(B) - P(A \cup B)$$

$$= \frac{1}{5} + \frac{2}{3} - \frac{4}{5} = \frac{3 + 10 - 12}{15} = \frac{1}{15}$$

By (9.6), $$P(A \mid B) = \frac{P(A \cap B)}{P(B)}$$

Substituting the value of $P(A \cap B)$ and $P(B)$,

We get, $$P(A \mid B) = \frac{1/15}{2/3} = \frac{1}{10}$$

Similarly, $$P(B \mid A) = \frac{P(A \cap B)}{P(A)}$$

$$= \frac{1/15}{1/5} - \frac{1}{3}$$

Example 9.8. There are 5 white and 7 red balls in a bag. Two balls are drawn from the bag in order that the ball drawn first is not replaced back in the bag. Find the probability of drawing a red ball in the second draw when the first ball drawn is white and not replaced.

Let A denote the event of drawing a white ball.

Let B denote the event of drawing a red ball.

Probability of drawing a white ball in first draw.

i.e. $$P(A) = \frac{5C_1}{12C_1} = \frac{5}{12}$$

Probability of getting a red ball in the second draw when the first is white and not replaced $= P(B \mid A) = \frac{7}{11}$.

Probability of getting a white ball and a red ball in that order under the condition of non-replacement means that A and B are dependent. Hence,

$$P(A \cap B) = P(B \mid A) \cdot P(A)$$
$$= \frac{7}{11} \times \frac{5}{12}$$
$$= \frac{35}{132}$$

Example 9.9. In a market survey of 125 households, an investigator gave the following information regarding owning a computer and also owning a car in the family.

	Having a car	*Having no car*	*Total*
Owning a computer	45	30	**75**
Not-owning a computer	20	30	**50**
Total	65	60	**125**

Find the probability of a household owning a computer when it is known that the household is having a car.

Let the two events be denoted as follows:

A: The household owns a computer.

B: The household has a car.

$$P(A) = \frac{75}{125} = \frac{3}{5}\ ;\ P(B) = \frac{65}{125} = \frac{13}{25}$$

The event that a household owning a computer is also having a car is $(A \cap B)$

From the table, $n(A \cap B) = 45$

$$\therefore \quad P(A \cap B) = \frac{45}{125} = \frac{9}{25}$$

Probability of owning a computer given that the household has a car amounts to finding the conditional probability of A given B.

$$\therefore \quad P(A \mid B) = \frac{P(A \cap B)}{P(B)} = \frac{9/25}{13/25} = \frac{9}{13}$$

Example 9.10. If the probability of a player X winning is $\frac{1}{4}$ and that of Y winning is $\frac{1}{5}$. Find the probability of (i) winning the game by X and Y both, (ii) losing the game by X and Y both, (iii) losing by X and winning by Y, (iv) winning by either X or Y.

Let the event X wins is denoted by A and Y wins by B.

Given that $P(A) = \frac{1}{4}$. $\quad \therefore$ P (*losing* by X) $= P(\bar{A}) = 1 - \frac{1}{4} = \frac{3}{4}$

Given that $P(B) = \frac{1}{5}$, $\quad \therefore P(\bar{B}) = 1 - \frac{1}{5} = \frac{4}{5}$

Winning or losing a game by A and B are independent.

i. P (winning by both X and Y) $= P(A \cap B)$

$$= P(A) \cdot P(B) = \frac{1}{4} \cdot \frac{1}{5} = \frac{1}{20}$$

ii. P (Losing by both X and Y) $= P(\bar{A} \cap \bar{B})$

$$= P(\bar{A}) \cdot P(\bar{B}) = \frac{3}{4} \times \frac{4}{5} = \frac{3}{5}$$

iii. P (Losing by X and winning by Y) $= P(\bar{A} \cap B)$.

$$= P(\bar{A}) \cdot P(B)$$

$$= \frac{3}{4} \cdot \frac{1}{5} = \frac{3}{20}$$

iv. P (winning either by X or Y) $= P(A \cap B)$

$$= P(A) + P(B) - P(A \cap B)$$

$$= \frac{1}{4} + \frac{1}{5} - \frac{1}{20} = \frac{8}{20} = \frac{2}{5}$$

Example 9.11. A bag contains 3 white and 5 black balls. One ball is drawn and its colour un-noted set aside. Again another ball is drawn. The probability that it is, (i) black, (ii) white, can be found as follows:

Total number of balls = 3 + 5 = 8

There can possibly be two situations. One is that first ball is white (W) and the other is that first ball is black. So we have to use conditional probability.

i. P (Black ball/1st ball is either white or black)

$$= P\text{ (1st } W) P \text{ (2nd } B/\text{ 1st } W) + P\text{ (1st } B) \cdot P \text{ (2nd } B/\text{1st } B)$$

$$= \frac{3}{8} \times \frac{4}{7} + \frac{5}{8} \cdot \frac{4}{7}$$

$$= \frac{3}{14} + \frac{5}{14} = \frac{8}{14} = \frac{4}{7}$$

ii. P (White ball/first ball is either white or black)

$$= P\text{ (1st } W) \cdot P \text{ (2nd } W/\text{1st } W) + P\text{ (1st } B) \cdot P \text{ (2nd } W/\text{1st } B)$$

$$= \frac{3}{8} \cdot \frac{2}{7} + \frac{5}{8} \cdot \frac{3}{7}$$

$$= \frac{6}{56} + \frac{15}{56} = \frac{21}{56} = \frac{3}{8}$$

Example 9.12. A person applies for a job in two firms, say X and Y. The probability of his being selected in firm X is 0.7 and being rejected in firm Y is 0.5. The probability of at least one of his applications being rejected is 0.6. The probability that he will be selected in one of the two firms can be calculated in the manner given below.

Let A and B denote the events that the person is selected in firms X and Y respectively.

Given that $P(A) = 0.7, \therefore P(\bar{A}) = 1 - 0.7 = 0.3$

$P(\bar{B}) = 0.5, \therefore P(B) = 1 - 0.5 = 0.5$

Also $P(\bar{A} \cup \bar{B}) = 0.6$

Again $P(\bar{A} \cup \bar{B}) = P(\bar{A}) + (\bar{B}) - P(\bar{A} \cap \bar{B})$

$0.6 = 0.3 + 0.5 - P(\bar{A} \cap \bar{B})$

i.e. $P(\bar{A} \cap \bar{B}) = 0.8 - 0.6 = 0.2$

By De-Margan's law, $\bar{A} \cap \bar{B} = 1 - A \cup B$

$\therefore$ $P(\bar{A} \cap \bar{B}) = 1 - P(A \cup B)$

$P(A \cup B) = 1 - P(\bar{A} \cap \bar{B})$

$= 1 - 0.2 = 0.8$

Example 9.13. A die is thrown twice. The probability of getting an even sum of spots when it is known the face at first throw shows up 3 spots can be worked out as follows:

Let A be the event that the die shows up 3 spots in first throw.

Let B denote the event that the sum of spots in two throws is even.

Total number of pairs of spots = 6^2 = 36.

$$P(A) = \frac{1}{6}$$

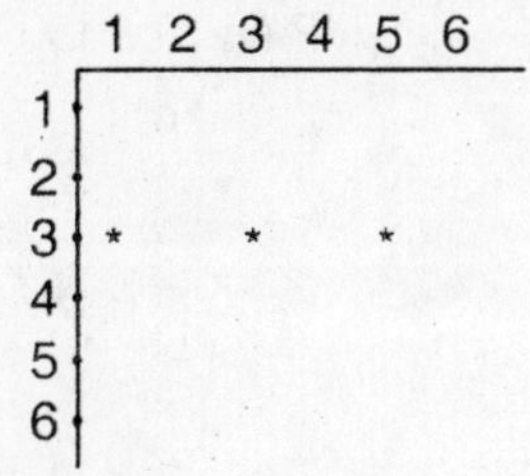

Event B has 18 pairs whose sum is even. Out of the 18 even pairs, there are only 3 pairs of spots whose first digit is 3, namely, (3, 1), (3, 3), (3, 5).

$\therefore \quad A \cap B = (3, 1), (3, 3), (3, 5)$

or $\quad n(A \cap B) = 3, \quad \therefore P(A \cap B) = \dfrac{3}{36}$

$$P(\text{Even sum/1st digit in 3}) = P(B \mid A)$$

$$= \frac{P(B \cap A)}{P(A)} = \frac{3/36}{1/6} = \frac{1}{2}$$

Example 9.14. A die is rolled once and it is known that the number of spots that comes up is greater than 4. Find the probability of the event that the die shows up an even number of spots.

Let the event A: Die shows up an even number of spots.

Let the event B: Number of spots is greater than 4.

$$\Omega : 1, 2, 3, 4, 5, 6$$

$$n(\Omega) = 6.$$

$$B: 5, 6 \,;\, n(B) = 2.$$

$$P(B) = \frac{n(B)}{n(\Omega)} = \frac{2}{6} = \frac{1}{3}$$

The required probability is $P(A \mid B)$

$A \cap B$ = Even no. of spots and > 4 is 6; $n(A \cap B) = 1$

$$P(A \cap B) = \frac{1}{6}$$

$$P(A \mid B) = \frac{P(A \cap B)}{P(B)} = \frac{1/6}{1/3} = \frac{1}{2}$$

Example 9.15. The chance of road accident is 10 in 50 in Bombay, 5 in 40 in Jaipur and 25 in 75 in Delhi every day. Find the probability that an accident occurs on a day, (i) all the three cities, (ii) at least in one of the three cities.

Suppose A, B, C are the events that the accidents occur in Bombay, Jaipur and Delhi respectively.

As per question, $P(A) = \dfrac{10}{50} = \dfrac{1}{5}$; $P(B) = \dfrac{5}{40} = \dfrac{1}{8}$; $P(C) = \dfrac{25}{75} = \dfrac{1}{3}$

Occurrence of accident in one city is independent of the accident in the other city.

i. Accident occurs in all the three cities = $A \cap B \cap C$

$$P(A \cap B \cap C) = P(A) \cdot P(B) \cdot P(C)$$

$$= \frac{1}{5} \cdot \frac{1}{8} \cdot \frac{1}{3} = \frac{1}{120}$$

ii. To find the probability of accident in at least one city is to calculate the probability of $A \cup B \cup C$.

$$
\begin{aligned}
P(A \cup B \cup C) &= P(A) + P(B) + P(C) - P(A \cap B) - P(A \cap C) - P(B \cap C) + P(A \cap B \cap C) \\
&= \frac{1}{5} + \frac{1}{8} + \frac{1}{3} - \frac{1}{5}\cdot\frac{1}{8} - \frac{1}{5}\cdot\frac{1}{3} - \frac{1}{8}\cdot\frac{1}{3} + \frac{1}{5}\cdot\frac{1}{8}\cdot\frac{1}{3} \\
&= \frac{24 + 15 + 40 - 3 - 8 - 5 + 1}{120} \\
&= \frac{64}{120} = \frac{8}{15}
\end{aligned}
$$

BAYES' THEOREM OF PROBABILITY

Thomas Bayes', a British mathematician in 1763 propounded a theorem of probability theory which made possible to revise the old (apriori) probability of an event in the light of additional information provided by the experimenter. New derived probability after making use of the additional knowledge about the event is known as *posteriori probability*. As a matter of fact this is an extension of the conditional probability.

Bayes' theorem

If $E_1, E_2, \ldots E_k$ are k mutually exclusive and exhaustive events in B with each $P(E_i) > 0$ where $i = 1, 2, \ldots, k$, and A is any other event in B which can occur such that $P(A) > 0$, then the probability of the event E_i given A can be computed by the formula given below.

$$P(E_i \mid A) = \frac{P(E_i \cap A)}{P(E_1 \cap A) + P(E_2 \cap A) + \ldots\ldots + P(E_k \cap A)} \tag{9.11}$$

where, $P(A) = P(E_1 \cap A) + P(E_2 \cap A) + \ldots + P(E_k \cap A)$
and $P(E_i \cap A) = P(E_i)\,P(A \mid E_i)$

In Bayes' theorem, probability of E_i is revised on the basis of post information. This is just the reverse case of conditional probability. Hence, Bayes' probability is also known as **Inverse probability**.

Example 9.16. Suppose E_1, E_2 and E_3 denote the events that three persons X, Y and Z can be appointed as managers in a company with probabilities 0.5, 0.3 and 0.2 respectively. Let A be an event that liberalization policy is introduced in the company. The probabilities of introducing liberalization with persons X, Y and Z are 0.4, 0.5 and 0.6 respectively. The liberalization policy has been introduced in the company. Find the probability that it is introduced by Mr X.

Given that, $P(E_1) = 0.5$, $P(E_2) = 0.3$, $P(E_3) = 0.2$

Also $P(A \mid E_1) = 0.4$, $P(A \mid E_2) = 0.5$ and $P(A \mid E_3) = 0.6$

$P(A \cap E_1) = P(E_1)\,P(A \mid E_1) = 0.5 \times 0.4 = 0.20$

$P(A \cap E_2) = P(E_2)\,P(A \mid E_2) = 0.3 \times 0.5 = 0.15$

$P(A \cap E_3) = P(E_3)\,P(A \mid E_3) = 0.2 \times 0.6 = 0.12$

$P(A) = P(A \cap E_1) + P(A \cap E_2) + P(A \cap E_3)$
$= 0.20 + 0.15 + 0.12 = 0.47$

$$P(E_1 \mid A) = \frac{P(E_1 \cap A)}{P(A)} = \frac{0.20}{0.47} = \frac{20}{47}$$

Example 9.17. A company has two plants to manufacture scooters. Plant I manufactures 80% of the scooters and plant II 20%. At plant I 85 out of 100 scooters are rated standard quality. At plant II, 65 out of 100 scooters are rated standard quality. What is the probability that a scooter selected at random came from, (i) plant I, (ii) plant II, if it is known that the scooter is of standard quality?

Let E_1 be the event of selecting the scooted produced by plant I.
Let E_2 be the event of selecting the scooter produced by plant II.
Suppose A is the event that the scooter is of standard quality produced by any plant.

$$P(E_1) = \frac{80}{100} = 0.80\ ;\ P(E_2) = \frac{20}{100} = 0.20$$

$$P(A \mid E_1) = \frac{85}{100} = 0.85;\ P(A \mid E_2) = \frac{65}{100} = 0.65$$

Also $P(A \cap E_1) = P(E_1)\ P(A \mid E_1) = 0.80 \times .85 = 0.68$
$P(A \cap E_2) = P(E_2)\ P(A \mid E_2) = 0.20 \times 0.65 = 0.13$

i. $$P(E_1 \mid A) = \frac{P(E_1 \cap A)}{P(E_1 \cap A) + P(E_2 \cap A)} = \frac{.68}{.68 + 13} = \frac{68}{81}$$

ii. $$P(E_2 \mid A) = \frac{0.13}{0.81} = \frac{13}{81}$$

Example 9.18. Urn I contains 3 black (B) and 5 white (W) balls and urn II contains 5 black (B) and 3 white (W) balls. A coin is tossed. If it turns head, 2 balls are drawn from the urn I and otherwise from urn II, in both the cases with replacement. What is the probability that, (i) urn I is used, (ii) urn II is used, when it is known that both the balls drawn are white?

A : The event that on tossing the coin, it turns up head.
E_1: Both the balls are white and drawn from urn I.
E_2: Both the balls are white and drawn from urn II.

$$P(A) = \frac{1}{2}, \quad P(\bar{A}) = 1 - \frac{1}{2} = \frac{1}{2}$$

$$P(E_1 \mid A) = \frac{5c_2}{8c_2} = \frac{10}{28} = \frac{5}{14}$$

$$P(E_2 \mid A) = \frac{3c_2}{8\,c_2} - \frac{3}{28}$$

$$P(E_1 \cap A) = \frac{1}{2} \cdot \frac{5}{14} = \frac{5}{28} \quad \text{and} \quad P(E_2 \cap \bar{A}) = \frac{1}{2} \cdot \frac{3}{28} = \frac{3}{56}$$

i. The required probability,

$$P(A \mid E_1) = \frac{5/28}{5/28 + 3/56} = \frac{10}{13}$$

Similarly,

ii. $$P(A \mid E_2) = \frac{3/56}{5/28 + 3/56} = \frac{3}{13}$$

Example 9.19. The production of bolts in a factory from machines A, B and C is 25%, 35% and 40% respectively. Out of total output from machines A, B and C, 4, 3 and 2 % are defective bolts in order. A bolt is picked randomly from the lot of bolts and it happens to be defective. Find the probability that it was manufactured by machine A. Also calculate probabilities whether the bolt was manufactured by the machine B, C.

Let E_1, E_2 and E_3 be the events that the bolt is manufactured by machines A, B, and C respectively. Thus,

$P(E_1) = 0.25$, $P(E_2) = 0.35$ and $P(E_3) = 0.40$

$$P(A \mid E_1) = \frac{4}{100} = 0.04,\ P(A \mid E_2) = \frac{3}{100} = 0.03,\ P(A \mid E_3) = \frac{2}{100} = 0.02$$

$P(A \cap E_1) = P(E_1)\, P(A \mid E_1) = 0.25 \times 0.04 = 0.0100$

Similarly $P(A \cap E_2) = 0.0105$; $P(A \cap E_3) = 0.0080$

$$P(E_1 \mid A) = \frac{P(E_1 \cap A)}{P(E_1 \cap A) + P(E_2 \cap A) + P(E_3 \cap A)}$$

$$= \frac{0.0100}{0.0100 + 0.0105 + 0.0080} = \frac{0.0100}{0.0285}$$

$$= \frac{100}{285} = \frac{20}{57}$$

Similarly,

$$P(E_2 \mid A) = \frac{0.105}{0.0285} = \frac{105}{285} = \frac{7}{19}$$

$$P(E_3 \mid A) = \frac{0.0080}{0.0285} = \frac{80}{285} = \frac{16}{57}$$

Example 9.20. The contents of three urns are as follows:

Urn I :	4 white,	2 Black,	4 Red balls
Urn II :	2 " ,	2 " ,	4 " "
Urn III :	3 " ,	4 " ,	5 " "

An urn is chosen and two balls are drawn from this urn. Out of these two balls, one is white and one is red.

What is probability whether the balls have come from urn III.

Suppose E_1, E_2 and E_3 are the respective events that urns I, II and III are chosen randomly. Let A be the event that two balls drawn from the chosen urn are white and red. All urns have equal chance of being chosen.

$$\therefore P(E_1) = \frac{1}{3}, P(E_2) = \frac{1}{3}, P(E_3) = \frac{1}{3}$$

Also
$$P(A \mid E_1) = \frac{4c_1 \times 4c_1}{10\,c_2} = \frac{16}{45}$$

$$P(A \mid E_2) = \frac{2c_1 \times 4c_1}{8\,c_2} = \frac{2}{7}$$

$$P(A \mid E_3) = \frac{3c_1 \times 5c_2}{12\,c_2} = \frac{5}{11}$$

$$P(A \cap E_1) = P(E_1)\, P(A \mid E_1) = \frac{1}{3} \times \frac{16}{45} = \frac{16}{135}$$

Similarly, $P(A \cap E_2) = \dfrac{2}{21}$ and $P(A \cap E_3) = \dfrac{5}{33}$

The required probability is to find $P(E_3 \mid A)$

By Bayes' formula,

$$P(E_3 \mid A) = \frac{P(E_3 \cap A)}{P(E_1 \cap A) + P(E_2 \cap A) + P(E_3 \cap A)}$$

$$= \frac{5/33}{\frac{16}{135} + \frac{2}{21} + \frac{5}{33}}$$

$$= \frac{0.15\,151}{0.11852 + 0.09524 + 0.15\,151}$$

$$= \frac{0.15\,151}{0.36\,527}$$

$$= 0.4148$$

PRACTICE QUESTIONS AND EXERCISES

1. Give addition law of probability and explain the events for which this law is applicable.
2. When two or more events are independent, which law of probability is to be used. Give two examples of the same.
3. Is multiplicative or additive law valid only for two events? Justify your answer by explaining the laws.
4. What do you understand by conditional probability? Explain its implications through practical examples.

5. If it is known that $P(E) = 0$, then what shall be the conditional probability of A given E.
6. If $P(A \mid B) = P(B \mid A)$, then what do you conclude?
7. If the events A and B are independent, then what is the value of $P(A \mid B)$?
8. Find the values of the following
   a. $P(\Omega \mid B)$ b. $P(B \mid \Omega)$ c. $P(\bar{A} \cap \bar{B})$
   when the events A and B are independent. Then find d. $P(A \mid \bar{B}) + P(\bar{A} \mid \bar{B})$ e. $P(\bar{A} \mid \bar{B}) + P(A)$ f. $P(\bar{A} \mid \bar{B})$
9. Find which of the following statements are true or false.
   a. $P(A) \leq P(A \cap B)$ b. $P(A) \leq P(A \cup B)$
   c. $P(A \cap B) \geq P(A) + P(B)$ d. $P(A) = P(A \cap \bar{B})$
10. When the events A, B and C are independent, examine the validity of the following statements.
    a. $P(A \cap B \cap C) = P(A) \cdot P(B) \cdot P(C)$ b. $P(A \mid B) = P(B)$
    c. $P(\bar{B} \mid A) = P(\bar{B})$ d. $P(\bar{B} \mid A) = P(A)$
11. What does apriori and posteriori probabilities mean?
12. Why Bayes's probability is called inverse probability?
13. State and give Bayes' theorem of probability.
14. If A and B are independent and their probabilities exist, then justify that A and B can not be mutually exclusive.
15. Prove that if two events A and B are independent, then their complements are also independent.
16. A bag contains 10 gold and 8 silver coins. Two successive drawing of 3 coins are made such that, (i) coins are replaced before the second draw, (ii) the coins are not replaced before the second draw. In each case find the probability that the first draw will give 3 gold and second 3 silver coins.
17. Let the events A and B be independent with $P(A) = 0.5$ and $P(B) = 0.8$. Find the probability that neither the event occurs.
18. Let A and B be two events such that $P(A) = 0.4$ and $P(A \cup B) = 0.7$ and $P(B) = p$. For what value of p, events A and B are independent?
19. Urn 1 contains 4 red and 6 black balls and urn 2 contains 6 red and 4 black balls. One urn is chosen at random and a ball is drawn from it. The colour of the ball drawn is black. What is the probability that it has been drawn from urn 1.
20. If two events A and B are not disjoint and are connected with a random experiment yielding the information $P(A) = \frac{1}{4}$, $P(B) = \frac{2}{5}$ and $P(A \cup B) = \frac{1}{2}$. Find the value of $P(B \mid A)$.
21. Find the value of $P(AB)$ when A and B are two equally likely, exhaustive and independent events.
22. A class consists of 25 students, out of whom the number of girls is 5. In the class 2 girls and 5 boys are rankers in the previous examination. If a student is selected at random and is found to be a rank holder, then what is the probability that the student selected is a girl?

23. The odds against an event are 5 to 2 and odds in favour of another independent event B are 6 to 5. Find the probability that at least one of the event will occur.
24. The subscribers of a newspaper A are 30%, of newspaper B 20% and of newspaper C 15%. Newspaper A and B are subscribed by 10%, B and C by 8% and A and C by 5%. Only 3% people subscribe all the three newspapers. A person is chosen at random. Find the probability that, (i) the person subscribes at least one news paper, (ii) does not subscribe any news paper, (iii) does not subscribe newspaper B.
25. The probability of diagnosing a disease X correctly by a doctor A is 0.70. The probability of the patient dying by his treatment after correct diagnosis is 0.40 and the chance of death by wrong diagnosis is 0.80. A patient coming to doctor A treated for disease X died. What is the probability that his disease was correctly diagnosed.
26. Given that $P(A \cup B) = \frac{5}{6}$, $P(A \cap B) = \frac{1}{3}$, $P(\bar{B}) = \frac{1}{2}$. Find $P(A)$ and $P(B)$. Also prove that A and B are independent.
27. Two fair dice are rolled in an experiment. Let A denote the event of an odd total, B be the event of one spot on the first dice and C the event of getting a total of seven. Prove that, (i) A and B are independent, (ii) A and C are not independent, (iii) B and C are independent.
28. If A and B are two mutually exclusive events and $P(A) = \frac{1}{4}$, $P(B) = \frac{2}{5}$ and $P(A \cup B) = \frac{1}{2}$, then find (i) $P(A \cap \bar{B})$ (ii) $P(\bar{A} \cup \bar{B})$.
29. A person is known to hit a target in 5 out of 8 shots whereas another person is known to hit the target in 3 out of 5 shots. Find the probability that the target will be hit at all when they both try.
30. The probability that a car holder stopping at a petrol pump will ask for checking his car's tyres is 0.15 and the probability of his asking for coolant checked is 0.30. Also the probability that he will ask for checking tyres and coolant both is 0.08. Find the probability that, (i) the person will get either his car's tyres checked or coolant checked, (ii) if he gets his car's tyres checked will also get his coolant checked, (iii) if he gets his coolant checked will also get the tyres checked.

OBJECTIVE TYPE QUESTIONS

Choose the correct answer from the given ones from each of the following problem.

31. Let there be two events A and B. It is required to obtain the probability of at least one of them to occur. Which law of probability would you use?
    a. Multiplicative law of probability b. Additive law of probability
    c. Conditional probability d. Law of independence of events
32. If A, B and C are three mutually exclusive events, then the probability of the union of A, B and C is:
    a. $P(A \cup B \cup C) = P(A) + P(B) + P(C) - P(A \cap B) - P(A \cap C) - P(B \cap C)$
    b. $P(A \cup B \cup C) = 1$
    c. $P(A \cup B \cup C) = P(A) + P(B) + P(C)$

d. $P(A \cup B \cup C) = P(A) + P(B) + P(C) - P(A \cap B) - P(A \cap C) - P(B \cap C) + P(A \cap B \cap C)$

33. Which of the following relation holds good?
a. $P(A) \geq P(A \cup B)$
b. $P(A \cap B) \leq P(B)$
c. $P(A \cup B) \leq P(A) + P(B)$
d. All of the above

34. If A and B are two independent events, then which of the following relations is correct?
a. $P(A \mid B) = P(B)$
b. $P(B \mid A) = P(B)$
c. $P(A \cap B) = P(A)/P(B)$
d. All of the above

35. If two events A and B are independent, then their complementary events $\bar{A}$ and $\bar{B}$ are:
a. Mutually independent
b. Mutually exclusive
c. Disjoint
d. None of the above

36. If A and B are independent events and $\bar{A}, \bar{B}$ are their respective complementary events, then find which of the following relation is not correct?
a. $P(\bar{A} \cap \bar{B}) = 1 - P(A \cup B)$
b. $P(\bar{A} \cap \bar{B}) = P(\bar{A}) \cdot P(\bar{B})$
c. $P(\bar{A} \mid \bar{B}) + P(A \mid \bar{B}) = 1$
d. $P(\bar{A} \mid \bar{B}) = P(A)$

37. Given that $P(A) = 1$, $P(B) = 1$ and $P(A \cap B) = 1$, then the probability $P(B \mid A)$ is:
a. 1
b. 1/2
c. 0
d. None of the above

38. A card is drawn from a well shuffled deck. What is the probability that either it is a heart or a spade?
a. 2/13
b. 1/2
c. 1/16
d. 7/16

39. Two dice are rolled simultaneously. What is the probability that the difference in the number of spots on the two dice is 1?
a. 5/36
b. 5/18
c. 5/12
d. None of the above

40. In a trial, a fair coin is tossed twice. Let us denote the event A as head on first throw, and B as head on second throw. Then $P(A \mid B)$ is:
a. 1/2
b. 1/4
c. 1
d. 1/8

41. A cricket match was to be played in a city of 10,000 people. 500 persons planned to purchase the ticket (A) to enjoy the play in the stadium. But actually only 350 persons purchased the ticket (B). What is the probability, a person purchased the ticket given that he had planned to purchase it?
a. 3/10
b. 7/10
c. 7/20
d. 3/20

42. Urn A contains 3 black and 5 white balls. Urn B contains 7 black and 1 white ball. A coin is tossed. If it turns up head, two balls will be drawn from urn A and otherwise from urn B. What is the probability that urn A is used given that both the balls drawn are black?
    a. 1/8 b. 3/56
    c. 3/28 d. 3/4
43. After conducting a random experiment, for two events A and B, it is found that $P(A) = \frac{2}{3}$, $P(B) = \frac{3}{5}$ and $P(A \cup B) = \frac{5}{6}$. Find the conditional probability $P(B \mid \bar{A})$.
    a. 5/12 b. 13/20
    c. 5/18 d. 1/2
44. For a given event A such that $P(A) > 0$, the conditional probability of an event E of empty set ϕ say, $P(E \mid A)$ is:
    a. 1 b. 0
    c. Can not be found out d. None of the above
45. If A and B are two independent events, then which of the following statement does not hold?
    a. $P(B \mid A)\, P(A) = P(A \mid B)\, (B)$ b. $P(B \mid A) + P(\bar{B} \mid A) = 1$
    c. $P(A \cap \bar{B}) = P(A) \cdot P(\bar{B})$ d. $P(\bar{A} \cup \bar{B}) = P(\bar{A}) + P(\bar{B})$

CHAPTER 10

Probability Distributions

BASIC CONCEPTS

This chapter is an advancement of probability theory for further usages. Probability of distribution is always given for the occurrence of value of a variable. So before discussing the distribution, it seems necessary to define random variable and its types. In common parlance, a variable may be described as a factor or character which can take different values. In statistics a more specific term is designated as **random variable** (*r.v.*).

RANDOM VARIABLE

A numerically valued function defined over a sample space is called a random variable. In simple words, it is a rule which assigns a numerical value to each outcome of a random experiment. A random variable may be **discrete** or **continuous.** A random variable is generally denoted by the capital letters like $X, Y, Z, \ldots$ and their values by lower case letters $x, y, z, \ldots$

DISCRETE RANDOM VARIABLE

If a variable can take on a finite number of values is called discrete random variable, generally, whole numbers are discrete variables. For instance, family size, number of heads in repeated tossings of a coin, number of spots turning up in rolling of a die or dice, number of accidents in a city, etc.

CONTINUOUS RANDOM VARIABLE

A variable which can take any value within a specified range is called a continuous random variable. For a one dimensional variable, these values can be marked on a straight line. For example, the height of persons, distance from a point to another point, strength of a wire, etc.

PROBABILITY OR THEORETICAL DISTRIBUTIONS

In consideration of a probability distribution, a conceptual experiment is assumed to serve as a model governed by a mathematical function which enables to calculate the probability of the occurrence of a variate value as an individual or in an interval. The probability multiplied by the total number of trials or population units, say N, yields the expected or theoretical frequency. So we obtain the variate values and their corresponding frequencies providing the frequency distribution. For instance, three coins are tossed simultaneously, then all possible outcomes are:

Outcomes	*No. of heads*
HHH	3
HHT	2
HTH	2
HTT	1
THH	2
THT	1
TTH	1
TTT	0

In the above trial, the variable is number of heads. Frequencies are obtained by second column. So the theoretical distribution is

No. of heads	*Frequency*
0	1
1	3
2	3
3	1

Such distribution can be developed theoretically with the help of probability as given forthwith

Note: A discrete variable follows discrete distribution and a continuous variable follows continuous distribution.

DISCRETE DISTRIBUTIONS

Bernoulli Trial

An experiment in which only two outcomes, say A and A', are possible at each performance (trial) such that the probability of the occurrence of A, i.e. $P(A)$ vis-a-vis $P(A')$ remains same at each repetition, is called a Bernoulli trial. Generally, one outcome is referred to as success and the other as failure. For example, in tossing a fair coin, the outcome is either a head or a tail. Also the probability of head or tail at each tossing is $\frac{1}{2}$. As another example, in throwing a true die, the probability of turning up either an even or odd number is $\frac{1}{2}$. Such experiments fall in the category of Bernoulli trials.

Bernoulli Distribution

This distribution is named after its inventor James Bernoulli. It was published in 1713, eight year after his death.

If a dichotomous variable x has a discrete distribution with constant probability p as,

$$p^x (1-p)^{1-x} \tag{10.1}$$

where $x = 0$ or 1
and $x = 1$ means the trial results in success
and $x = 0$ means the trial results in failure,

than x is said to follow Benoulli's distribution. Also $(1 - p)$ is called the probability of a failure and is usually denoted by q, i.e. $1 - p = q$ or $p + q = 1$.

As an illustration, in tossing a true coin, if it turns up with head, $x = 1$, $p = \frac{1}{2}$

$$P(x = 1) = \left(\frac{1}{2}\right)^1 \left(1 - \frac{1}{2}\right)^{1-1} = \frac{1}{2}$$

Properties: The mean of Bernoulli distribution is p and variance is equal to pq.

Binomial Distribution

The credit of inventing this distribution goes to James Bernulli, a Swiss mathematician, who discovered it in 1700 but it was published in 1713. He extended the idea of Bernoulli trial to repeated trials a number of times. If a Bernoulli trial can be repeated n times with probability of success p and failure $q = 1 - p$, then the probability of x successes out of n trials is given by the probability function,

$$p(x, n, p) = nc_x\, p^x\, q^{n-x} \tag{10.2}$$

for $x = 0, 1, 2, ..., n$

The probability function given by (10.2) is known as binomial distribution of the variable x. It has two parameters, n and p, it is denoted as $b(n, p)$.

Properties: 1. The mean of binomial distribution = np
2. Variance of binomial distribution = npq.

This implies that S.D. = $\sqrt{npq}$

Special Case

When $n = 1$, the function (10.2) reduces to $p^x q^{1-x}$, i.e. the Bernoulli distribution. This has tremendous use in calculating the probabilities in a large number of trials which have outcomes into two categories only. Some popular type of cases are put forth through examples.

Expected Value

In simple words, expected value can be defined as the average value of a probability distribution.

Let x be a discrete random variable with probability function $p(x)$, then the expected value of x is given as,

$$E(x) = \Sigma x p(x) \tag{10.3}$$

where, Σ is the sum over all values of x, i.e. $\Sigma x p(x)$ is the sum of the cross product of the values of x and its probability of occurrence $p(x)$.

Example 10.1. Six fair coins are tossed simultaneously. Find the probability of obtaining

i. 3 heads

ii. at least four heads.

As per question, $n = 6$, prob. of a head, $p = \frac{1}{2}, q = \frac{1}{2}$

i. Probability of obtaining 3 heads means $P(x = 3)$.

By the formula (10.2),

$$P(x=3) = 6\,C_3 \left(\frac{1}{2}\right)^3 \left(\frac{1}{2}\right)^{6-3}$$

$$= \frac{6.5.4}{3.2.1} \cdot \left(\frac{1}{2}\right)^3 \left(\frac{1}{2}\right)^3$$

$$= 20 \cdot \frac{1}{2^6} = \frac{20}{64} = \frac{5}{16}$$

ii. Probability of obtaining at least 4 heads means, $x = 4$, 5 and 6.

$$P(x \geq 4) = 6\,C_4 \left(\frac{1}{2}\right)^4 \left(\frac{1}{2}\right)^{6-4} + 6\,C_5 \left(\frac{1}{2}\right)^5 \left(\frac{1}{2}\right)^{6-5} + 6C_6 \left(\frac{1}{2}\right)^6 \left(\frac{1}{2}\right)^{6-6}$$

$$= \frac{1}{2^6}(6\,C_4 + 6\,C_5 + 6\,C_6)$$

$$= \frac{1}{64}\left(\frac{6.5}{2.1} + 6 + 1\right) = \frac{22}{64} = \frac{11}{32}$$

[Recall : $nC_r = nC_{n-r}$ $\therefore$ $6\,C_4 = 6\,C_2$; $6\,C_5 = 6\,C_1$]

Example 10.2. Past experience reveals that Mr Rana can hit the target 3 times out of 5 shots. Find the probability of hitting the target,

i. 4 times out of six shots

ii. at least 2 times out of six shots

iii. not more than once out of six shots.

As per question, $n = 6, p = \frac{3}{5}, q = 1 - \frac{3}{5} = \frac{2}{5}$

i. Probability of 4 successes out of 6 shots is,

$$P\,(x = 4) = 6\,C_4 \left(\frac{3}{5}\right)^4 \left(\frac{2}{5}\right)^{6-4}$$

$$= \frac{6.5}{2.1} \times \frac{1}{5^6} \times 3^4 \times 2^2$$

$$= \frac{15 \times 81 \times 4}{125 \times 125} = \frac{972}{3125}$$

ii. Probability of hitting at least 2 times amounts to finding [1 – P (0) – P (1)]

$$P\,(X \geq 2) = 1 - 6\,C_0 \left(\frac{3}{5}\right)^0 \left(\frac{2}{5}\right)^{6-0} - 6\,C_1 \left(\frac{3}{5}\right)^1 \left(\frac{2}{5}\right)^{6-1}$$

$$= 1 - \left(\frac{2}{5}\right)^6 - 6 \cdot \frac{3}{5}\left(\frac{2}{5}\right)^5$$

$$= 1 - 0.0041 - 0.03686$$

$$= 0.9590$$

iii. Probability of not more than 1 success means to find the sum of probabilities for $x = 0, 1$.

$$P(X \leq 1) = 6\,C_0 \left(\frac{3}{5}\right)^0 \left(\frac{2}{5}\right)^{6-0} + 6\,C_1 \left(\frac{3}{5}\right)^1 \left(\frac{2}{5}\right)^{6-1}$$

$$= \frac{1}{5^6}[2^6 + 6 \times 3 \times 2^5]$$

$$= \frac{1}{5^6}[64 + 576]$$

$$= \frac{640}{125 \times 125} = \frac{128}{3125}$$

Example 10.3. Following information is available about the binomial distribution of a discrete variable x. Mean of the binomial distribution = $\frac{16}{3}$ and variance = $\frac{16}{9}$. Find the distribution.

The probability function of the binomial distribution involves two parameters n and p.

Also $p + q = 1$

Given that $np = \frac{16}{3}$ and $npq = \frac{16}{9}$

Putting the value of np in npq, we get,

$$\frac{16}{3}q = \frac{16}{9} \quad \text{or} \quad q = \frac{1}{3}$$

$$p = 1 - \frac{1}{3} = \frac{2}{3}$$

Again, $$n \cdot \frac{2}{3} = \frac{16}{3} \quad \text{or} \quad n = 8$$

Thus, the binomial distribution is $8C_x \left(\frac{2}{3}\right)^x \left(\frac{1}{3}\right)^{8-x}$

Example 10.4. Five coins are tossed simultaneously 320 times. Find the frequency distribution of the number of heads. Also find the expected value of x.

In the given question, $n = 5$, $p = \frac{1}{2}$, $q = \frac{1}{2}$ and $N = 320$. First, the probabilities of 0 to 5 heads are calculated. Next on multiplying these probabilities by N, theoretical frequencies are obtained. Writing the number of heads with corresponding frequencies, the frequency distribution is displayed.

No. of heads (x)	*Probability* p	*Expected Frequency* NP
0	$5C_0 \left(\frac{1}{2}\right)^0 \left(\frac{1}{2}\right)^{5-0} = \frac{1}{32}$	$320 \times \frac{1}{32} = 10$
1	$5C_1 \left(\frac{1}{2}\right)^5 = \frac{5}{32}$	$320 \times \frac{5}{32} = 50$
2	$5C_2 \left(\frac{1}{2}\right)^5 = \frac{10}{32}$	$320 \times \frac{10}{32} = 100$

3	$5C_3\left(\frac{1}{2}\right)^5 = \frac{10}{32}$	$320 \times \frac{10}{32} = 100$
4	$5C_4\left(\frac{1}{2}\right)^5 = \frac{5}{32}$	$320 \times \frac{5}{32} = 50$
5	$5C_5\left(\frac{1}{2}\right)^5 = \frac{1}{32}$	$320 \times \frac{1}{32} = 10$

So the frequency distribution is,

No. of heads; x:	0	1	2	3	4	5
Frequency; f:	10	50	100	100	50	10

Example 10.5. From a standard deck of cards, four cards are drawn randomly. Find the probability of getting, (i) 2 red cards, (ii) all the four red cards, (iii) at least 3 red cards, (iv) no red card, (v) one or less red card.

In a standard deck of cards, there are 26 red cards and 26 black. So the probability of getting a red card, $p = \frac{1}{2}$ and of a black card $q = \frac{1}{2}$. Also given that $n = 4$. since there are only two possible out comes, i.e., either a red card or a black card, probabilities will be calculated by the formula (10.2)

i. Probability of exactly 2 red cards is,

$$P(x = 2) = 4C_2\left(\frac{1}{2}\right)^2\left(\frac{1}{2}\right)^{4-2}$$

$$= \frac{4 \times 3}{2 \times 2} \cdot \frac{1}{2^4} = 6 \cdot \frac{1}{16} = \frac{3}{8}$$

ii. Probability of all the red cards is,

$$P(x = 4) = 4C_4\left(\frac{1}{2}\right)^4\left(\frac{1}{2}\right)^{4-4}$$

$$= \frac{1}{16}$$

iii. Probability of at least 3 red cards means, there may be 3 or 4 red cards. So the required probability is,

$$P(x \geq 3) = P(x = 3) + P(x = 4)$$

$$= 4C_3\left(\frac{1}{2}\right)^3\left(\frac{1}{2}\right)^{4-3} + 4C_4\left(\frac{1}{2}\right)^4\left(\frac{1}{2}\right)^{4-4}$$

$$= 4 \cdot \frac{1}{16} + 1 . \frac{1}{16} = \frac{5}{16}$$

iv. Probability of no red card means $x = 0$, Hence,

$$P(x = 0) = 4C_0 \left(\frac{1}{2}\right)^0 \left(\frac{1}{2}\right)^{4-0}$$

$$= 1 \times \frac{1}{16} = \frac{1}{16}$$

v. Probability of one or less red cards means, the probability of either one or no red card.

$$P(x \le 1) = P(x = 0) + P(x = 1)$$

$$4C_0 = 4C_0 \left(\frac{1}{2}\right)^0 \left(\frac{1}{2}\right)^{4-0} + 4C_1 \left(\frac{1}{2}\right)^1 \left(\frac{1}{2}\right)^{4-1}$$

$$= 1 \times \frac{1}{16} + 4 \times \frac{1}{16} = \frac{5}{16}$$

Example. 10.6. A die is rolled four times. If the number of dots on the die show up 5 or 6, it is considered a success, otherwise a failure. What is the probability of obtaining, (i) two successes, (ii) no success.

Given that $n = 4$. Since the possible outcomes are 1, 2, 3, 4, 5 and 6, i.e. six outcomes. Only two of them, 5 and 6 lead to success.

Therefore, $P = \frac{2}{6} = \frac{1}{3}$, $q = 1 - \frac{1}{3} = \frac{2}{3}$

i. Probability of two success is

$$P(x = 2) = 4C_2 \left(\frac{1}{3}\right)^2 \left(\frac{2}{3}\right)^{4-2}$$

$$= \frac{4 \times 3}{2 \times 1} \cdot \frac{1}{9} \times \frac{4}{9} = \frac{8}{27}$$

ii. Probability of no success is,

$$P(x = 0) = 4C_0 \left(\frac{1}{3}\right)^0 \left(\frac{2}{3}\right)^{4-0}$$

$$= 1 \times 1 \times \frac{16}{81} = \frac{16}{81}$$

Example 10.7. A box contains 20 capacitors, 4 of which are defective. Five capacitors are selected randomly. What is the chance that

a. 3 out of 5 selected capacitors are defective?
b. there is no defective capacitors among these 5?
c. there is at least one defective?

Given that $p = \frac{4}{20} = \frac{1}{5}, q = 1 - \frac{1}{5} = \frac{4}{5}$ and $n = 5$

a. Probability of three defective is,

$$P(x=3) = 5C_3\left(\frac{1}{5}\right)^3\left(\frac{4}{5}\right)^{5-3}$$

$$= \frac{5.4.3}{3.2.1}\cdot\frac{1}{125}\cdot\frac{16}{25}$$

$$= \frac{32}{625}$$

b. Probability of no defective is,

$$P(x=0) = 5C_0\left(\frac{1}{5}\right)^0\left(\frac{4}{5}\right)^{5-0}$$

$$= 1\times 1\times\left(\frac{4}{5}\right)^5 = \frac{1024}{3125}$$

c. To obtain the probability of at least one defective, subtract the probability of no defective from 1, i.e.,

$$P(x\geq 1) = 1 - P(x=0)$$

$$= 1-\frac{1024}{3125} = \frac{2101}{3125}$$

Example 10.8. A bomber can hit the enemy's atomic reactor 3 times out of 7 attempts. The bomber made 6 attempts. What is the probability that the reactor will be hit once.

Give that $p = \frac{3}{7}, q = 1-\frac{3}{7} = \frac{4}{7}$; and $n = 6$

Probability of hitting the bomber once out of 6 attempts is,

$$P(x=1) = 6C_1\left(\frac{3}{7}\right)^1\left(\frac{4}{7}\right)^{6-1}$$

$$= 6\times\frac{3\times 4^5}{7^6}$$

$$= \frac{18432}{117649}$$

Example. 10.9. If for binomial variable x with usual notations, $n = 6$ and $9\,P(x=4) = P(x=2)$, then find p.

According to the given condition,

$$9\,P(x=4) = P(x=2)$$

$$9\times 6C_4\,(p)^4(1-p)^{6-4} = 6C_2\,(p)^2(1-p)^{6-2}$$

$$9p^2 = (1-p)^2 \qquad \because\ 6C_4 = 6C_2$$

$$9P^2 = 1 - 2p + p^2$$
$$8p^2 + 2p - 1 = 0$$
$$(4p - 1)(2p + 1) = 0$$

$2p + 1 = 0$ implies that $p = -\frac{1}{2}$ which is impossible

$\therefore \quad 4p - 1 = 0$ or $p = -\frac{1}{4}$ which is acceptable.

Example 10.10. Two players *A* and *B* play a game. The chance of winning the game by *A* is 60%. The game is played in a set of 5 games. What per cent chance is there that *A* wins 3 or more times.

It is given that, $n = 5$, $p = \frac{60}{100} = \frac{3}{5}$, $\therefore \quad q = 1 - \frac{3}{5} = \frac{2}{5}$

Probability of *A* winning the game 3 or more times,

$$P(x \geq 3) = 5C_3\left(\frac{3}{5}\right)^3\left(\frac{2}{5}\right)^{5-3} + 5C_4\left(\frac{3}{5}\right)^4\left(\frac{2}{5}\right)^{5-4} + 5C_5\left(\frac{3}{5}\right)^5\left(\frac{2}{5}\right)^{5-5}$$

$$= \frac{1}{5^5}\left[\frac{5.4.3}{3.2.1} \times 27 \times 4 + 5 \times 81 \times 2 + 243\right]$$

$$= \frac{1}{3125}[1080 + 810 + 243]$$

$$= \frac{2133}{3125}$$

POISSON DISTRIBUTION

In binomial distribution, the number of trials *n* (sample size) is finite and it is possible to enumerate the number of times an event can occur. But the question arises what to do when such a situation does not exist. Basic reason for this is that the probability of occurrence of certain events is very low and unpredictable. For instance, number of suicides per month in a city, number of false telephone calls on a call centre, number of aeroplane accidents per year of an airline, number of printing errors per page of a new book, etc. In all these cases, the number of trials is not known. To deal with such situations, Simon Denis Poisson, a French mathematician and physicist, developed a probability distribution and published it in 1837 and thereby **Poisson distribution** is an eponym.

Poisson distribution is a limiting case of binomial distribution in which *n*, the number of trials is indefinitely large, i.e., $n \to \infty$ and *p*, the constant probability of occurrence of an event under each trial is extremely small, i.e. $p \to 0$. This distribution has only one parameter, say *m*, which is the mean of the occurrence of an event, obtained on the basis of existing knowledge. The probability function of a Poisson variable X for $X = x$ successes with mean m is as given below.

$$P(X = x) = \frac{e^{-m} \cdot m^x}{\lfloor x} \qquad (10.4)$$

Usually $np = m$ is finite. Also e is the base of natural logarithm. Value of e^{-m} can be obtained by log-tables or directly by a scientific calculator. In the examination paper, the value of e^{-m} is traditionally provided with the question.

Properties: 1. Poisson distribution has only one parameter m, i.e. the mean of the variable x.

2. This is the only distribution in which mean and variance of the variable are equal, i.e. mean = m; variance. = m.

Note : In algebra exponential series is given as

$$e = \frac{1}{\lfloor 0} + \frac{1}{\lfloor 1} + \frac{1}{\lfloor 2} + \cdots + \frac{1}{\lfloor n} + \cdots$$

$$= 1 + 1 + 0.5 + 0.1667 + \ldots = 2.71828$$

Again, $$e^m = 1 + \frac{m}{\lfloor 1} \frac{m^2}{\lfloor 2} + \frac{m^3}{\lfloor 3} + \cdots + \frac{m^n}{\lfloor n} + \cdots$$

Also $$e^{-m} = \frac{1}{e^m}$$

A few numerical examples are solved so as to intensify the concepts about the usages of Poisson distribution in real life.

Example 10.11. The first print of a new book consisting of 750 pages has on an average 1 error in five pages. Find the number of pages which have 0, 1, 2, 3 errors per page in the whole book. [Give that $e^{-0.2} = 0.8187$]

The variable, number of errors per page, follows Poisson distribution.

Also given that, $m = \frac{1}{5} = 0.2$

The probability function of Poisson variate with $m = 0.2$ is,

$$P(X = x) = \frac{e^{-0.2} \cdot (0.2)^x}{\lfloor x}$$

for $x = 0, 1, 2, 3$

Putting the values of x, the probabilities will be calculated for 0, 1, 2, 3 errors. Multiplying these probabilities by 750, expected number of pages having 0, 1, 2 and 3 errors are worked out. Also put $e^{-0.2} = 0.8187$ in the above formula.

		Prob.	Expected no. of pages
$P(x = 0)$ =	$\dfrac{0.8187 \times (0.2)^0}{\lfloor 0}$	= 0.8187,	0.8187 × 750 = 614
$P(x = 1)$ =	$\dfrac{0.8187 \times (0.2)^1}{\lfloor 1}$	= 0.1637,	0.1637 × 750 = 123
$P(x = 2)$ =	$\dfrac{0.8187 \times (0.2)^2}{\lfloor 2}$	= 0.01637,	0.01637 × 750 = 12
$P(x = 3)$ =	$\dfrac{0.8187 \times (0.2)^3}{\lfloor 3}$	= 0.0011,	0.0011 × 750 = 1

Thus, the distribution of errors is,

X :	0	1	2	3
No. of pages :	614	123	12	1

Example 10.12. Last few years record reveals that on an average 4 accident occur per week in a city. Find the probability that in a chosen week not more than 2 accidents shall occur. [Given : $e^{-4} = 0.0183$]

The variable number of accidents per week follows Poisson distribution.

In this question, $m = 4$.

First, the probabilities for $x = 0, 1, 2$ are calculated by the formula (10.4) and then added to get the required probability.

$$P(X = 0) = \frac{e^{-4} \times 4^0}{\lfloor 0} = 0.0183$$

$$P(X = 1) = \frac{e^{-4} \times 4^1}{\lfloor 1} = 0.0183 \times 4 = 0.0732$$

$$P(X = 2) = \frac{e^{-4} \times 4^2}{\lfloor 2} = 0.0183 \times 8 = 0.1464$$

Probability of not more than 2 accidents in a chosen week is,

$$P(X \le 2) = P(X = 0) + P(X = 1) + P(X = 2)$$
$$= 0.0183 + 0.0732 + 0.1464$$
$$= 0.2379$$

Example 10.13. A match Box producing company produces 5% defective match boxes. Find the probability of not having more than three defective match-boxes in a packet of 10 match-boxes.

[Given $e^{-0.5} = 0.6065$]

Given that proportion of defectives, $p = \frac{5}{100} = 0.05$. In a packet of 10 match-boxes, the average number of defective match-boxes, $n = 10 \times 0.05 = 0.5$. To find the probability of not more than 3 defective match-boxes, find the probabilities of $x = 0, 1, 2, 3$ by Poisson probability function (10.4). In this case,

$$P\,(X = x) \;=\; \frac{e^{-0.5}(.5)^x}{\lfloor\underline{x}}$$

$$P(X = 0) \;=\; \frac{e^{-.5}(.5)^0}{\lfloor\underline{0}} = 0.6065$$

$$P(X = 1) \;=\; \frac{e^{-.5}(.5)^1}{\lfloor\underline{1}} = 0.6065 \times .5 = 0.3032$$

$$P(X = 2) \;=\; \frac{e^{-.5}(.5)^2}{\lfloor\underline{2}} = \frac{0.6065 \times .25}{2} = 0.0758$$

$$P(X = 3) \;=\; \frac{e^{-.5}(.5)^3}{\lfloor\underline{3}} = \frac{0.6065 \times 0.125}{6} = 0.0126$$

Probability of not having more than 3 defective match-boxes is,

$$\begin{aligned} P\,(X \le 3) &= P\,(X = 1) + P\,(X = 2) + P\,(X = 3) \\ &= 0.6065 + 0.3032 + 0.0758 + 0.0126 \\ &= 0.9981 \end{aligned}$$

Example 10.14. A razor blade manufacturing company has a chance of 1 defective blade in 500 blades. The blades are marketed in packets of 5 blades. One hundred packets are supplied to a retailer. Find the number of packets which are likely to have no, 1 or 2 defective blades.

Proportion of defective = $\frac{1}{500} = 0.002$

Average number of defective blades in a packet of 5 blades,
$m = np = 5 \times 0.002 = 0.01$. Also $N = 100$
From the table we get, $e^{-0.01} = 0.99$
No. of packets with no defective blade,

$$N.\,P\,(X = 0) \;=\; 100 \times \frac{e^{-0.01} \times (.01)^0}{\lfloor\underline{0}} = 100 \times .99 = 99$$

No. of packets with one defective blade,

$$N.\,P\,(X = 1) \;=\; 100 \times \frac{e^{-0.01} \times (.01)^1}{\lfloor\underline{1}} = 100 \times .99 \times .01 = 0.99 = 1$$

No. of packets with two defective blades.

$$N.\ P\ (X = 2) = 100 \times \frac{e^{-0.01} \times (.01)^2}{\lfloor 2} = \frac{100 \times .99 \times .0001}{2} = 0.001 = 0$$

Example 10.15. Fit in the Poisson distribution to the following observed frequency distribution.

Variable,	X:	0	1	2	3	4	5
Frequency,	f:	88	35	28	23	18	8

Also find the expected value of X.

To fit in the Poisson distribution, first find the mean of X by the formula, $\frac{\Sigma fx}{\Sigma f}$.

$$m = \frac{88 \times 0 + 35 \times 1 \times 28 \times 2 \times 23 \times 3 + 18 \times 4 + 8 \times 5}{88 + 35 + 28 + 23 + 18 + 8}$$

$$= \frac{272}{200} = 1.36$$

From the table, $e^{-1.36} = 0.2567$ and given N = 200

To fit in Poisson distribution, find Poisson probabilities by the formula (10.4) and on multiplying these probabilities by $N = 200$, we get the expected frequencies. These frequencies arranged corresponding to the variate values provide the fitted Poisson distribution

$$P\ (X = x) = \frac{e^{-1.36}\ (1.36)^x}{\lfloor x}$$

$P\ (X = x)$	*Expected freq.* $N \times P\ (x)$
$P\ (X = 0) = \frac{e^{-1.36} \cdot (1.36)^0}{\lfloor 0} = 0.2567$	$200 \times 0.2567 = 51.34 = 51$
$P\ (X = 1) = \frac{e^{-1.36} \cdot (1.36)^1}{\lfloor 1} = 0.3491$	$200 \times 0.3491 = 69.82 = 70$
$P\ (X = 2) = \frac{e^{-1.36} \cdot (1.36)^2}{\lfloor 2} = 0.2374$	$200 \times 0.2374 = 47.48 = 48$
$P\ (X = 3) = \frac{e^{-1.36} \cdot (1.36)^3}{\lfloor 3} = 0.1076$	$200 \times 0.1076 = 21.52 = 22$
$P\ (X = 4) = \frac{e^{-1.36} \cdot (1.36)^4}{\lfloor 4} = 0.0366$	$200 \times 0.0366 = 7.32 = 7$

$$P(X=5) = \frac{e^{-1.36} \cdot (1.36)^5}{\lfloor 5} = 0.0010 \qquad 200 \times 0.0010 = 2$$

Check : Confirm that the sum of expected frequency is 200. Expected value of X can be found by the formula,

$$E(X) = \Sigma x p(x).$$

$$E(X) = 0 \times .2567 + 1 \times .3491 + 2 \times .2374 + 3 \times .1076 + 4 \times .0366 + 5 \times .0010$$

$$= 1.298 = 1.3.$$

PRACTICE QUESTIONS AND EXERCISES

1. Define and discuss a random variable.
2. Distinguish between discrete and continuous random variables.
3. What do you understand by probability distribution?
4. What is the difference between observed and theoretical distribution of a variable.
5. Explain Bernoulli's trial vis-a-vis Bernoulli's distribution.
6. How Bernoulli's distribution is extended to binomial distribution?
7. Give the probability function of binomial distribution and its properties.
8. Under what conditions does a discrete variable follow Poisson distribution?
9. What are the advantages of Poisson distribution over binomial distribution?
10. Give probability function of Poisson distribution and its properties.
11. Give three examples where it will be appropriate to use Poisson's probabilities.
12. In what manner does a probability distribution helps to find the theoretical distribution of a discrete variable?
13. After a clinical trial, it is claimed that 60% patients of a particular disease cured by administering a drug X. Five patients are treated by this drug. What is the probability that four patients will be cured?
14. A fair coin is tossed six times. What is the probability that the coin will show at least 4 heads in six tosses?
15. Find the probability of obtaining 4 times odd sums of pairs of spots in rolling two dice simultaneously five times.
16. Four coins are tossed simultaneously 128 times. Find the frequency distribution of the number of heads (X). Also find the expected value of X.
17. Five dice are thrown 96 times. If 4, 5 or 6 are shown up by the dice, then it is considered a success and otherwise a failure. Find the frequency distribution of the successes. Also find the mean and variance of the binomial distribution.

18. 4% items produced by a machine are defective. A simple of 5 items from a lot of 120 items is selected randomly. Find the probability that
    i. 3 items are defective.
    ii. no item is defective
    iii. not less than 4 items are defective. [Given that $e^{-4.8} = 0.0082$]
19. On a telephone booth, every hour on an average, three callers enter. What is the probability that in a particular hour five callers will enter the booth. [Given that $e^{-3} = 0.0498$]
20. A book of 300 pages has 300 mistakes. Calculate the chance that a randomly selected page contains at least two mistakes. [Given that $e^{-1} = 0.3679$]
21. In rolling a true dice five times, find the probability of obtaining,
    i. exactly one dot,
    ii. exactly twice one dot
    iii. at least once a single dot.
    [**Hint :** Use binomial probabilities]
22. In a city there are 1 percent left handed people. Find the probability of having at least four left handed persons in a locality of 200 people.
    [**Hint :** $m = 2$, $P(X \geq 4) = 1 - P(0) - P(1) - P(2) - P(3)$]
23. All the 52 cards of a deck are distributed one by one among four players. Find the probability that the player sitting in the north has exactly 2 red cards by using binomial distribution.
24. The probability of hitting the bull's-eye by a shooter is $\frac{2}{5}$. Ten shots are fired independently. Find the probability that the bull's-eye will be hit exactly six times.
25. Assume that the probability of a male birth is same as that of female birth. What is the chance that a family with eight children has four boys and four girls.

OBJECTIVE TYPE QUESTIONS

Sort-out the correct answer from the given ones for each statement.

26. A Bernoulli variate can:
    a. Take only two discrete values
    b. Be dischotmous
    c. Result either in a success or a failure
    d. All of the above
27. Relation between mean and variance of Bernoulli's distribution is:
    a. Mean > variance b. Mean < variance
    c. Mean = variance d. All of the above
28. The parameters of the binomial distribution are:
    a. p and q b. n, p
    c. n, q d. n, p and q

29. The probability of r successes in n Bernoulli's trials can be calculated by the probability function:

a. $np^r q^{1-r}$
b. $\binom{n}{r} p^r q^{n-r}$
c. $np^r (1-p)^{n-r}$
d. $\binom{n}{r} p^n q^{r-n}$

30. The mean of a binomial distribution is 3 and its variance is 2. The values of n, p and q are,

a. $n=5, p=\frac{3}{5}, q=\frac{2}{5}$
b. $n=6, p=\frac{1}{2}, q=\frac{1}{2}$
c. $n=9, p=\frac{1}{3}, q=\frac{2}{3}$
d. All of the above

31. A fair coin is tossed four times. The probability of obtaining 3 heads is:

a. $\frac{1}{2}$
b. $\frac{1}{4}$
c. $\frac{3}{8}$
d. $\frac{1}{8}$

32. In a trial, two successes follow a single failure. If the trial is repeated six times, then the probability of no success is:

a. $\frac{1}{729}$
b. $\frac{64}{729}$
c. $\frac{1}{64}$
d. $\frac{63}{64}$

33. A binomial variate follows poisson distribution when:

a. p is large, n is small
b. n and p are large
c. p is small and n is large
d. p and q are large

34. Poisson distribution with mean μ having n trials with probability of success p, has the parameter(s):

a. n and μ
b. n and p
c. n
d. μ

35. Probability function of the Poisson distribution with mean m for r successes is:

a. $\frac{e^m \cdot m^r}{\underline{|r}}$
b. $\frac{e^{-m} \cdot m^r}{\underline{|r}}$
c. $\frac{e^{-m} \cdot m^r}{r}$
d. None of the above

36. If X is a Poisson variate with mean m such that $P(X=3) = P(X=4)$, the value of m is:

a. 3
b. 4
c. 2
d. 6

37. If the mean of a Poisson variate X is 6.25, then the standard deviation of X is:

a. 2.5
b. 6.25
c. 39.0625
d. 3.75

38. Three per cent watch cells produced by a factory were defective. A lot of 200 cells had been supplied to a watches' showroom. If a cell is taken from this lot, then the probability of its being defective is:

a. 0.03	b. 0.015
c. 0.205	d. 0.15

39. If X is a poisson variate such that $P(X = 1) = P(X = 2)$, then $P(X = 3)$ is:

a. 0.1280	b. 0.1202
c. 0.1804	d. None of the above

40. Name of the discrete distribution for which mean is greater than its variance.

a. Binomial	b. Bernoulli's distribution
c. Both a. and b.	d. Neither a. nor b.

CHAPTER 11

Continuous Distributions

GENERAL DISCUSSION

There is a long list of continuous, probability distributions. To name a few, normal, Cauchy, Beta, Gama, exponential, etc., are continuous distributions. Out of all continuous distributions, normal distribution is a most frequently used distribution. It has deep roots in statistics. So this distribution is discussed appropriately without mathematical derivations and proof.

Besides theoretical continuous probability distributions, there are other continuous distributions which are classified as **sampling distributions.**

Definition:

"The distribution of the values of statistic obtainable from all possible distinguishable samples that could be randomly drawn from a population is known as sampling distribution".

Under this category, only three sampling distributions namely, χ^2, *t and F shall be succinctly delineated as they are extensively used in testing of hypotheses*

NORMAL DISTRIBUTION

The probability density function (pdf) of the normal distribution as first formulated by De-Moivre, an English mathematician in 1733. He applied this distribution in the game of chance. It was also discovered independently by Laplace in 1774 and by Karl Friedrich Gauss in 1809 as the distribution of errors in astronomy. Some people give full credit to Gauss for the invention of normal distribution. This sort of controversy still exists. But it has hardly any effect on its tremendous usage in a large number of statistical problems.

Definition:

A continuous random variable X is said to follow normal distribution with mean μ *and variance* σ^2, *if its probability density function f (x) is given by the equation.*

$$f(x) = \frac{1}{\sigma\sqrt{2\pi}} e^{-\frac{1}{2\sigma^2}(x-\mu)^2} \tag{11.1}$$

Where, $-\infty < x < \infty, -\infty < \mu < \infty, \sigma^2 > 0$.

μ and σ^2 are called the parameters of the normal distribution and it is conventionally denoted as $N(\mu, \sigma^2)$.

SHAPE OF THE NORMAL CURVE

Normal curve is a perfectly symmetrical ball shaped curve. It is symmetrical about the ordinate at the mean as shown in figure given below.

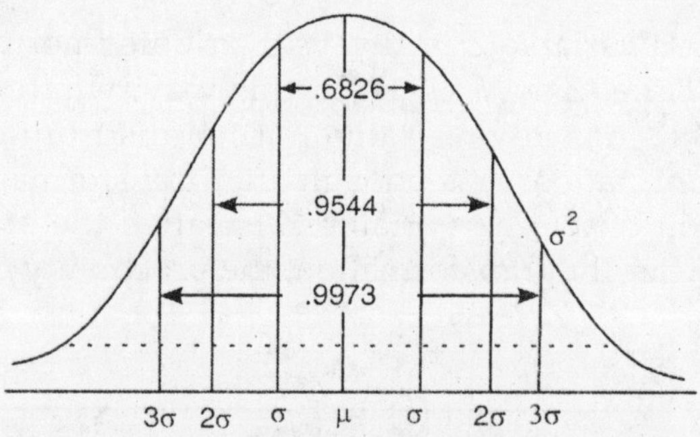

Fig. 11.1: Normal curve

The shape of the curve depends on the values of μ and σ^2. But it is unique for any given values of μ and σ^2.

Properties

1. Mean, median and mode of a normal distribution are always same, i.e. mean = median = mode.
2. It has only one mode which is at the top of the bell shaped curve just above the mean.
3. The ordinate at the mean divides frequency curve of the normal distribution into two equal halves.
4. The total area under the normal curve is unity. In this way, the area to the left of the ordinate at μ is equal to the area on its right, i.e. on both sides the area is 0.5.
5. Normal distribution is unimodal.
6. The tails of the curve never touch the *X*-axis.
7. The area under the normal curve between $(\mu - \sigma)$ and $(\mu + \sigma)$ = 0.6826. It means 68.26% of the total population lies in this area.

Similarly, area between ($\mu \mp 2\sigma$) = 0.9544 or 95.44% population lies in this area. Also area between ($\mu \mp 3\sigma$) = 0.9973, i.e. 99.73 population is covered in this region as shown in fig. (11.1).

It is to emphasize that the area gives the probability of a variable lying in an internal. The area (probability) multiplied by 100 provides the percentage of population lying in the specified region.

Nota bene: In case of continuous distribution, the proability is attached to an interval. The probability, at a point is zero.

Z-TRANSFORMATION

As already given, the shape of the normal curve changes as the values of μ and/or σ vary. To cope with this problem, a transformation is made as,

$$Z = \frac{X - \mu}{\sigma} \tag{11.2}$$

The transformed variable Z is always distributed normally with mean 0 and variance 1, i.e. $Z \sim N\,(0, 1)$. In this way, whatever may be the parameters of X, Z has always same normal distribution $N\,(0, 1)$ and hence only one normal curve is enough after transformation irrespective of the distribution of X. The variable Z is called the **standard normal deviate** (SND). After the transformation, the probability density function of the SND-Z is,

$$f(z) = \frac{1}{\sqrt{2\pi}} e^{-\frac{1}{2}z^2} \tag{11.3}$$

for $-\infty < z < \infty$.

Note : Table for area under standard normal curve are either provided in the examination or the values are given in the paper itself.

Some application of normal distribution are illustrated through the following examples.

Example 11.1. The effective life of dry battery cell is considered to be distributed with mean 20 hours and standard deviation 5 hours. In a consignment of 100 battery cells, how many cells are expected to have life, (i) less than 15 hours, (ii) between 8 and 16 hours, (iii) more than 15 hours, (iv) between 15 and 25 hours, (v) more than 30 hours.

[From the table of the area under the normal curve for $Z \sim N\,(0, 1)$, we have area 0 to 1 = 0.34134, 0 to 2.4 = 0.49180, 0 to 0.8 = 0.28814, 0 to 2 = 0.47725]

Given, $\mu = 20$ and $\sigma = 5$

i. For X less than 15 hours, $Z = \dfrac{15-20}{5} = -1$

The shaded area from 0 to 1, A = 0.34134.

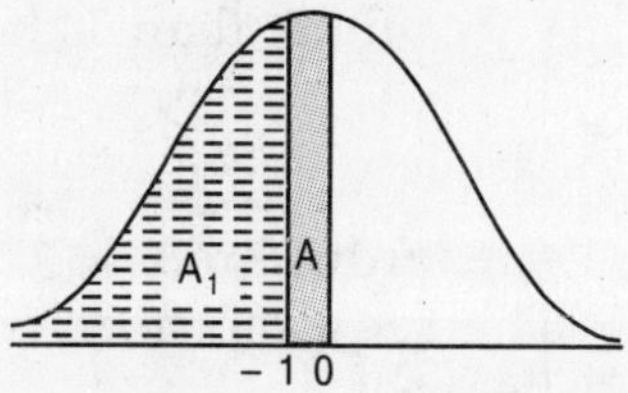

The required area is to the left of the ordinated at –1 indicate as A_1.

$\therefore A_1 = 0.5 - A = 0.5 - 0.34134 = 0.15866$

On multiplying the area A_1, i.e. the probability of the cell having life less than 15 hours is obtained, i.e. no. of cells = 100 × .15886 = 15.88 = 16 cells

ii. To know the number of cells with life between 8 and 16 hours, find Z_1 and Z_2 as,

$$Z_1 = \frac{8-20}{8} = \frac{-12}{5} = -2.4;\ Z_2 = \frac{16-20}{5} = \frac{-4}{5} = -0.8$$

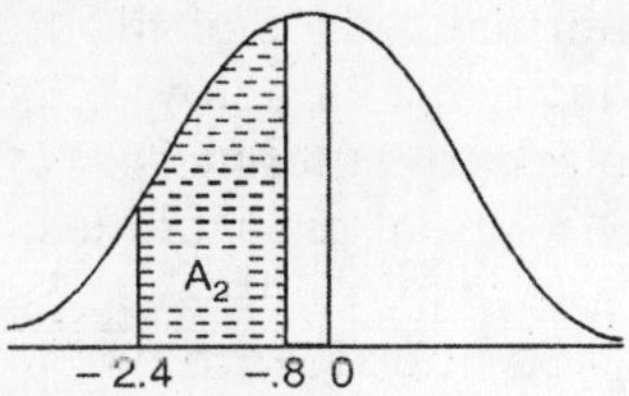

Here the required area is A_2. To find the area of A_2, find the area from 0 to 2.4 and 0 to 0.8. Subtract smaller area from the larger area.

Area from 0 to 2.4 = 0.49180

Area from 0 to 0.8 = 0.28814

$\therefore \quad A_2 = 0.49180 - 0.28814 = 0.20366$

No. of cells having life between 8 and 16 hours

= 100 × 0.20366 = 20.366 =20 cells

iii. For more than 15 hours,

$$Z = \frac{15-20}{5} = -1$$

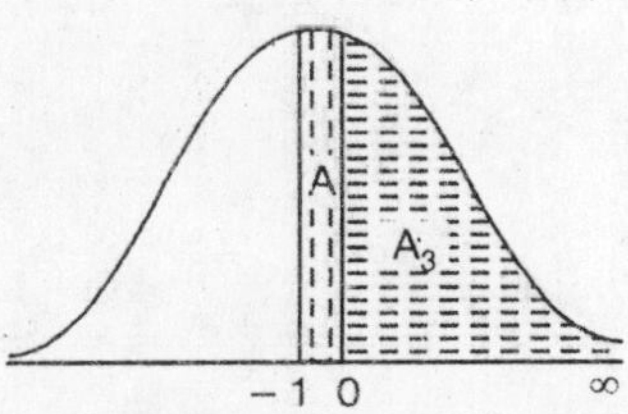

Area from 0 to –1 = 0.34134 = A (say)

Area from 0 to ∞ = 0.5

The required area A_3 = A + 0.5

$\therefore \quad A_3 = 0.34134 + 0.5$

= 0.84134

No. of cells = 100 × 0.84134 = 84.134 = 84 cells

iv. For the number of cells having life between 15 and 25 hours,

$$Z_3 = \frac{15-20}{5} = -1,\ Z_4 = \frac{25-20}{5} = 1$$

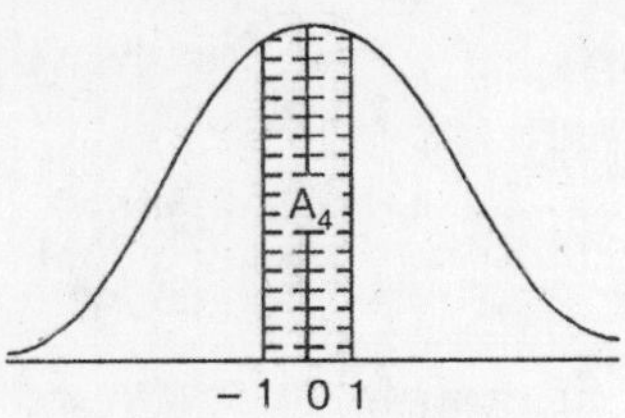

Area from 0 to 1 = Area from 0 to – 1

= 0.34134.

The required Area, A_4 = 0.34134 + 0.34134

= 0.68268

No. of cells having life between 15 and 25 hours = 1000 × 0.68268 = 68.268 = 68 cells

v. For more than 30 hours

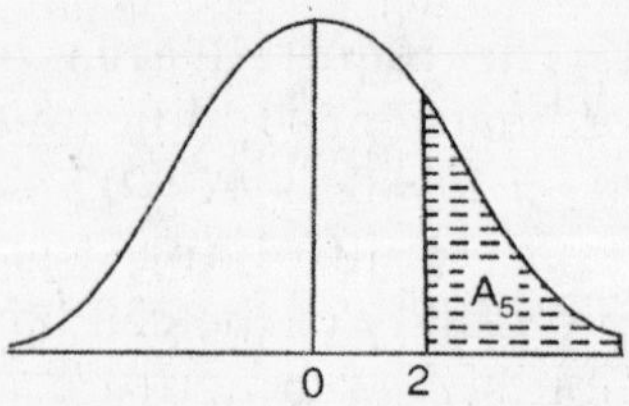

$$Z_5 = \frac{30-20}{5} = 2.0$$

Area from 0 to 2 = 0.47725

The required area is to the right of the ordinate at Z = 2.

$$\therefore \quad \text{Area, } A_5 = 0.5 - 0.47725 = 0.02275$$

Hence, the number of cells having life more than 30 hours

$$= 100 \times 0.02275 = 2.275 = 2 \text{ cells.}$$

Example 11.2. Assuming that the marks of students are distributed normally, 15% of the students have marks under 40 and 80% students have marks below 65. Find the mean and standard deviation of the marks of students.

Normal probabilities as per question are,

$$p(X \le 40) = 0.15,\ P(X < 65) = .80,\ P(X > 65) = 0.20.$$

So the area from 0 to z_1 = 0.35 and from 0 to z_2 = 0.30.

Now from the table, one has to find the values of z_1 and z_2 for the given area.

From the table, $Z_1 = 1.04$ and $Z_2 = 0.84$

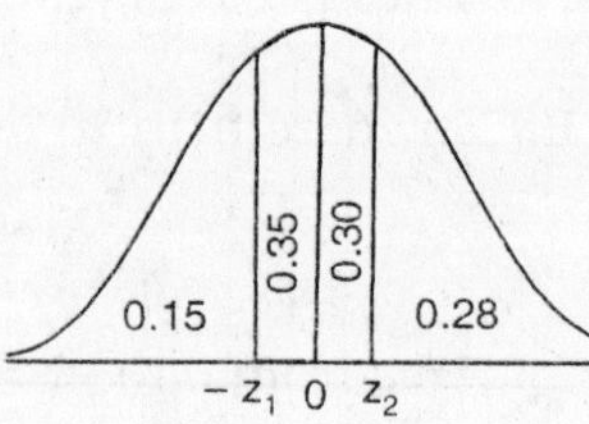

From (11.2), $Z = \frac{X-\mu}{\sigma}$

$$\text{Again,} \quad -Z_1 = \frac{40-\mu}{\sigma} = -1.04$$

$$Z_2 = \frac{65-\mu}{\sigma} = 0.84$$

$$-1.04\,\sigma + \mu = 40 \quad \text{... i}$$

$$0.84\,\sigma + \mu = 65 \quad \text{... ii}$$

Solving the equations i and ii, we get the values of μ and σ.

$$-1.88\,\sigma = -25$$

or
$$\sigma = \frac{25}{1.88} = 13.3$$

and
$$-1.04 \times 13.3 + \mu = 40$$

or
$$\mu = 53.82$$

Example 11.3. Probability density function of a random variable x is given as,

$$f(x) = \frac{1}{5\sqrt{2\pi}} e^{-\frac{1}{50}(x^2-50x+625)}$$

Find the mean and variance of the given distribution

Given p.d.f. can be rewritten as,

$$f(x) = \frac{1}{5\sqrt{2\pi}} e^{-\frac{1}{2}\left(\frac{x-25}{5}\right)^2}$$

The given p.d.f. is that of a normal distribution.
So on comparing, $\mu = 25$, $\sigma = 5$ and $\sigma^2 = 25$.

CHI-SQUARE DISTRIBUTION

consider a large population divided into k classes $C_1, C_2, \ldots.., C_k$ and let p_i be the probability that an element of the population belongs to C_i for $i = 1, 2, , \ldots\ldots k$. Suppose a random sample of size n is drawn from the population and f_i is the observed number of individuals in the sample that belong to C_i. Obviously the expected number of individuals in the class C_i is np_i. As a measure of total deviation of the class frequencies in the sample from their respective expected frequencies, Karl Pearson defined a quantity given by

$$\chi^2 = \sum_{i=1}^{m} \frac{(f_i - np_i)^2}{np_i} \quad (11.4)$$

$$= \sum_{i=1}^{k} \frac{f_i^2}{np_i} - n \quad (11.4.1)$$

The quantity given by (11.4) is known as Pearsonion χ^2. To find out the limit distribution, i.e. when $n \to \infty$, let us define a variable,

$$\chi_i = \frac{f_i - np_i}{\sqrt{np_i}} \quad (11.5)$$

Substituting the value of χ_i from (11.5) in (11.4), we get

$$\chi^2 = \sum_{i=1}^{k} \chi_i^2 \quad (11.6)$$

The relation (11.6) clearly reveals that the sum of squares of k independent variates χ_i is distributed as chi-square.

The probability density function of chi-square distribution is,

$$f(\chi^2) = \frac{1}{2^{k/2}\sqrt{\frac{k}{2}}} (\chi^2)^{\frac{k}{2}-1} e^{-\chi^2/2} \quad (11.7)$$

where $0 \le \chi^2 < \infty$

The distribution of χ^2 was first given by Helmert in 1876 and later independently given by Karl Pearson in 1900.

Properties of χ^2-distribution

1. Whole of the chi-square distribution curve lies in the first quadrant as χ^2 is never negative.

2. Chi-square distribution has only one parameter, i.e. k. k is known as the degrees of freedom. The number of independent variate values in a set of observation is known as degree of freedom for x^2.
3. The shape of the probability density curve solely depends on the degrees of freedom k. For five values of k, the curves are shown below.

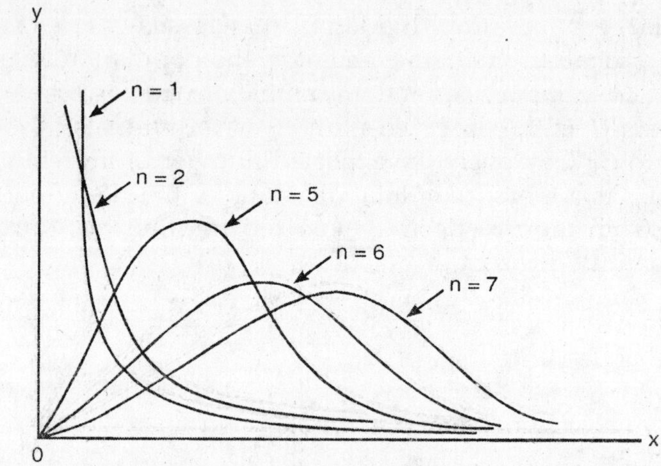

Fig. 11.2: Chi-square distribution curves

From the above figure of the χ^2-distribution curves, it is apparent that for degrees of freedom 1 and 2, the shape of the curve is that of hyperbola. Further, as the degrees of freedom increases the curve is convex with single peak. The peakedness decreases with the increase in degrees of freedom for chi-square.

4. Chi-square distribution curve is highly positive skewed.
5. Mean of chi-square distribution is k and variance is 2k.
6. chi-square distribution is unimodal.
7. If $x \sim \chi^2_{k_1}$ and $y \sim \chi^2_{k_2}$, then $x + y$ is also distributed as chi-square with $(k_1 + k_2)$ degree of freedom.

STUDENT-*t* DISTRIBUTION

William S. Gosset Published a paper entitled 'The probable error of the mean' under pseudonym 'student' in 1908 providing t distribution. Later in 1926, R.A. Fisher gave a rigorous proof for its sampling distribution.

Consider two independent variables ξ and η, where ξ follows as standard normal distribution and η is distributed as chi-square with k degrees of freedom. Define a variable,

$$t = \frac{\xi}{\sqrt{\eta/k}} \tag{11.8}$$

If x_1 x_2, ... , x_n are n sample values with $\bar{x}$ as its mean, s the standard deviation.

Let μ_0 be an assumed value of population mean. The distribution of $t = \frac{\bar{x} - \mu_0}{s_{\bar{x}}}$ is known as student t- distribution. The probability density function of t is,

$$f(t) = \frac{1}{\sqrt{k}} \cdot \frac{1}{B\left(\frac{k}{2}, \frac{1}{2}\right)} \cdot \frac{1}{\left(1 + \frac{t^2}{k}\right)^{\frac{k+1}{2}}} \tag{11.9}$$

where $k = n - 1$. Also $-\infty < t < \infty$

Further, $B\left(\frac{k}{2}, \frac{1}{2}\right) = \frac{\Gamma_{k/2}\ \Gamma_{1/2}}{\Gamma_{\frac{k+1}{2}}}$ and $\sqrt{\pi} = \Gamma_{1/2}$

t has k degree of freedom.

Properties of t- distribution

1. t- distribution is unimodal
2. Probability distribution curve of t is a bell shaped curve but more peaked than a normal curve as shown below.

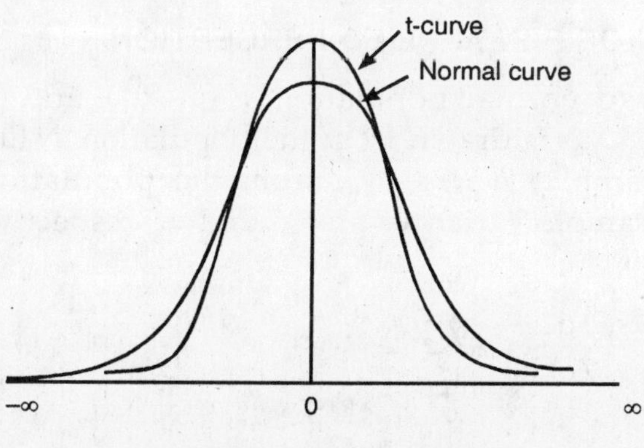

Fig. 11.3: t-distribution curve

3. Sample size n should not be more than 30. In case, n is greater than 30, student t-distribution tends to normal distribution.
4. Mean of t-distribution is zero for $k \geq 2$.
5. Variance of t-distribution is $\frac{k}{(k-2)}$ for $k \geq 3$.

F-DISTRIBUTION

Given any two independent chi-square variates say, u with k_1 degrees of freedom and v with k_2 degrees of freedom, the ratio of the variables $\left(\frac{u}{k_1}\right) / \left(\frac{v}{k_2}\right)$ follows F-distribution. Distribution of F was propounded by G.W. Snedecor. Let us denote,

$$F = \frac{u/k_1}{v/k_2} \quad (11.10)$$

$$= \frac{k_2 u}{k_1 v} \quad (11.10.1)$$

The probability density function of F is,

$$f(F) = \frac{1}{B\left(\frac{k_1}{2}, \frac{k_2}{2}\right)} \left(\frac{k_1}{k_2}\right)^{k_1/2} \frac{F^{\frac{k_1}{2}-1}}{\left(1 + \frac{k_1}{k_2} F\right)^{(k_1+k_2)/2}} \quad (11.11)$$

$0 \leq F < \infty$

F has degrees of freedom (k_1, k_2)

DISTRIBUTION OF F IN APPLIED PERCEPTION

Let there be two normal population $N(\mu_1, \sigma_1^2)$ and $N(\mu_2, \sigma_2^2)$. A sample $x_1\ x_2, \ldots\ldots x_{n_1}$ is drawn from the population $N(\mu_1, \sigma_1^2)$ and an independent sample $y_1\ y_2, \ldots\ldots y_{n_2}$ from the population $N(\mu_2, \sigma_2^2)$. Suppose their sample variances are s_1^2 and s_2^2 respectively. Then the statistic

$$\frac{s_1^2/\sigma_1^2}{s_2^2/\sigma_2^2} = \frac{\chi_1^2/k_1}{x_2^2/k_2} \quad (11.12)$$

$$= F_{k_1,k_2} \quad (11.13)$$

where $k_1 = n_1 - 1$ and $k_2 = n_2 - 1$.

In the expression (11.12), if it is assumed that $\sigma_1^2 = \sigma_2^2$, then the ratio of two sample variances follows F-distribution. This amelioration has made F-distribution practically viable.

PROPERTIES OF F-DISTRIBUTION

1. Statistic F is always positive and h nce F-distribution curve fully lies in the first quadrant.
2. F-distribution has two parameters (k_1, k_2).

3. The shape of F-distribution curve depends on the degrees of freedom (k_1, k_2). F-distribution curves for degrees of freedom (25, 4) and (3, 15) are displayed below.
4. F-distribution is unimodal and its mode lies at the point $\text{F} = \dfrac{k_2\,(k_1 - 2)}{k_1\,(k_2 + 2)}$ value of F is always less than 1 provided $k_1 > 2$.
5. F-distribution curves is positive skewed and this skewness increases with the decrease in the value of k_2.

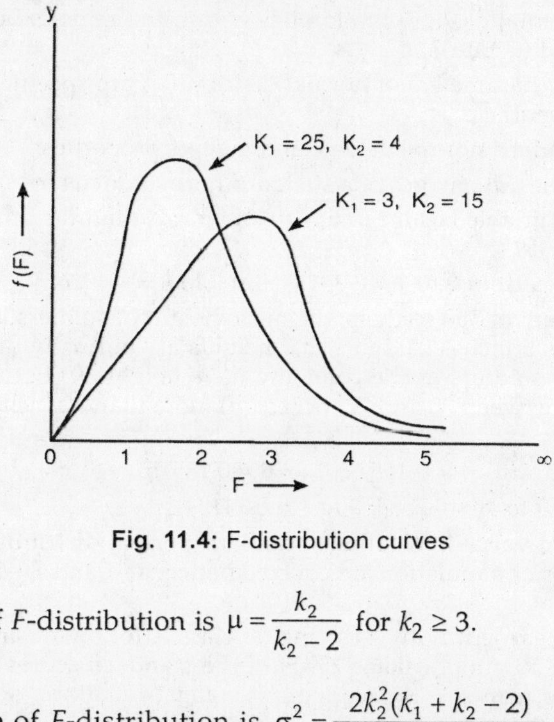

Fig. 11.4: F-distribution curves

6. Mean of F-distribution is $\mu = \dfrac{k_2}{k_2 - 2}$ for $k_2 \geq 3$.
7. Variance of F-distribution is $\sigma^2 = \dfrac{2k_2^2(k_1 + k_2 - 2)}{k_1(k_2 - 2)^2(k_2 - 4)}$ for $k_1 \geq 3$ and $k_2 \geq 5$.
8. Analysis of variance utilizes maximally F-statistics.

CONCLUDING REMARK

The use of sampling distributions is made in the chapter on testing of hypotheses. The statistic given for each distribution shall be used as such without explanation. The readers should also make clear the normal distribution and these three sampling distributions as they are the backbone of applications of statistics.

PRACTICE QUESTIONS AND EXERCISES

1. Give historical background of the normal distribution.
2. What is the main difference between a continuous and discrete distribution in working?
3. Give the probability density function of a continuous normal variable.
4. Show graphically the normal curve and discuss its main features.
5. What is the relation between mean, median and mode of a normal distribution?
6. What does the area under the normal curve provides and how does it help in dealing with different problems?
7. What percentage of population lies within the regions between ($\mu \pm \sigma$), ($\mu \pm 2\sigma$) and ($\mu \pm 3\sigma$)?
8. How many parameters of normal distribution are specified and what do they represent?
9. Define standard normal deviate and give its properties.
10. What are the advantages of a standard normal deviate?
11. A normal variable has mean $\mu = 10$ and $\sigma = 2$. Find the area between $x_1 = 12$ and $x_2 = 18$.
    [Given: Area from 0 to 1 = 0.34134 and 0 to 3 = 0.49865]
12. In a company of 300 soldiers, the mean height of soldiers is 68 inches and their S.D. is 5 inches. Assume that heights are normally distributed. Find how many soldiers in the company have heights (*i*) between 65 and 70 inches (*ii*) between 70 and 72 inches (*iii*) more than 72 inches (*iv*) less than 63 inches
    [Given area: 0 to .4 = 0.15542; 0 to .6 = 0.22575;
    0 to .8 = 0.2884; 0 to 1 = 0.34134]
13. If a random variable X follows standard normal distribution, then what percentages of papulation are covered between –1 and 1, –2 and 2, – 3 and 3?
14. The scores earned by the students of class X follow normal distribution with mean 50 and variance 25. Find the standard scores if the students have scored marks
    a. 40 b. 50 c. 75 d. 90.
15. If a set of variate values is distributed normally, then what proportion of values differs, from mean by, (i) more than $\sigma/4$, (ii) less than $\sigma/2$. [Given: Area between 0 and 0.25 = 0.09871 and Area between 0 to 0.5 = 0.19146]

[Hint : i. $-p\left(\mu - \frac{\sigma}{4} \le X \le \mu + \frac{\sigma}{4}\right) = 1 - p\left(-\frac{1}{4} \le \frac{X-\mu}{\sigma} \le \frac{1}{4}\right)$

$= 1 - 2 \times 0.0987 = 0.80258$

ii. $p\left(\mu - \frac{\sigma}{2} \le X \le \mu + \frac{\sigma}{2}\right) = p\left(-\frac{1}{2} \le \frac{X-\mu}{\sigma} \le \frac{1}{2}\right)$

16. If the mean scores in an examination are 64 with S.D. 9. If top 10% students will be awarded grade A, then what minimum scores should a student achieve so that he earns A grade?
    [Given that area from 0 to 1.28 = 0.4]
    [Hint. $Z = \frac{X - 64}{9} = 1.28$]
17. If the mean weight of students of a college is 62 kg. and variance 9 kg^2, then find the probability of students who weigh, (i) less than 55 kg, (ii) between 55 and 65 kg, (iii) more than 65 kg.
    [Given areas: 0 to 2.33 = 0.4901, 0 to 1 = 0.34134]
18. In a normal population, 10% values are below 15 and 30% are above 25. Find the mean and standard deviation of the normal population.
    [Given : Area from 0 to 1.28 = 0.4; 0 to .52 = 0.2]
19. If 35% population lies between mean 65 and a value X = 80, then find the value of σ.
    [Given : $P(0 \leq Z \leq 1.04) = 0.35$]
    [Hint : $Z = \frac{80 - 65}{\sigma} = \frac{15}{\sigma}$, *i.e.* $P\left(0 \leq Z \leq \frac{15}{\sigma}\right) = 0.35 \therefore \frac{15}{\sigma} = 1.04$]
20. In a standard normal curve, find the area (i) to the left of Z = 0.6, (ii) to the right of Z = 0.6, (iii) in between Z = 0.6 and Z = 1.3.
    [Given : Area from 0 to .6 = 0.22575 and 0 to 1.3 = 0.40320]
21. Discuss chi-square variate and give its probability density function.
22. Who are credited for discovering and enhancing *t*-distribution?
23. Discuss the variable which follows *t*-distribution and also give its probability density function.
24. Compare *t*-distribution with a standard normal curve.
25. Enunciate the properties of a chi-square distribution curve.
26. Give the parameter(s) of chi-square distribution and also its mean and variance.
27. In what manner, F-distribution is related to chi-square statistics?
28. Write down the probability density function of the distribution of F and also explain the terms involved in it.
29. How the ratio of two sample variances is considered to be distributed as F.
30. Who discovered chi-square distribution and in which year(s)?
31. What type of variable is involved in chi-square distribution and what is the basis of this distribution?
32. Give the mean and variance of *t*-distribution and their limitations.
33. How does the degrees of freedom of F-statistic influence the shape of F-distribution curve?
34. At what point, mode of F-distribution exists?
35. What restriction is imposed for a variable to follow t-distribution and why?

36. Give the mean and variance of F-distributions and the conditions under which they exist.

CONCLUDING REMARK

Numerical problems on Z, χ^2, t and F tests are not given in this chapter. Reason being that they are extensively dealt with in the Chapter 14 on Testing of Hypothesis.

Continuous distributions delineated inside are some most popular and useful distribution and these are very judiciously covered. Rest of the continuous distributions are kept out of the scope of this book as they are covered in advance courses.

OBJECTIVE TYPE QUESTIONS

Select the most appropriate option out of the provided four options for each problem/question.

37. The shape of the normal frequency distribution curve depends on:
    a. The variance σ^2 b. The mode of the distribution
    c. The mean μ d. The mean μ and variance σ^2
38. A standard normal curve is always:
    a. Symmetric b. Properly peaked
    c. Symmetric and properly packed d. None of the above
39. If a normal curve is properly peaked, than it is called:
    a. Mesokurtic b. Playkurtic
    c. Leptokurtic d. Any one of the above
40. Value of measure of skewness (J) for a normal curve is:
    a. $J = 1$ b. $J = 0$
    c. $J > 0$ d. $J < 0$
41. If the income of 500 persons follows normal distribution and the area between two stand normal variate values for the incomes 5.25 and 7.05 lacs is 0.006234, then the number of persons having an income between 5.25 and 7.05 lacs is almost:
    a. 31 b. 22
    c. 24 d. None of the above
42. Sum of squares of the n normal deviates follows:
    a. Chi-square distribution b. t-distribution
    c. Normal distribution d. F-distribution
43. The mean and variance of chi-square distribution with k degrees of freedom are:
    a. Mean = k, variance = k^2 b. Mean = k, variance = $2k$
    c. Mean = $2k$ and variance = $2k$ d. None of the above
44. A standard normal deviate has the frequency distribution,
    a. $\frac{1}{\sigma\sqrt{2\pi}} e^{-\frac{1}{2}\frac{z^2}{\sigma^2}}$ b. $\frac{1}{\sqrt{2\pi}} e^{-\frac{1}{2}(z-\mu)^2}$

c. $\frac{1}{\sqrt{2\pi}} e^{-\frac{1}{2}z^2}$

d. $\frac{1}{\sqrt{2\pi}\,\sigma} e^{-\frac{1}{2}(z-\mu)^2}$

45. A variate as the ratio of a normal variate and underroot chi-square follows:
    a. F-distribution
    b. Standard normal distribution
    c. *t*-distribution
    d. Binomial distribution
46. chi-square statistic defined by Karl Pearson for *k* classes with usual notations is,
    a. $\sum_{i=1}^{k} \frac{f_i^2}{np_i} - n$
    b. $\sum_{i=1}^{k} \frac{(f_i - np_i)^2}{np_i}$
    c. Both a. and b.
    d. Neither a. nor b.
47. A normal distribution has the property that:
    a. The values of mean and median are always same
    b. Median, mean and mode coincide
    c. Mode is always greater than mean
    d. Median is always less than mode
48. Chi-square distribution curve is:
    a. Negatively skewed
    b. Skew on either side
    c. Symmetrical
    d. Positively skewed
49. Which of the statistic follows F-distribution?
    a. The ratio of two independent chi-squares
    b. The ratio of two sample variances
    c. Both a. and b.
    d. None of a. and b.
50. Mean of the t-distribution:
    a. Does not exist
    b. Does exist but it is zero
    c. Does exist but it is one
    d. Is always negative
51. A biparametric discrete distribution is:
    a. Poisson distribution
    b. F-distribution
    c. Normal distribution.
    d. Binomial distribution
52. Mean of F-distribution, when $k_1 > 3$, is:
    a. Zero
    b. Less than 1
    c. Greater than 1
    d. Undefined
53. With increase in sample size, t-distribution tends to:
    a. Normal distribution
    b. Poisson distribution
    c. Positive skewness
    d. More peakedness
54. Probability density curve of t-distribution is:
    a. Normally peaked
    b. Less peaked than normal
    c. More peaked than normal
    d. Any of the above
55. For an sample of size 15, degrees of freedom for student-t are:

a. 15 b. 14

c. 16 d. 13

56. which one of the following is a uniparametric distribution?

a. Poisson distribution b. Binomial distribution

c. F-distribution d. Normal distribution

57. In case of standard normal curve, the area covered within the interval $\mu-2\sigma$ and $\mu + 2\sigma$ is:

a. 99.7% b. 95.4%

c. 68.3% d. 50.0%

58. Variance of *t*-distribution with 5 degrees of freedom is:

a. Not existing b. $\frac{3}{5}$

c. $\frac{5}{3}$ d. 4

59. For a $N(\mu, \sigma^2)$ distribution, within which interval the area of the normal curve is correctly given?

a. $-\infty$ to μ is 0.5 b. μ to ∞ is 0.5

c. $-\infty$ to ∞ is 1.0 d. All of these

60. If a variable X is distributed as χ_1^2 with 6 d.f, and another variable Y is distributed as χ_2^2 with 8 d.f., then the distribution of $(X + Y)$ is:

a. *F*-distribution with 6 and 8 *d.f* b. *t*-distribution with 14 d.f

c. χ^2 distribution with 14 *d.f.* d. χ^2 distribution with 3 d.f

61. Given the following probability density function, $\frac{i}{5\sqrt{2\pi}} e^{-\frac{1}{2}\left(\frac{x-5}{5}\right)^2}$. What is the value of coefficient of variation?

a. 20% b. 100%

c. 223.6% d. 44.7%

62. Skewness of F_{k_1,k_2} distribution curve increase when:

a. k_1 *d.f.* decrease b. k_2 *d.f.* increase

c. k_1, k_2 *d.f.* increase d. k_2 *d.f.* decrease

63. Modal value M_0 of F_{k_1,k_2} - distribution is:

a. Lying within the range $0 \le M_0 < 1$ b. $M_0 > 1$

c. Within the range $-1 \le M_0 < 1$ d. Within the range $-\infty < M_0 < \infty$

64. Range of the value of F is:

a. 0 to 1 b. 0 to ∞

c. $-\infty$ to ∞ d. -1 to 1

65. Student's t-distribution is known as sampling distribution, because:

a. It is based on small sample

b. It was given under the pseudonym 'student'

c. Statistic-t is a function of sample values only

d. It is used to test the null hypothesis

CHAPTER 12

Sampling Methods

This is very important to know at the outset, what is a sample. So, sample is defined.

Definition:

A sample is a part of the population consisting of a few units of it which represents the whole population.

POPULATION

In statistics population is an aggregate of certain units, individual or objects which possess specified characteristics. A population may be finite or infinite. For example, students of a university, households in a city, trees in an orchard, all even numbers, etc.

SAMPLING UNIT

The units or individuals of a population meant to be selected in a sample and on which the observations are to be taken are called **sampling units.** Each student of a university, every household in a locality, each tree in a grove, are a few examples of sampling units.

SAMPLING

It is a device by which a sample is drawn from a population so as to represent the population as truly as possible.

In the book, **Basic Statistics** by B.L. Agarwal, it has been written in the beginning of chapter on sampling **Sampling in Statistics is as common and important as salt in the food.** From this statement, it is clear that there is hardly any statistical technique which does not involve sampling. Sampling is not only important in statistics but it is used in daily life without any thinking. For instance, in the homes, ladies take a grain or two from the cooking pan and test whether the food article is cooked or not. When one goes to the market to purchase wheat or rice, he takes a handful of wheat (rice) and judges the quality of wheat in the heap or in the bag. A doctor takes a little quantity of blood and finds the deficiencies of whole blood in the body. All these examples reveal that in sampling one selects a small number of units (quantity) from a population which enables to know about all its units or contents.

Advantages of Sampling

There are many advantages of sampling as compared to study the population as a whole. Some main advantages are delineated here.

1. Saving in time. Generally a population consists of large number of units. Study of the whole population will take lot of time in taking the observations on each and every sampling unit. But on taking a sample, only a few units are to be measured which naturally consumes less time. The results obtained by a sample stand for the whole population which are reasonably reliable.

2. Reduction in expenditure. To study a large number of units comprising the population require too many personnel in the team. There will be lot of expenditure on travelling, salaries, taking readings, equipment, etc. But, when a few units are under study, one needs a small number of trained personnel and other expenses will also be limited. On the whole a lot of money is saved.

3. Enables to study an infinite population. If a population consists of an infinite number of units, the process of taking observation will never come to an end. Hence, there is no alternative except to take sample and study it.

4. Survey of perishable items. In a number of studies, items are destroyed during the process of taking observation or otherwise. If all the population units are tested, they all will be perished and nothing will be left to use. For instance, a battery cell producing company wishes to know the average life of cells. If all cells will be tested for their life, then no cell will be left to sell in the market. Hence, sampling is inevitable in this case.

5. Availability of results in time. All studies are to be completed within a specified time so as to make the results available at the time of requirement. But studying the whole population rules out such a possibility. For example, a disease is spreading in a city. If all the patients taken for investigation, it will take lot of time to find the cause of the disease. So, a sample of a limited number of patients is selected and investigations are made. This will quickly provide the solution to the problem otherwise, many patients would have died.

Uses of sampling

Sampling makes possible to draw a sample which truly represents a population from which the sample is selected. From the study of the sample, one estimates the population parameters like mean, variance, correlation, etc. With the help of sample(s), it is possible to perform a test to confirm whether a claimed value of a population parameter is true or not. Also, parameters of two or more populations can be compared. Further, in a way, advantages of sampling are uses of sampling as well.

Census versus sample studies

Census means taking observations on each and every unit of the population or counting each unit. This is also termed as **complete enumeration.** Such type of studies are presently made about two things—(i) to know the population of the country, every head is counted, (*ii*) to know the number of tax-payers. But census studies are very expensive and time consuming. So they are avoided. On the contrary, sample studies are simple and less expensive in terms of time and money. So these are preferred.

Some people believe that the results obtained from a sample are not reliable. They will not give the true picture of the population. Their belief is absolutely wrong. If a proper sample is drawn from a population, it sometimes gives better results than census studies. The reasons for this may be given as follows.

1. There are greater chances of errors of observation in census studies.
2. Recording of values vary from person to person as many investigators change the meaning and senses of a question asked from the respondents.
3. There are more chances of errors in tabulation and analysis of data in a large scale study.
4. Many times respondents deliberately supply wrong information regarding their age, income, etc. This type of error increases in complete enumeration.
5. Experiments can not be conducted on all animals, plants, human beings, etc. Hence, sample study is the only way where census studies are not possible.
6. Sample contains a small number of units as compared to population. Therefore, a more detailed study can be made on any subject of enquiry. In this way, a sample results into more information than census studies.

Simple Random Sampling

In this type of sampling, each and every sampling unit has same chance of being included in the sample. Hence, there remains no preference for any unit to be included or not to be included in the sample. If a sample of adequate size is selected from a population by the method of simple random sampling (SRS), it is a true representative of the population. In this situation, the results obtained from the sample hold good for the population.

SELECTION METHODS

A sample by the method of simple random sampling can be selected by two methods, (*i*) lottery method (*ii*) with the help of random number tables.

i. **Lottery method.** In this method, N population units are numbered serially 1 to N and then N chits are prepared numbered from 1 to N. These chits are kept in a container or bag and thoroughly mixed. Now as many chits are drawn one by one as the size of sample, say n. The numbers found on the chits are noted. The units of the population on serial numbers corresponding to the numbers on the selected chits are included in the sample. This type of random sampling is known as **simple random sampling without replacement** (srswor). As an instance, suppose there are ten units in the population and are numbered. Let them be denoted as, U_1, U_2, U_3, U_4, U_5, U_6, U_7, U_8, U_9, U_{10}.

A sample of three units is to be drawn. Ten chits bearing the numbers from 1 to 10 are placed in a container and shaked well. Now three chits are drawn with closed eye from it one by one. Let these chits bear numbers 3, 5 and 8. So select the units U_3, U_5 and U_8 for the sample.

Sampling using Random Number Table

Chit system becomes cumbersome if the population size is enough large. Also this is not completely free from human bias, so use of random number tables is always preferred. In this selection process also, the units are numbered serially from 1 to N. Random number tables contain large number of columns having natural numbers 0 to 9. First see how many digits are there in N. Take as many columns of a random number table as the number of digits in N. Select numbers from these columns conjointly one after the other. Select a number if it lies from 1 to N, otherwise reject it. Continue the process of selecting numbers till the sample of required size is selected. If a number is repeated, it is rejected in sampling without replacement and accepted in case of **sampling with replacement**. It should be beared in mind that in sampling with replacement, a unit can occur any number of times in the sample. Sampling with replacement is less preferred as compared to srswor.

Now the procedure of selection is practically explained. Part of a two digited random number table is given on next page.

As a matter of fact, these tables have hundreds of columns and each column contains a large number of integers 0 to 9. Here a few are given so as to acquaint the young readers.

Suppose there is a population of sixty units. So the units are serially numbered from 1 to 60. Suppose a sample of 6 units to be selected. It means it is required to select random numbers from Table 12.1. Since 60 is a two digited figure, start from column (1). Select six random number from 1 to 60 which are 15, 30, 19, 10, 23, 39.

Table 12.1: Random number table

Columns				
(1)	(2)	(3)	(4)	(5)
15	00	41	92	25
30	92	91	45	51
19	94	30	67	48
10	70	49	92	05
23	13	67	95	07
63	71	54	50	06
19	29	11	23	27
39	79	77	28	94
86	47	35	55	33
51	26	02	96	29
07	21	49	84	48
86	33		90	21

In the process of selecting random numbers, the number 19 occurring second time is omitted. Also number 63 is omitted as it is greater than 60. Thus, select the units placed at serial numbers, 15, 30, 19, 10, 23, 33, 39.

FORMULAE

Let $x_1, x_2, \ldots, x_n$ be the n values obtained from n sample units.

Let sample mean be denoted by $\overline{x}$. The formula for **sample mean** is,

$$\overline{x} = \frac{\sum_i x_i}{n} \tag{12.1}$$

$$\text{for } i = 1, 2, \ldots, n.$$

$$= \frac{\text{Sum of all sample values}}{\text{Number of values}} \tag{12.1.1}$$

$$= \frac{x_1 + x_2 + \cdots + x_n}{n} \tag{12.1.2}$$

Formula for **sample variance** is,

$$s^2 = \frac{1}{n-1}\sum_{i=1}^{n}(x_i - \overline{x})^2 \tag{12.2}$$

$$= \frac{1}{n-1}\left\{\sum_i x_i^2 - \frac{(\sum_i x_i)^2}{n}\right\} \tag{12.2.1}$$

where, s^2 denotes the sample variance.

FORMULA FOR STANDARD DERIVATION

The positive square root of sample variance is the sample standard deviation, i.e.,

$$\text{S.D or s.d.} = \sqrt{s^2} = +s \tag{12.3}$$

STANDARD ERROR OF MEAN

It is apparent that the mean varies from sample to sample even though the sample size is kept fixed. As a matter of fact from a population of size N, NC_n sample of size n can be selected. In this way one gets a series of means $\overline{x}$ and thus $\overline{x}$ behaves as random variable. The standard deviation of $\overline{x}$ is called **standard error of mean.** It is denoted as S.E. ($\overline{x}$). Formula for standard error of mean is,

$$\text{S.E.}(\overline{x}) = \frac{s}{\sqrt{n}} \tag{12.4}$$

Lesser the value of standard error, more reliable is the sample as a representative of the population.

ESTIMATE OF POPULATION TOTAL

If $\overline{x}$ is sample mean and N is number of unit in the population, the estimate of population total $\hat{X}$ is

$$\hat{X} = N\overline{x} \tag{12.5}$$

Example 12.1. Six observations from a sample of six units are as given below.

x: 7, 12, 6, 4, 3, 10

Find the sample mean, variance and standard error.

Sample mean by the formula (12.1) is,

$$\overline{x} = \frac{7+12+6+4+3+10}{6}$$

$$= \frac{42}{6} = 7.0$$

To calculate the variance by the formula (12.2), the deviation from mean $\overline{x} = 7$ are:

$(x-\overline{x})$: (7 – 7), (12 – 7), (6 – 7), (4 –7), (3 – 7), (10 – 7)

Deviation : 0, + 5, – 1, – 3, – 4, 3

$(x-\overline{x})^2$: 0, 25, 1, 9, 16, 9

$\sum(x-\overline{x})^2$ = 0 + 25 + 1 + 9+ 16 + 9 = 60

$\therefore$ The sample variance, $s^2 = \dfrac{60}{6-1} = \dfrac{60}{5} = 12.0$

Note : Check that sum of the deviation from mean is always zero. In this example, $\sum(x_i - \bar{x}) = 8 - 8 = 0$

The standard error by the formula (12.4) can be worked out. The standard deviation, $s = \sqrt{12} = 3.464$

$$\therefore \quad S.E.(\bar{x}) = \frac{3.464}{\sqrt{6}} = \frac{3.464}{2.449} = 1.414$$

Example 12.2. Following are the test scores of nine students of class IX out of 20 marks in first terminal. Find the variance of the test scores.

Scores x : 12, 9, 14, 16, 10, 7, 18, 11, 15

$$\Sigma x = 12 + 9 + 14 + 16 + 10 + 7 + 18 + 11 + 15 = 112$$

$$\bar{x} = \frac{112}{9} = 12.44$$

Since $\bar{x}$ is not a round figure, it is preferable to use the formula (12.2.1) for variance. It is easy to work out with it and also provides accurate value of the variance.

x^2 : 144, 81, 196, 256, 100, 49, 324, 121, 225

$\Sigma x^2 = 144 + 81 + 196 + 256 + 100 + 49 + 324 + 121 + 225 = 1496$

By (12.2.1),
$$s^2 = \frac{1}{9-1}[1496 - \frac{(112)^2}{9}]$$

$$= \frac{1}{8}[1496 - 1393.78]$$

$$= \frac{102.22}{8} = 12.78$$

N.B.: Formulae (12.2) and (12.2.1) are two forms of the same formula for variance. Both of them yield the same value of variance. One can use either of them as per convenience.

PURPOSIVE SAMPLING

In this type of selection method, units are selected by the researcher which possess certain characteristics and are conveniently available to him. This method of selection is a non-probability procedure. This type of sampling is also called **judgement sampling** or **convenient** sampling. Consequently this method is not suitable for estimating parameters. Also there is no control on the magnitude of sampling errors.

CONCLUDING REMARK

Sample random sampling is the foremost method of sampling and is most frequently used in statistics. Besides this method some other methods of sampling are also popular because of their superiority in a variety of situations. Stratified sampling, systematic sampling, cluster sampling, multi-stage sampling, etc. are some other popular methods of sampling. But all these methods of sampling are kept out of scope of this book.

PRACTICE QUESTIONS AND EXERCISES

1. What are the advantages of sampling as compared to complete enumeration?
2. Distinguish between sampling and a sample.
3. Discuss population in the context of statistics.
4. Define sampling unit and discuss its importance.
5. Discuss two situations where census is absolutely necessary.
6. Explain the method of selecting a sample from a finite population with the help of random number tables.
7. Define simple random sampling and give formulae for sample mean and variance.
8. Given a population of 12 values as.

   11, 3, 9, 12, 10, 7, 6, 8, 7, 3, 5, 2

   Draw a random sample of five values with the help of random number table inside this chapter and calculate its variance.

   [**Hint:** Selected values of x : 3, 6, 5, 3, 10]
9. Given the income ('000 Rs) per month of 12 workers, find the variance of income.

   8.3, 7.4, 5.4, 3.2, 4.5, 6.5, 7.8, 12.6, 16.1, 17.8, 9.6, 10.6
10. Define and discuss standard error of mean.
11. Given the sample variance of marks of fifteen students as 46.6, find the standard error of mean.
12. For the following set of sample values,

    10.6, 7.3, 8.9, 12.6, 5.3, 14.4, 11.8, 9.4, 13.1

    Calculate standard error of mean
13. The means of four samples of size three from a population of 4 units are given below.

    10.6, 11.1, 9.8, 10.2

    Find the standard error of mean.
14. Do the errors in sample studies are always greater than complete enumeration? Justify your answer.
15. Differentiate between sampling with replacement and without replacement. Which is likely to give more precise results in general?
16. Compare census versus sample survey studies.
17. Why lottery system is not preferred for selecting a sample?

18. What are other types of sampling methods besides simple random sampling?
19. Two terms A and B scored the following number of goals in seven matches.

    Team A : 3, 2, 5, 6, 4, 5, 3

    Team B : 1, 5, 4, 3, 2, 3, 5

    Find which team has less variability in its performance?
20. How can you estimate the population total for a variable character X?

OBJECTIVE TYPE QUESTIONS

Given the four answer-choices for each statement or problem, select the best one.

21. Sampling study is inevitable because:
    a. It is not possible to study an infinite population
    b. It is not possible to test all units of the population if they are perished under observation
    c. A population study requires too much time and resources
    d. All of the above
22. Sampling is a procedure for:
    a. Studying a known population
    b. Knowing about an unknown population
    c. Gathering information about a part of unknown population
    d. None of the above
23. Standard error is concerned with:
    a. Error in sampling method
    b. Error in survey method
    c. Standard deviation of means of all possible samples
    d. Error of measurement
24. Precision of an estimate is measured by:
    a. Sample variance   b. Sample standard deviation
    c. Sample size   d. Standard error
25. Sampling unit is a term related to:
    a. Population   b. Sample
    c. Measurement of unit   d. Unit of measurement
26. Simple random sampling is a procedure in which:
    a. Some units possessing desired qualities are selected
    b. Investigator selects some units convenient to him
    c. Each unit is likely to be selected with equal probability
    d. Some units are preferred over the other
27. As the sample size increases, standard error (S.E):
    a. Decreases   b. Increases
    c. Tends to zero
    d. No certainty about increase or decrease in S.E

28. From a well shuffled pack of cards, a card is drawn blindly. Its colour is noted and not replaced. This process is continued five times. This type of sampling is known as:
    a. Sampling with replacement
    b. Sampling without replacement
    c. Convenient sampling
    d. Nonrandom sampling
29. If a doctor wants to assess the efficacy of a drug on the patients of gastroentitis, then which sampling procedure should he follow?
    a. Simple random sampling with replacement
    b. Simple random sampling without replacement
    c. Purposive sampling
    d. None of the above
30. From a population of 10 units, how many distinct random sample of size 3 can be drawn?
    a. 720
    b. 1000
    c. 60
    d. 120
31. Sample mean of the values 12, 9, 11, – 4, 0, 8, 14, 19, and 21 is:
    a. 10.0
    b. 11.25
    c. 10.9
    d. None of the above
32. For the data given is question 31, the standard deviation of the sample is:
    a. 7.63
    b. 8.65
    c. 8.093
    d. 7.239
33. The mean and variance of a set of values are 12.56 and 18.74 respectively. The coefficient of variation is:
    a. 290.13 %
    b. 34.47 %
    c. 149.20 %
    d. 122.15 %
34. Homogeneity of a sample is measured by:
    a. Standard deviation
    b. Sample size
    c. Standard error
    d. All of the above
35. Census study involves:
    a. 50 percent subjects of the population
    b. Each and every subject comprising the population
    c. Any number of subjects
    d. None of the above

CHAPTER 13

Correlation and Regression

IMPORTANCE

Often the need arises to study two or more variables simultaneously. In this chapter, the mater is confined to two variables only. For example, one may be interested to know relation between height and weight of persons, age of wife and husband at the time of marriage, input of fertilizer and production of a crop, pressure and volume of a gas, income and expenditure of households, etc.

Studies of two variables conjointly may be of two types. Someone may either be interested to measure the covariation between two variables or may like to establish the cause and effect relationship between them as a function of one variable in terms of the other. In this case, one variable is classified as dependent variable and the other as independent variable. Simply measuring covariation between two variables leads to correlation whereas establishing a functional relationship between two variables leads to regression.

SIMPLE CORRELATION

In the study of two of variables jointly, many times an investigator is interested to know the degree or extent of dependence between them. Actually one wants to know whether the relation between two variables is of high, moderate or low degree. If the two variables have no relation, it means the change in one variable has no impact about the change in the other. In this case, two variables are said to be **independent.**

Definition:
Correlation is a measure of extent or degree of mutual dependence between two variables.

METHODS OF DETERMINING CORRELATION

Graphical method

The extent of relation between two variable can roughly be judged by plotting the pairs of observations as points on a graph paper. These points are spread in different patterns and as such these are called scatter diagrams. Larger the number of points in a straight line, greater is the degree of relationship between them. Following seven scatter diagrams shown in Figs 13.1a to g depict the clear picture.

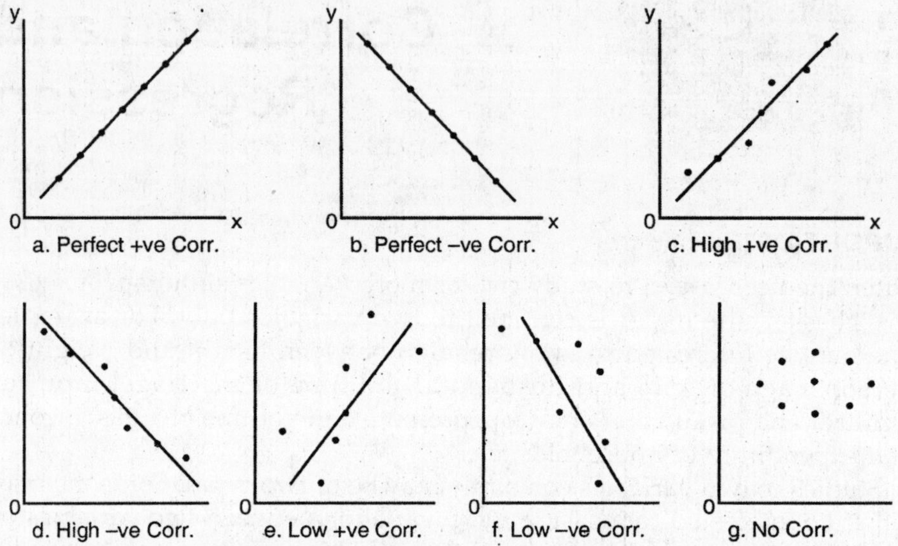

Figs 13.1a to g: Scatter diagrams

Figure 13.1a shows that there is a perfect positive linear relationship between *X* and *Y*, i.e., the variable is proportional to *Y* and vice-versa. In this case the line flows from lower left side to upper right side. All the points lie on the line.

Figure 13.1b divulge the same phenomenon but in opposite direction, i.e., if *X* increases, then *Y* decreases. In this situation, the line runs from upper left to right bottom side.

Figures 13.1c and d delineated high positive and negative correlation respectively as most of the points lie near the straight lines or lie on them.

Figures 13.1e and f displaying the same phenomena as c and d except that in the these figures, the points lie farther from the lines indicating a low degree of correlation between the variables.

In Fig. 13.1g hardly any line can be drawn about which all the points concentrate. It means there is no correlation between the variables.

MATHEMATICAL MEASURE

A graph provides a rough idea about the type and extent of correlation between two variables. But more exactly the correlation can be measured numerically by calculating **coefficient of correlation.** This is known as numerically by calculating **coefficient of correlation.** This is known as Pearson's coefficient of correlation and the formula for it was developed by Karl Pearson, a British biometrician. This is based on three assumptions as follows:

1. The variables X and Y are distributed normally.
2. The relationship between X and Y is linear.
3. There is a cause and effect relationship between X and Y.

If from a bivariate population there are n pairs of values of the variables X and Y as, (x_1, y_1), (x_2, y_2), (x_3, y_3), ..., (x_n, y_n). Then the formula for coefficient of correlation is,

$$r_{XY} = \frac{\Sigma_i(x_i - \bar{x})(y_i - \bar{y})}{\sqrt{\Sigma_i(x_i - \bar{x})^2 \, \Sigma_i(y_i - \bar{y})^2}} \qquad (13.1)$$

for $i = 1, 2, ..., n$

where,

r_{XY} – correlation coefficient between X and Y. But mostly suffix XY is omittled due to inconvenience.

$\Sigma_i (x_i - \bar{x})(y_i - \bar{y})$ – Sum of the cross product of deviations from their respective means.

$\Sigma_i (x_i - \bar{x})^2$ – Sum of squares of deviation from mean of x-values.

$\Sigma_i (y_i - \bar{y})^2$ – Sum of squares of deviation from mean of y-values.

Elaborately,

$$\Sigma_i (x_i - \bar{x})(y_i - \bar{y}) = (x_1 - \bar{x})(y_1 - \bar{y}) + (x_2 - \bar{x})(y_2 - \bar{y}) + \cdots + (x_n - \bar{x})(y_n - \bar{y})$$

$$\Sigma_i (x_i - \bar{x})^2 = (x_1 - \bar{x})^2 + (x_2 - \bar{x})^2 + \cdots + (x_n - \bar{x})^2$$

$$\Sigma_i (y_i - \bar{y})^2 = (y_1 - \bar{y})^2 + (y_2 - \bar{y})^2 + \cdots + (y_n - \bar{y})^2$$

ALTERNATIVE FORMULA

Often taking deviations from mean increases the labour of calculation, consumes more time and also introduces some inaccuracy particularly when means are not exact and whole numbers. Therefore, the formula given in the following alternative form removes all these difficulties and provides the exact value of r.

$$r = \frac{\Sigma_i x_i y_i - \frac{(\Sigma_i x_i)(\Sigma_i y_i)}{n}}{\sqrt{\left\{\Sigma_i x_i^2 - \frac{(\Sigma_i x_i)^2}{n}\right\}\left\{\Sigma_i y_1^2 - \frac{(\Sigma_i x_i)^2}{n}\right\}}} \qquad (13.2)$$

Putting $x_i - \bar{x} = u_i$ and $y_i - \bar{y} = v_i$, the formula (13.1) reduces to the form,

$$r = \frac{\Sigma_i u_i v_i}{\sqrt{\Sigma_i u_i^2 \cdot \Sigma_i v_i^2}} \tag{13.3}$$

This formula can also be written as,

$$r = \frac{\Sigma_i u_i v_i}{(n-1) s_x \cdot s_y} \tag{13.4}$$

where,
s_x – standard deviation of x
s_y – standard deviation of y.
n – number of paired values.

Properties

1. The value of coefficient of correlation lies between –1 and 1.
2. The value of r indicates perfect, high, moderate, low positive or negative and nil degree of correlation as per the values of r given in the table below

Degree of correlation	*Positive corr. coeff.*	*Negative corr. coeff.*
Perfect	$r = +1$	$r = -1$
High	$0.75 \le r < 1$	$-1 < r \le -0.75$
Moderate	$0.25 \le r < 0.75$	$-0.75 \le r \le -0.25$
Low	$0 < r < 0.25$	$-0.25 < r < 0$
Nil	0	0

3. Coefficient of correlation has no unit as it is a pure ratio.
4. **Coding of data:** If a constant value ***a*** is added or substracted from each value of x and ***b*** from each value of y and also each value of x is divided (multiplied) by a constant ***c*** and y by ***d***, the value of correlation coefficient calculated from coded values is same as that of original value. It means coding of data does not affect the value of r.
5. If X and Y are independent, then the correlation coefficient between them is zero, but the converse is true. The method of calculation of correlation coefficient is demonstrated through the following solved examples.

Example 13.1. Marks of seven students in Physics and Mathematics in an hourly test out of 10 were as follows:

Students:	I	II	III	IV	V	VI	VII
Marks in Maths (x):	7	9	10	6	5	4	8
Marks in physics (y):	9	6	5	4	3	2	6

Find the correlation coefficient between the marks scored in the two subjects.

To calculate r, do the following calculations.

$$\bar{x} = \frac{7+9+10+6+5+4+8}{7} = \frac{49}{7} = 7.0$$

$$\bar{y} = \frac{9+6+5+4+3+2+6}{7} = \frac{35}{7} = 5.0$$

$$\begin{aligned}
\Sigma(x_i - \bar{x})(y_i - \bar{y}) &= (7-7)(9-5) + (9-7)(6-5) + (10-7)(5-5) \\
&\quad + (6-7)(4-5) + (5-7)(3-5) + (4-7)(2-5) \\
&\quad + (8-7)(6-5) \\
&= 0 \times 4 + 2 \times 1 + 3 \times 0 + (-1)(-1) + (-2)(-2) + \\
&\qquad (-3)(-3) + 1 \times 1 \\
&= 0 + 2 + 0 + 1 + 4 + 9 + 1 = 17 \\
\Sigma(x_i - \bar{x})^2 &= (7-7)^2 + (9-7)^2 + (10-7)^2 + (6-7)^2 + (5-7)^2 \\
&\qquad + (4-7)^2 + (8-7)^2 \\
&= 0 + 4 + 9 + 1 + 4 + 9 + 1 = 28 \\
\Sigma(y_i - \bar{y})^2 &= (9-5)^2 + (6-5)^2 + (5-5)^2 + (4-5)^2 + (3-5)^2 \\
&\qquad + (2-5)^2 + (6-5)^2 \\
&= 16 + 1 + 0 + 1 + 4 + 9 + 1 = 32
\end{aligned}$$

By the formula (13.1),

$$\begin{aligned}
r &= \frac{17}{\sqrt{28 \times 32}} \\
&= \frac{17}{\sqrt{896}} = \frac{17}{29.93} \\
&= 0.568
\end{aligned}$$

Since the value of r is little more than 0.5, it can be interpreted that the correlation between marks in mathematics and physics is moderate.

Example 13.2. The ages of wives and their husbands at marriage are given below.

	Age in years					
Wife (X) :	20	21	17	23	27	18
Husband (Y) :	23	23	20	24	32	22

Calculate the coefficient of correlation between ages of wives and husbands.

The value of r can easily be obtained by the formula (13.1)

$$\bar{x} = \frac{20+21+17+23+27+18}{6} = \frac{126}{6} = 21$$

$$\bar{y} = \frac{23+23+20+24+32+22}{6} = \frac{144}{6} = 24$$

$$\begin{aligned}\Sigma(x_i - \bar{x})(y_i - \bar{y}) &= (20-21)(23-24) + (21-21)(23-24) \\ &\quad + (17-21)(20-24) + (23-21)(24-24) \\ &\quad + (27-21)(32-24) + (18-21)(22-24) \\ &= (-1)(-1) + 0 \times (-1) + (-4)(-4) + 2 \times 0 + 6 \times 8 \\ &\quad + (-3)(-2) \\ &= 1 + 0 + 16 + 0 + 48 + 6 = 71\end{aligned}$$

$$\begin{aligned}\Sigma(x_i - \bar{x})^2 &= (20-21)^2 + (21-21)^2 + (17-21)^2 + (23-21)^2 \\ &\quad + (27-21)^2 + (18-21)^2 \\ &= 1 + 0 + 16 + 4 + 36 + 9 = 66\end{aligned}$$

$$\begin{aligned}\Sigma(y_i - \bar{y})^2 &= (23-24)^2 + (23-24)^2 + (20-24)^2 + (24-24)^2 \\ &\quad + (32-24)^2 + (22-24)^2 \\ &= 1 + 1 + 16 + 0 + 64 + 4 = 86\end{aligned}$$

The coefficient of correlation by the formula (13.1)

$$\begin{aligned} r &= \frac{71}{\sqrt{66 \times 86}} = \frac{71}{75.34} \\ &= 0.94\end{aligned}$$

The value of r is greater than 0.9, it confirms a high degree positive relationship between the ages of wives and husbands.

Example 13.3. Calculate Pearson's coefficient of correlation between price of items (X) and demand of items (Y).

X:	13	14	16	10	14	12	15	12	8	12	27
Y:	9	8	14	6	5	7	4	9	6	5	2

First, find the mean of x and y values

$$\Sigma x_i = (13 + 14 + \ldots + 12 + 27) = 153; \ \bar{x} = \frac{153}{11} = 13.91$$

$$\Sigma y_i = (9 + 8 + \ldots + 5 + 2) = 75; \ \bar{y} = \frac{75}{11} = 6.82$$

It is to be noted that the mean values of x and y are not whole numbers. In this situation, it will be convenient to use the formula (13.2) so, further calculate $\Sigma x^2, \Sigma y^2$ and Σxy

$$\Sigma_i x_i^2 = 13^2 + 14^2 + \ldots + 12^2 + 27^2 = 2367$$

$$\Sigma_i y_i^2 = 9^2 + 8^2 + \ldots + 5^2 + 2^2 = 613$$

$$\Sigma_i x_i y_i = 13 \times 9 + 14 \times 8 + \ldots + 12 \times 5 + 27 \times 2 = 997$$

$$\therefore \quad r = \frac{997 - \dfrac{153 \times 75}{11}}{\sqrt{\left(2367 - \dfrac{153^2}{11}\right)\left(613 - \dfrac{75^2}{11}\right)}}$$

$$= \frac{997 - 1043.18}{\sqrt{238.91 \times 101.64}}$$

$$= \frac{-46.18}{155.83}$$

$$= -0.296$$

r has a low negative valve. This indicates that as the price of items increase, there is little decline in demand.

Example 13.4. Height and weights of 9 soldiers of a battalion are as follows:

Height (x) : *(in inches)*	63	62	66	68	72	73	65	69	67
Weight (y): *(in kgs)*	68	65	70	72	81	78	66	71	68

Calculate the correlation coefficient between height and weight of soldiers.

Since the variate values are of large magnitude, it will be appropriate to subtract 60 from each value of x and 65 from each value of y. Then the value of r is calculated from the coded values say x' and y'

coded value are:

x' :	3	2	6	8	12	13	5	9	7
y' :	3	0	5	7	16	13	1	6	3

Calculate the values as below,

$$\Sigma x' = 65, \; \bar{x}' = \frac{65}{9} = 7.22$$

$$\Sigma y' = 54, \; \bar{y}' = \frac{54}{9} = 6.00$$

Since $\bar{x}'$ for price is not a whole number, nor an exact value, it is better to use the formula (13.2).

$$\Sigma x'^2 = 3^2 + 2^2 + \ldots\ldots + 7^2 = 581$$

$$\Sigma y'^2 = 3^2 + 0^2 + \ldots\ldots + 3^2 = 554$$

$$\Sigma x'y' = 3 \times 3 + 2 \times 0 + \ldots.\ 7 \times 3 = 536$$

$$r = \frac{536 - \dfrac{65 \times 54}{9}}{\sqrt{\left(581 - \dfrac{65^2}{9}\right)\left(554 - \dfrac{54^2}{9}\right)}}$$

$$= \frac{536 - 390}{\sqrt{(581 - 469.44)\,(554 - 324)}}$$

$$= \frac{146}{\sqrt{111.56 \times 230}}$$

$$= \frac{146}{160.18} = 0.91$$

$r = 0.91$ affirms a high degree of correlation between the height and weight of soldiers.

Example 13.5. Given the following partial calculations $n = 10$, $\Sigma x = 2$, $\Sigma x^2 = 2414$, $\Sigma y = 26$, $\Sigma y^2 = 150$, $\Sigma xy = 266$.

Calculate the coefficient of correlation.

$$\text{By (13, 2),} \quad r = \frac{266 - \dfrac{(2 \times 26)}{10}}{\sqrt{\left(2414 - \dfrac{2^2}{10}\right)\left(150 - \dfrac{26^2}{10}\right)}}$$

$$= \frac{260.8}{\sqrt{2413.6 \times 82.4}}$$

$$= \frac{260.8}{445.96} = 0.585$$

RANK CORRELATION

At many occasions, units are not measured for certain characteristics but are ranked according to some criteria. In such situations, a certain number of units are ranked according to two criteria or the units are ranked for a single criterian by two different judges or investigators independently. For example, the students of a class are ranked according to their marks in physics and mathematics, index of production and index of export, years of service and performance of sales executives, etc. In this situation it is worked out whether there is a correlation between ranks under two criteria. The other situation is in which some contestants in a beauty competition are ranked by two judges. Players of a team, competitors in a singing or dancing contest are judges by two selectors for their performance, etc. In this situation it is to measure what extent of agreement is there between the ranks awarded by two judges. Rank correlation was given by **Spearman.** It is named after him and in general called as **Spearman's rank correlation.** Also it is denoted by r_s.

Spearman's formula for rank correlation is as follows:

Let there be n units which are ranked as per two criteria or by two judges.

Units : u_1 u_2 .... u_i ..... u_n
Criterion (judge) 1: 2 3 ...... i 1
Criterion (judge) 2: 5 3 ...... i' 7
Difference d_1 d_2 ...... d_i ...... d_n

Rank correlation,

$$r_s = 1 - \frac{6\Sigma_i d_i^2}{n(n^2 - 1)} \tag{13.5}$$

for $i = 1, 2, \ldots n$

The range of r_s is , $-1 \le r_s \le 1$.

Example 13.6. Nine competitors in a musical contest were ranked by two judges as follows:

Competitors :	C_1	C_2	C_3	C_4	C_5	C_6	C_7	C_8	C_9
Judge – A :	3	1	4	7	8	9	2	6	5
Judge – B :	4	2	3	6	5	8	1	7	9

Find the rank correlation between the ranks given by the judges.

In this problem, $n = 9$

Difference d_i :	– 1	– 1	1	1	3	1	1	– 1	– 4
d_i^2 :	1	1	1	1	9	1	1	1	16

$$\Sigma d_1^2 = 1 + 1 + 1 + 1 + 9 + 1 + 1 + 1 + 16 = 32$$

By the formula (13.5),

$$r_s = 1 - \frac{6 \times 32}{9(9^2 - 1)}$$

$$= 1 - \frac{192}{720}$$

$$= 1 - 0.267 = 0.733$$

The value of r_s is greater than 0.5. Hence; it is concluded that there is a fair degree of agreement between the ranks awarded by two judges.

Example 13.7. Marks of 12 top students in mathematics and chemistry are given below

Students	*Marks in maths*	*Marks is chemistry*
1	78	76
2	65	68
3	72	70
4	84	69
5	67	63
6	56	58
7	63	66
8	70	71
9	81	77
10	49	52
11	88	80
12	57	55

Rank the marks in both the subjects from lower to higher side.

Ranks		*Difference*	
Maths	*Chem*	d_i	d_i^2
9	10	–1	1
5	6	–1	1
8	8	0	0
11	7	4	16
6	4	2	4
2	3	– 1	1
4	5	– 1	1
7	9	– 2	4
10	11	– 1	1
1	1	0	0
12	12	0	0
3	2	1	1

$$\Sigma_i d_i^2 = 1 + 1 + 0 + 16 + 4 + 1 + 1 + 4 + 1 + 0 + 0 + 1 = 30$$

Rank correlation by the formula (13.5),

$$r_s = 1 - \frac{6 \times 30}{12\,(12^2 - 1)}$$

$$= 1 - \frac{180}{12 \times 143}$$

$$= 1 - 0.105 = 0.895$$

The value of r_s is almost 0.9. So there is a high degree of closeness between the marks in maths and chemistry.

REGRESSION LINE

When a graph between two variable is drawn, it can take any shape—a straight line, a curve or a zig-zag figure. A straight line or a curve indicates a definite relationship between the two variables. In this chapter, the study is restricted to straight line only. On the basis of sample data, an equation of a line is established. This line is called **simple regression line** in the sense that one estimates the value of a dependent variable. The concept of regression was propounded by Sir Francies Galton in a study of inheritance of stature in human beings. Here he found the regression between height of fathers and their sons. The regression between heights and weights is also very common.

EQUATION OF LINE OF REGRESSION

The equation of a line of regression is given as,

$$y = \alpha + \beta x + e \tag{13.6}$$

This is known as the regression line of Y on X. In equation (13.6), Y is dependent variable and X is an independent variable. Also α and β are two parameters and e is an error term. To determine the regression line, one has to estimate α and β in such a way that error is minimized, preferably zero. Let the estimates of α and β be a and b respectively. The estimated equation is,

$$\hat{Y} = a + bX \tag{13.7}$$

Suppose there are n pairs of values of X and Y as,
$(x_1, y_1), (x_2, y_2), (x_3, y_3), \ldots\ldots, (x_n, y_n)$.

Find the values of $\overline{x}$ and $\overline{y}$ and calculate the quantities $\Sigma_i (x_i - \overline{x})(y_i - \overline{y})$, $\Sigma_i (x_i - \overline{x})^2$ and $\Sigma_i (y_i - \overline{y})^2$ as in case of coefficient of correlation. The value of b can be obtained by the formula,

$$b = \frac{\Sigma_i (x_i - \overline{x})(y_i - \overline{y})}{\Sigma_i (x_i - \overline{x})^2} \tag{13.8}$$

Supposing that $x_i - \overline{x} - u_i$, $y_i - \overline{y} = v_i$.
Formula (13.8) can be written as,

$$b = \frac{\Sigma_i u_i v_i}{\Sigma_i u_i^2} \tag{13.9}$$

b can directly be calculated without taking deviations from means for the same reason as given in case of correlation by the formula,

$$b = \frac{\Sigma_i x_i y_i - \dfrac{(\Sigma x_i)(\Sigma y_i)}{n}}{\Sigma_i x_i^2 - \dfrac{(\Sigma x_i)^2}{n}} \tag{13.10}$$

Value of regression coefficient b in terms or r, s_x, s_y is,

$$b_{yx} = r\frac{s_y}{s_x} \tag{13.11}$$

Value of a is obtained by the formula,

$$a = \overline{y} - b\overline{x} \tag{13.12}$$

Thus, the equation of the estimated regression line is

$$\hat{Y} = (\overline{y} - b\overline{x}) + bX$$
$$= \overline{y} + b(X - \overline{x}) \tag{13.13}$$

Crow (^) over Y indicates that Y is estimated through regression equation for any value of X. Regression equation in terms of r, s_x, s_y is,

$$\hat{Y} = \bar{y} + r\frac{s_y}{s_x}(X - \bar{x}) \qquad (13.14)$$

b in full form is written as b_{YX} to connote that it is the regression coefficient of y on x. YX is omitted for the sake of convenience. But it has to be whenever required to specify.

β_{YX} or its estimated value b_{YX} is known as regression coefficient.

Definition:

Regression coefficient b_{yx} (β_{yx}) is the measure of change in dependent variable Y corresponding to an unit change in independent variable X.

Note: Substituting the value of a and b in equation (13.7) and obtaining the regression equation is also known as **fitting of regression line.**

Regression of X on Y

In may situations X can also depend on Y besides Y-depends on X. It means there can be two regression lines namely, Y on X and X on Y. But same equation can not represent both since the mode of dependence of Y on X is not the same as that of x on y.

Let the regression equation of x on y be.

$$\hat{X} = a_1 + b_1 Y \qquad (13.15)$$

where,

$$b_1 = \frac{\Sigma_i (x_i - \bar{x})(y_i - \bar{y})}{\Sigma_i (y_i - \bar{y})^2} \qquad (13.16)$$

$$= \frac{\Sigma_i x_i y_i - \dfrac{(\Sigma x_i)(\Sigma y_i)}{n}}{\Sigma y_i^2 - \dfrac{(\Sigma y_i)^2}{n}} \qquad (13.17)$$

$$= r\frac{s_x}{s_y} \qquad (13.18)$$

and $a_1 = \bar{x} - b_{XY}\,\bar{y}$ where $b_{XY} = b_1$ (13.19)

Hence, the regression line of x on y is,

$$\hat{X} = (\bar{x} - b_1\,\bar{y}) + b_1 Y$$

$$= \bar{x} + b_1 (Y - \bar{y}) \qquad (13.20)$$

Regression equation in terms of r, s_x, s_y is,

$$\hat{X} = \bar{x} + r\frac{s_x}{s_y}(Y - \bar{y}) \qquad (13.21)$$

Point of Intersection of Two Regression Lines

It should be remembered that the regression lines of Y on X and X on Y intersect each other at the point $(\bar{x}, \bar{y})$. It means, if the two regression equations are solved for X and Y, the resulting value of $X = \bar{x}$ and $Y = \bar{y}$.

Properties of Regression Coefficient

1. The value of b lies between $-\infty$ and ∞, i.e., $-\infty < b < \infty$.
2. It has unit of measurement. For instance, in case of regression of weight on height, the unit of b is kg/inch or cm.
3. The sign of r, b_{YX} and b_{XY} is always same.
4. If $b_{YX} \geq 1$, then $b_{XY} \leq 1$ and vice-versa.
5. If a constant value is subtracted from each x-value and same or other constant value from y, the value of b remains unaltered.
6. On dividing each value of x and y by the same constant, b remains unchanged. But if the divisors of x and y are different, b is affected and has to be adjusted.

Relation between Correlation and Regression Coefficients

Correlation coefficient is the geometric mean of regression coefficient of y on x and x on y. The sign of r will be same as that of regression coefficients. Symbolically, the relation between r, b_{YX} and b_{XY} is,

$$r = \sqrt{b_{YX} \cdot b_{XY}} \tag{13.22}$$

Following solved examples will further elucidate the method of fitting of regression line and allied problems.

Example 13.8. For the following pairs of observations,

x :	8,	4,	12,	6,	10
y :	7,	9,	3,	6,	5

Fit in the regression line $\hat{y} = a + bx$.

First calculate the following quantities required for obtaining the values of a and b.

$$\Sigma x_i = 8 + 4 + 12 + 6 + 10 = 40, \ \bar{x} = \frac{40}{5} = 8.0$$

$$\Sigma y_i = 7 + 9 + 3 + 6 + 5 = 30, \ \bar{y} = \frac{30}{5} = 6.0$$

$$\begin{aligned}\Sigma(x_i - \bar{x})(y_i - \bar{y}) &= (8-8)(7-6) + (4-8)(9-6) + (12-8)(3-6) \\ &\quad + (6-8)(6-6) + (10-8)(5-6) \\ &= 0 \times 1 + (-4)(+3) + (4)(-3) + (-2) \times 0 + 2 \times (-1) \\ &= 0 - 12 - 12 + 0 - 2 = -26\end{aligned}$$

$$\begin{aligned}\Sigma x_i^2 &= (8-8)^2 + (4-8)^2 + (12-8)^2 + (6-8)^2 + (10-8)^2 \\ &= 0 + 16 + 16 + 4 + 4 = 40\end{aligned}$$

By (13.8), $b = \dfrac{-26}{40} = -0.65$

By (13.12), $a = 6 - (-0.65) \times 8$

$= 6 + 5.20 = 11.20.$

Hence, the regression line is,

$$\hat{Y} = 11.20 - 0.65\,X$$

Example 13.9. For the following set of paired observations,

x :	4,	3,	6,	9,	4,	10
y :	2,	4,	5,	7,	3,	9

obtain the regression line of Y on X and estimate the value of Y for given value of $X = 5$.

Calculate the following quantities.

$$\bar{x} = \frac{4+3+6+9+4+10}{6} = \frac{36}{6} = 6.0$$

$$\bar{y} = \frac{2+4+5+7+3+9}{6} = \frac{30}{6} = 5.0$$

$$\begin{aligned}\Sigma(x_i - \bar{x})(y_i - \bar{y}) &= (4-6)(2-5) + (3-6)(4-5) + (6-6)(5-5) \\ &\quad + (9-6)(7-5) + (4-6)(3-5) + (10-6)(9-5) \\ &= (-2) \times (-3) + (-3) \times (-1) + 0 \times 0 + 3 \times 2 \\ &\quad + (-2)(-2) + 4 \times 4 \\ &= +6 + 3 + 0 + 6 + 4 + 16 = 35\end{aligned}$$

$$\begin{aligned}\Sigma(x_i - \bar{x})^2 &= (4-6)^2 + (3-6)^2 + (6-6)^2 + (9-6)^2 + (4-6)^2 \\ &\quad + (10-6)^2 \\ &= 4 + 9 + 0 + 9 + 4 + 16 = 42\end{aligned}$$

$$b = \frac{35}{42} = 0.83$$

$$\begin{aligned}a &= 5 - 0.83 \times 6 \\ &= 5 - 4.98 = 0.02\end{aligned}$$

Thus, the equation of regression line of Y on X is,

$$\hat{Y} = 0.02 + 0.83\,X$$

For $X = 5$, $\hat{Y} = 0.02 + 0.83 \times 5$

$$\hat{Y} = 0.02 + 4.15 = 4.17$$

Example 13.10. Given the following data of expenditure on advertising in lac of rupees (x) and profits in lac of rupees (y) of nine items,

Items :	**1**	**2**	**3**	**4**	**5**	**6**	**7**	**8**	**9**
Advt. (x) :	7	12	9	14	18	10	6	15	20
Profit (y) :	11	15	14	17	22	13	8	21	26

i. plot the scatter diagram.
ii. fit the regression equations of Y on X.
iii. find the coefficient of correlation between X and Y.
iv. predict the profit when Rs 30 lac are spent on advertising.

i. Scatter diagram is shown below. The plot shows that the points are almost in a line. So a straight line will be a good fit.

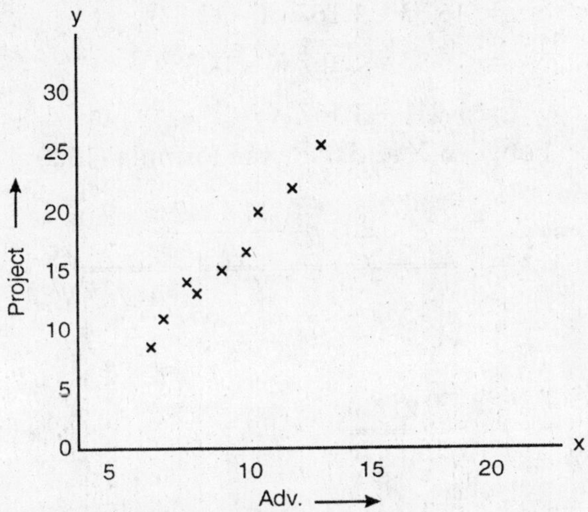

Fig. 13.10: Scatter diagram

ii. $\Sigma x = 111,\ \bar{x} = \dfrac{111}{9} = 12.33;\ \Sigma y = 147,\ \bar{y} = \dfrac{147}{9} = 16.33$. Since $\bar{x}$ and $\bar{y}$ are in fraction and also not exact values, it will be appropriate to apply the formula (13.10) for b. To calculate b and later r, prepare the following calculation table.

Items	x	y	xy	x^2	y^2
1.	7	11	77	49	121
2.	12	15	180	144	225
3.	9	14	126	81	196
4.	14	17	238	196	289
5.	18	22	396	324	484
6.	10	13	130	100	169
7.	6	8	48	36	64
8.	15.	21	315	225	441
9.	20	26	520	400	676
Total	**111**	**147**	**2030**	**1555**	**2665**

By (13.10),
$$b = \frac{2030 - \dfrac{111 \times 147}{9}}{5555 - \dfrac{111^2}{9}}$$

$$= \frac{2030 - 1813}{1555 - 1369}$$

$$= \frac{217}{186} = 1.167$$

Regression equation of Y on X is,

$$\hat{Y} = 16.33 + 1.167\,(X - 12.33)$$

$$\hat{Y} = 16.33 + 1.167\,X - 14.389$$

$$\hat{Y} = 1.941 + 1.167\,X$$

iii. corr. coeff. between X and Y by the formula (13.2)

is,
$$r = \frac{2030 - \dfrac{111 \times 147}{9}}{\sqrt{\left(1555 - \dfrac{111^2}{9}\right)\left(2265 - \dfrac{147^2}{9}\right)}}$$

$$= \frac{217}{\sqrt{186 \times 264}}$$

$$= \frac{217}{221.59} = 0.979$$

Since r is almost 1, there is a high degree of relationship between expenditure on advertising and profit.

Note: A high value of r also affirms that the regression line is a good fit.

iv. Equation of regression line from part ii. is,

$$\hat{Y} = 1.941 + 1.167X$$

Put $X = 30$ in the above equation to estimate Y.

$$\hat{Y} = 1.941 + 1.167 \times 30$$
$$= 1.941 + 35.01$$
$$= 36.951$$

This leads to the conclusion that on spending 30 lac of rupees on advertising, there will be a profit of Rs. 36.951 lac.

Example. 13.11. Given the following information,

No. of pairs of observations, $n = 12$

Average of values of x series, $\bar{x} = 25.0$

Average of values of y series, $\bar{y} = 20.0$

SD: $(x) = 4.0$, SD: $(y) = 3.0$

Sum of cross product of x and y values taking deviations from respective means, $\Sigma\, u_i\, v_i = 125.0$

i. Find the coefficient of correlation between X and Y.

ii. Find the regression line of X on Y.

iii. Find the regression line of Y on X.

i. Using the formula (13.4), the value of r is,

$$r = \frac{125}{12 \times 4 \times 3} = \frac{125}{144} = 0.868$$

ii. By the formula (13.18), obtain the value of b_1

$$b_1 = 0.868 \times \frac{4}{3} = 1.157$$

Regression line of X and Y.

$$\hat{X} = 25 + 1.157\,(Y - 20)$$

$$\hat{X} = 25 + 1.157\,Y - 23.14$$

$$\hat{X} = 1.86 + 1.157\,y$$

Similarly using (13.11), the regression equation of Y on X is,

$$\hat{Y} = 20 + 0.868 \cdot \frac{3}{4}(X - 25)$$

$$\hat{Y} = 20 + 0.651\,X - 16.275$$

$$\hat{Y} = 3.725 + 0.651\,X$$

Example 13.12. Given the two regression lines,

$$3X + 2Y = 26 \qquad (1)$$

$$6X + Y = 31 \qquad (2)$$

i. Identify which of the regression equation out of (1) and (2) represent the regression equation of Y on X and the other X on Y.

ii. Find the coefficient of correlation between X and Y.

iii. Find the mean values of X and Y.

iv. Given $s_x = 5$, find the value of s_y.

i. On trial and error basis, choose $6x + y = 31$ as the regression equation of y on x. So, $b_{yx} = 46$, the other equation will be of x on y_1, i.e.

$X = \frac{-2}{3}Y + 13$. So, $b_{XY} = \frac{-2}{3}$

By the relation (13.22), $r = \sqrt{-6 \times \frac{-2}{3}} = \sqrt{4} = -2$, which is impossible as r lies between – 1 and 1. Taking equation (1) as the regression line of Y on X, $b_{YX} = \frac{-3}{2}$ and from equation (2), $b_{XY} = -\frac{1}{6}$.

So, $r = \sqrt{\left(\frac{-3}{2}\right) \times \left(-\frac{1}{6}\right)} = \sqrt{\frac{1}{4}} = -\frac{1}{2}$ since the value of r is acceptable, equation (1) is the regression equation of Y on X and equation (2) of X on Y.

ii. As given in part (*i*), $b_{YX} = \frac{-3}{2}$ and $b_{XY} = \frac{-1}{6}$.

$$r = \sqrt{\left(-\frac{3}{2}\right) \times \left(\frac{-1}{6}\right)} = \sqrt{\frac{1}{4}} = -\frac{1}{2}$$

The sign of r is to be negative as b_{YX} and b_{XY} are negative.

iii. Solving equation (1) and (2), the values of X and Y will be their mean values.

$$3X + 2Y = 26$$
$$12X + 2Y = 62$$

or $$-9X = -36, \; X = \frac{-36}{-9} = 4$$

Again $$3 \times 4 + 2Y = 26 \quad \text{or} \quad 2Y = 14$$

or $$Y = \frac{14}{2} = 7$$

$\therefore \quad \bar{X} = 4, \quad \bar{Y} = 7$

iv. It is known that

$$b_{YX} = r\frac{s_Y}{s_X}$$

Putting the values of b_{YX}, r and s_X.

we get $$\frac{-3}{2} = \frac{-1}{2} \cdot \frac{s_Y}{5}$$

or $$s_Y = 15$$

CONCLUDING REMARK

Besides Karl Pearson's coefficient of correlation and rank correlation, there are other types of correlations also, e.g. bi-serial correlation, auto-correlation, etc. In the same way, there are curvilinear regression, multiple regression, etc. But the advances in correlation and regression are kept out of the scope of this book as this covers only preliminary statistics.

PRACTICE QUESTIONS AND EXERCISES

1. What do you understand by correlation?
2. Give the equation of regression line and formulae for finding a and b.
3. What is the basic difference between correlation and regression?

4. Give the properties of correlation coefficient.
5. When do you call the correlation between two variables of moderate, low and high degree?
6. When there is a need to calculate rank correlation?
7. Given the following seven pairs of values of x and y,

x :	8	10	12	14	16	20	18
y :	6	8	9	10	12	13	12

   Find

   i. The correlation between X and Y. Also interpret the value of r.

   ii. The regression lines of Y on X and X on Y.

8. Find the rank correlation between the ranks awarded by A and B to nine contestants.

Ranks

A :	1	2	3	4	5	6	7	8	9
B :	9	8	7	6	5	4	3	2	1

9. Find the regression line of Y on X for the following paired observations.

x :	3	5	7	9	11
y :	8	12	4	10	6

   Also calculate the coefficient of correlation.

10. Give the relation between correlation coefficient and regression coefficients.
11. Why can there be two regression line in case of simple regression?
12. Give five properties of regression coefficient.
13. A student reported the following results,

$$r = \sqrt{\frac{3}{4}},\ b_{YX} = \frac{-4}{3} \quad \text{and} \quad b_{XY} = \frac{-9}{16}$$

   Are these values compatible?

14. Given that $b_{YX} = \frac{3}{4}$, $r = 0.72$, $s_X = 6$, find s_Y^2.
15. What is a scatter diagram and how does it explain the correlation between two variables?
16. Distinguish between positive and negative correlation.
17. Scores of eight students in the final examination out of 60 and in an internal test out of 40 are given below.

Students :	S_1	S_2	S_3	S_4	S_5	S_6	S_7	S_8
Final Exam :	27	42	28	31	26	41	19	25
Internal Exam :	35	27	30	34	30	36	28	38

   Find Spearman's rank correlation between the scores in the final examination and internal test.

18. The table below gives the mean and standard deviation of the prices of two companies shares in an stock exchange.

Shares	*Mean (Rs)*	*S.D. (Rs)*
Company A	45.4	12.8
Company B	51.7	18.4

The corr. coeff. between the prices of two shares is 0.46.

Find the regression equations of share prices of *B* on *A* and *A* on *B*.

19. Discuss the effect of coding of data on correlation coefficient and regression coefficient.

20. Following are height of father and their sons.

Father's Height : *(inches)*	66	65	70	72	67	74	64	58
Son's Height : *(inches)*	67	68	72	71	71	70	65	60

i. Find regression equation of son's height on father's height.

ii. Estimate the height of son if father's height is 68".

OBJECTIVE TYPE QUESTIONS

Out of given four alternative for each problem, select the most appropriate one answer.

21. If the pairs of values of variables *X* and *Y* plotted on a graph paper show a trend from lower left to upper right, then the correlation between *X* and *Y* is:

a. Positive b. Negative

c. Zero d. Any of the above

22. If all the plotted points in a scatter diagram lie on a line from upper left to lower right, then the correlation between two variables is:

a. 1 b. – 1

c. 0.5 d. – 0.5

23. If the linear relation between x and y is, $2x + y - 5 = 0$, the correlation between x and y is:

a. – 1 b. 0

c. 1 d. – 0.5

24. If the variables x and y are not linearly related, then the correlation between x and y is:

a. 0 b. – 1

c. 1 d. 0.5

25. If the pairs of subjects are judged on the basis of certain attribute, then degree of relationship is measured by:

a. Pearsonian correlation b. Regression coefficient

c. Spearman's correlation d. Any of the above

26. If the coefficient of correlation between X and Y is around 0.5, then the degree of correlation is considered as:
    a. Perfect | b. High
    c. Moderate | d. Low
27. If individuals in all pairs receive same rank, then the value of r_s is:
    a. 1 | b. – 1
    c. 0 | d. None of the above
28. Simple linear regression line means:
    a. Only two variables are involved
    b. There is one dependent and one independent variable
    c. There is cause and effect relationship between two variables
    d. All of the above
29. The effect of coding of data on correlation coefficient is:
    a. The value of r increases | b. The value of r decreases
    c. The value of r reduces to zero | d. Nil
30. The range of Spearman's correlation coefficient is:
    a. 0 to 1 | b. 0 to ∞
    c. – 1 to 1 | d. – 1 to 0
31. Range of Pearsonian correlation coefficient is:
    a. 0 to 1 | b. – 1 to 1
    c. – 1 to 0 | d. $-\infty$ to ∞
32. Scatter diagram is a device to know:
    a. Roughly the extent of relationship | b. The nature of correlation
    c. Spread of points | d. All of the above
33. If $r = 0.6$, $b_{YX} = 2.4$, $s_X = 1.8$, then s_Y is in equal to:
    a. $\frac{1}{3}$ | b. 7.2
    c. 0.45 | d. 3.6
34. If $b_{YX} = -\frac{1}{6}$, $b_{XY} = \frac{-2}{3}$, then the value of r is:
    a. $\frac{1}{3}$ | b. $\frac{1}{9}$
    c. $-\frac{1}{3}$ | d. $-\frac{1}{9}$
35. Two lines of regression between variables X and Y intersect at the point:
    a. (0, 0) | b. (1, 1)
    c. (0, 1) | d. $(\bar{X}, \bar{Y})$
36. If $r = 0$, then lines of regression:
    a. Will be indentical | b. Will not exist
    c. Will be different | d. Will interest each other

37. The regression coefficients b_{YX} and b_{XY} hold the property that:
a. If $b_{YX} > 1$, then $b_{XY} < 1$
b. b_{YX} and b_{XY} have same sign
c. $b_{YX} \cdot b_{XY} = r^2$
d. All of the above

38. The range of regression coefficient is:
a. $-\infty$ to ∞
b. 0 to ∞
c. -1 to 1
d. 1 to ∞

39. If a production manager wishes to estimate the production of coming months on the basis of the records of production and working hours of the previous months, then the should find:
a. Correlation coefficient
b. Regression line of working hours on production
c. Regression line of production on working hours
d. None of the above

40. If the two regression lines are $2x + 3y = 13$ and $3x - 5y + 9 = 0$, then they intersect at the point:
a. $\left(\frac{1}{2}, 4\right)$
b. (3, 2)
c. (2, 3)
d. (5, 3)

41. The correlation between the age of person at the time of taking a life insurance policy and the premium is:
a. Highly positive
b. Highly negative
c. Zero
d. Vague

CHAPTER 14

Estimation and Hypothesis Testing

GENERAL NOTION

Almost in all situations our interest lies in determining some constant values of the population pertaining to certain characteristic. These constant values are termed as parameters. So let us define a parameter.

PARAMETER

Any statistical constant which serves to label a population is called a parameter, e.g. population mean 'μ', population variance 'σ^2, population median 'M_d', etc.

A population may have number of parameters. But in practice one is confined to those parameters which are involved in Probability distribution function of a variable. Most commonly used parameters are mean (μ) and variance (σ^2). As a matter of fact, parameter values are not known and thus they are estimated from the sample values as already given in chapter 12 on sampling methods. For example, mean μ is estimated by sample mean $\bar{x}$ and σ^2 by sample variance s^2. Here three more terms are defined.

STATISTIC

A function of the sample variate values $x_1, x_2, ... x_n$ which can be used for estimating a parameter or testing of hypothesis is called a *statistic.*

For example, $\bar{x}$ is obtained from $\left(\frac{\Sigma x_i}{n}\right)$ and s^2 by $\frac{\Sigma(x_i - \bar{x})^2}{(n-1)}$. These functions of observed values are statistic. Professor R.A. Fisher termed $\bar{x}$ and s^2 as statistic.

ESTIMATE

On substituting the values $x_1, x_2, ... x_n$ in statistic, a single value is obtained that is called an *estimate.* The value of a sample mean $\bar{x}$ is in an estimate of μ and a single value s^2 is an estimate of population variance σ^2. Such an estimation is known as *point estimation.*

INTERVAL ESTIMATION

If instead of estimating a single value of a statistic, two values are determined giving the range in which the parameter value can lie with certain probability is called *interval estimation.*

ESTIMATOR

The function of the sample variate values, which can be used to estimate a population constant and is itself a variable because its value varies from sample to sample. Such a function is called an *estimator.* There is a hair line difference between statistic and an estimator. The term estimator is used only in reference to estimation of a parameter whereas statistic is used in general sense, i.e. for estimation and testing of hypothesis as well.

UNBIASED ESTIMATION

If the expected value of an estimator is equal to the parameter value, then it is called an unbiased estimate. If $T(\mathbf{x}) = T(x_1, x_2 ...., x_n)$ is an estimator of a parameter θ, then $T(\mathbf{x})$ will be called an unbiased estimator of θ provided,

$$E[T(\mathbf{x})] = \theta \qquad ... (14.1)$$

Again, if $E[T(\mathbf{x})] = \theta + K$, then K is called the *bias* of the estimator $T(\mathbf{x})$.

ESTIMATION OF POPULATION MEAN μ

If $x_1, x_2 ....., x_n$ is a random sample from a normal population, then $\bar{x}$ is the unbiased estimate of μ. As already given in the chapter-12, the formula for $\bar{x}$ is

$$\bar{x} = \frac{x_1 + x_2 + ... + x_n}{n} \qquad ...(14.2)$$

$$= \frac{\Sigma x_i}{n} \qquad ... (14.2.1)$$

If the data are given in the form of frequency distribution such as,

x: $x_1, \quad x_2, \; ......, x_k$
f: $f_1, \quad f_2, \; ...., f_k$

then $$\bar{x} = \frac{f_1x_1 + f_2x_2 + ... + f_kx_k}{f_1 + f_2 ..... + f_k} \quad ... (14.3)$$

$$= \frac{\Sigma f_i x_i}{\Sigma f_i} = \frac{\Sigma f_i x_i}{n} \quad ... (14.3.1)$$

where $\Sigma f_i = n$

If data are given in groped frequency distribution as follows:

Classes	*Class Mid-values*	*Frequency*
$x_1 - x_2$	y_1	f_1
$x_2 - x_3$	y_2	f_2
⋮	⋮	⋮
$x_i - x_{i+1}$	y_i	f_i
⋮	⋮	⋮
$x_k - x_{k+1}$	y_k	f_k

where, $y_i = \frac{x_i + x_{i+1}}{2}$

The formula for sample mean is,

$$\bar{x} = \frac{f_1y_1 + f_2y_2 + ... + f_ky_k}{f_1 + f_2 ..... + f_k} \quad ... (14.4)$$

$$= \frac{\Sigma f_i y_i}{\Sigma f_i} = \frac{\Sigma f_i y_i}{n} \quad ... (14.4.1)$$

ESTIMATION OF MEAN AND VARIANCE OF PROPORTIONS

Consider a dichotomous population consisting of two classes C_1 and C_2 to which the units belongs. Suppose N_1 units belong to C_1 and N_2 units to C_2 in the population. Obviously $N_1 + N_2 = N$. Let P_1 be the proportion of units falling in C_1 and Q be the proportion of units falling in C_2.

Naturally, $P = \frac{N_1}{N}$ and $Q = \frac{N_2}{N}$, i.e. $Q = \frac{N - N_1}{N} = 1 - \frac{N_1}{N} = 1 - P$ or $P + Q = 1$. Suppose a random sample of size n is drawn from the population. In this sample, let n_1 be the number of units belonging to C_1 and n_2 to C_2. Again, $n_1 + n_2 = n$. Let the sample proportion of units in C_1 be denoted by p and that of units belonging to C_2 be q, i.e. $p + q = 1$. If the observations are coded in the manner that if the unit belongs to C_1, it is given a value 1 and if it belongs to C_2, it is given the value 0. Thus, the mean,

$$\bar{x} = \frac{\Sigma x_i}{n} = \frac{n_1}{n} = p \qquad \text{... (14.5)}$$

or

$$n_1 = np \qquad \text{... (14.5.1)}$$

Since in $x_1, x_2, ..., x_n$, there are only n_1 x's which receive a value 1 and rest of the x's receive a value 0. Hence, the estimate of the proportion is p.

ESTIMATE OF THE VARIANCE

We know that the sample variance is the estimate of the population variance and is obtained by the formula,

$$s^2 = \frac{1}{n-1}\left[\sum_i x_i^2 - \frac{(\Sigma x_i)^2}{n}\right] \qquad \text{... (14.6)}$$

$$s^2 = \frac{1}{n-1}\left[\sum_i x_i^2 - n(\bar{x})^2\right] \qquad \text{... (14.6.1)}$$

Let us workout Σx_i^2

$$\begin{aligned} \Sigma x_i^2 &= x_1^2 + x_2^2 + ... + x_n^2 \\ &= 1^2 + 1^2 + 0^2 .... 1^2 \\ &= 1 + 1 + 0 + ... + 1 = n_1 \end{aligned}$$

$$\begin{aligned} s^2 &= \frac{1}{n-1}(np - np^2) \\ &= \frac{np}{n-1}(1-p) \\ &= \frac{n}{n-1}pq \end{aligned} \qquad \text{... (14.7)}$$

It is to point out that p is an unbiased estimate of P.

HYPOTHESIS TESTING

Testing of hypothesis is the strongest and most used tool in applied statistics. It may be defined as-

"A procedure by which a decision can be taken on the basis of data collected from sample or trail, about an asserted or plausible value of a population parameter; to affirm a relationship between parameters of two or more populations or a hypothesis about the nature of a distribution, is called testing of hypothesis".

In short, by testing of hypothesis it is measured that how close the sample value is to the value under null hypothesis.

There are a large number of statistical tests available in the literature for testing various statistical hypotheses. But the author has confined to the four tests only in this chapter which shall make use of the theoretical distributions given in chapters 12 and 13. Before applying the tests, it is better to understand various steps of tests procedure in general. Thereupon the terminology, which will be used during the application of tests, is explicated. Then, ultimately various statistical tests will be dealt with and exemplified.

GENERAL PROCEDURE FOR HYPOTHESIS TESTING

Usually the following steps are to be followed in hypothesis testing.

1. First specify null hypothesis H_0 and alternative hypothesis H_1.
2. Collect and arrange the data obtained through a proper sample or experiment.
3. Choose the basic analysis procedure and the test statistic for analysis of data.
4. Decide about the level of significance 'α' prior to applying the tests.
5. Calculate the value of the test statistic by substituting the value of each term involved in it.
6. Find the critical value of test statistic from the parent probability distribution table at significance level α.
7. To decide about the rejection or acceptance of H_0 vis-a-vis H_1, compare the calculated value of the statistic with the critical value obtained from the table.
8. If calculated value of the statistic is greater than the critical value, then reject H_0 and if less, accept H_0.
9. If H_0 is rejected, obviously H_1 is accepted and vice-versa.
10. After decision about H_0, physical interpretation is given by the researcher in a pragmatic manner.

CONCEPT AND TERMINOLOGY

A test procedure involves many statistical terms as mentioned heretofore. It is necessary to understand them conceptually so as the make proper use of the same.

NULL HYPOTHESIS

It is an assertion or a statement of no difference or no effect about a factor or parameter value. The null hypothesis always bears an equality sign. Professor R.A. Fisher defined null hypothesis as,

"Null hypothesis is the hypothesis which is tested for possible rejection under the assumption that it is true".

For instance, suppose θ is a parameter, whose value θ_0 is considered to be a possible value. In this situation, the null hypothesis is, $H_0: \theta = \theta_0$.

ALTERNATIVE HYPOTHESIS

A hypothesis that contradicts the null hypothesis is called alternative hypothesis. In a way, it is an statement of some difference or some refutation from the claimed value. For instance, $H_1: \theta \neq \theta_0$ or $H_1: \theta < \theta_0$ or $\theta > \theta_0$.

As a consequence of testing of H_0 versus H_1, in case the null hypothesis is accepted, then one is to maintain the status quo. On the other hand, it the alternative hypothesis is accepted, then one is required to change the existing state of affair.

SIMPLE VERSUS COMPOSITE HYPOTHESIS

When a decision is to be taken out of two plausible values θ_0 and θ_1 of a parameter θ, of which θ_0 is considered more likely value of θ, i.e. establish $H_0 : \theta = \theta_0$ against less likely value θ_1 of θ, i.e. $H_1 : \theta = \theta_1$, then such a hypothesis is said to be a simple hypothesis versus simple hypothesis. In such a case, θ has two fixed known postulated values. On the contrary, if θ can take an indefinite value under H_1, then this is known as *composite hypothesis* e.g., $H_1: \theta \neq \theta_0$ or $H_1 : \theta > \theta_0$ or $H_1: \theta < \theta_0$. In such a situation, H_0 versus H_1 will be called as simple versus composite hypothesis.

TWO TYPES OF ERRORS

Type I error

This is an error which occurs when H_0 is rejected that is in fact true. For instance, a person admisnistered a medicine that is in fact effective. But it is changed considering that the medicine is not effective. This is type I error. Probability of committing type I error is denoted by α.

Type II error

This is an error which occurs when accept H_0 that is in fact false. For example, a person is administered a medicine that is in fact affecting adversely but it is taken to have good effect. Then it is type II error. Probability of commiting type II error is denoted by β.

If we consider the consequences of two type of errors, type II error is more severe than type I error. In view of this fact, in making a decision about H_0, type II error is minimized even at certain risk of type I error. This is reason, benefit of doubt is always given to the batsman in cricket.

LEVEL OF SIGNIFICANCE

This the amount of risk of type I error which we are ready to tolerate in making a decision. It is usually given in percentage as 100 α per cent. If $\alpha = 0.05$, then the level of significance is 5 per cent. Probability of type I error 'α' is known as the size of the test.

POWER OF A TEST

It is apparent that lesser the type II error, better it is. For a given test, if β is the probability of type II error, then $1 - \beta$ is is known as the power of the test.

DEGREES OF FREEDOM

Every test is based on sample observations. So the role of number of observations can not be ignored. The value of a test statistic varies with sample size. Hence, the sample size is involved in the form of degrees of freedom.

Definition:

The number of independent observations, on which a test is based, is known as degrees of freedom of the test statistic.

In general, there are n sample values from which a value of the test statistic is calculated, only $(n - 1)$ values are independent. Since we know the sum of values and any $(n - 1)$ value, the remaining one value can always be determined. Thus, the degrees of freedom are $(n - 1)$.

ONE TAILED AND TWO TAILED TEST

Once a test has been applied and a value of the test statistic is worked out, then one has to decide about the rejection or not rejection of the null hypothesis. For such a decision, some criteria is to be fixed. We know that the probability density curve of the test statistic contains all parametric values within its range. But in hypothesis testing, one is to know whether a hypothetical value or relation is justified or not. For this, total under the probability distribution curve is divided into two types of regions, the acceptance region and the rejection region (critical region). If the alternative hypothesis H_1 leads to two regions of rejection on both the tails of the curve, then it is called two tailed test and if H_1 leads to one rejection region on one tail only on either side, then it is known as one tailed test. Always the area of the region (*s*) of rejection is equal to level of significance α.

ONE TAILED TEST

If alternative hypothesis is one directional, then it leads to one tailed test. For instance, one is to test $H_0 : \mu = 40$ vs. $H_1 : \mu > 40$. It mean any value beyond 40 is not acceptable. In order to minimize type II error, a slightly larger value than 40 may be accepted at risk α. So the probability density curve is divided into two regions as shown in Fig. 14.1.

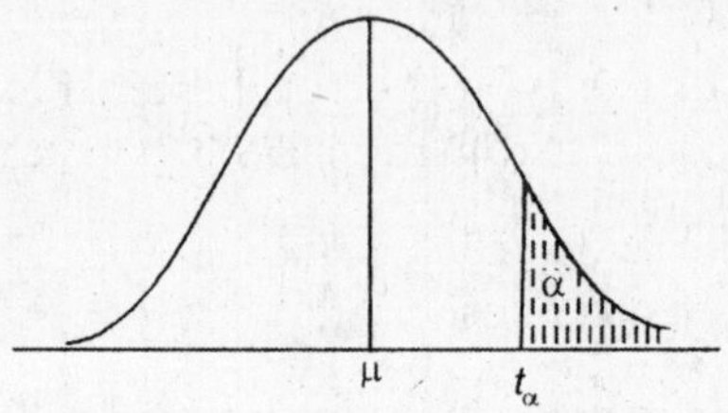

Fig. 14.1: Right sided one tailed test

Similarly if we test, $H_0 : \mu = 40$ vs. $H_1: \mu < 40$ then the region of rejection lies on the left tail as shown in Fig. 14.2.

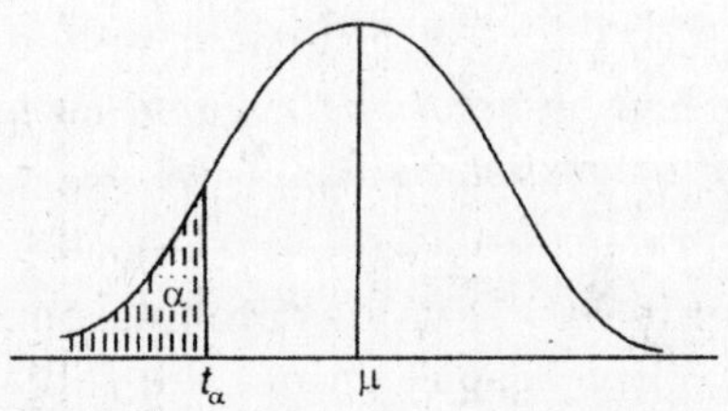

Fig. 14.2: Left sided one tailed test

TWO TAILED TESTS

If the alternative hypothesis is not specifically one directional, i.e. it may be either smaller or greater than a hypothetical value, then it is called two tailed test. In this situation, the region of rejection lies on both the tails of the density curve as shown in Fig. 14.3. The total area under the curve of both the regions of rejection is α. An area equal to $\alpha/2$ lies on the left tail and an area equal to $\alpha/2$ lies on the right tail.

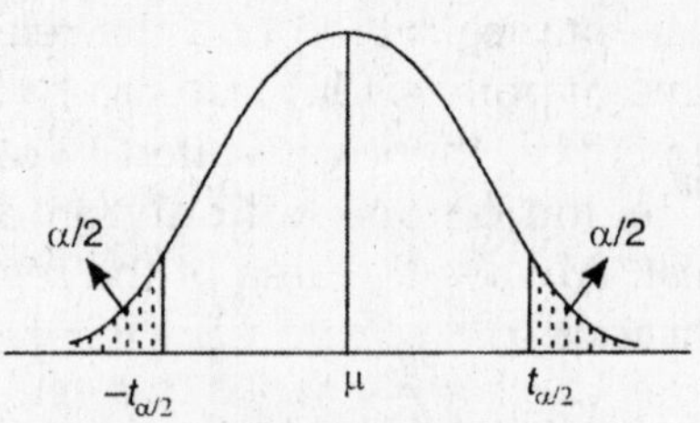

Fig. 14.3: Two tailed test

DECISION CRITERION

To decide about H_0, one has to compare the calculated value of the test statistic with the critical value obtained from the the table of the distribution of the corresponding test statistic at the pre-decided level of significance α and corresponding degrees of freedom.

Z and t distributions are symmetrical. Therefore, to avoid the complexity of sign, it is easier to consider the absolute value of the statistic Z or t. Hence, compare $|Z|$ or $|t|$ with t_α or $t_{\alpha/2}$, and Z_α or $Z_{\alpha/2}$, as the case may be. If cal $|SV|$ > critical value, reject H_0, if less then accept H_0. Where SV denotes the statistic value.

Note bene: The test procedure for one tailed and two tailed tests remains same. The only change occurs while comparing the calculated statistic value with the tabulated value. In one tailed test the tabulated value is consulted for the area of the critical region equal to α and for two tailed test for $\alpha/2$. If tables are provided for two tailed test, then for one tailed test, the table is consulted for 2α level of significance and vice-versa.

STUDENTS'S t-TEST

t-tests is used to test the hypothesis about a single population mean or the equality of two population means. Also significance of certain population constant like correlation coefficient, regression coefficient etc., is tested.

Definition:

Statistic t is the deviation of estimated mean from hypothesized value of population mean under H_0 expressed in terms of standard error.

If some asserted value of μ say, μ_0 is given and no other information is given, then test $H_0 : \mu = \mu_0$ vs. $H_1 : \mu \neq \mu_0$. To simply test whether a mean value is significant or not, the value of μ_0 is taken to be zero. In this situation, test $H_0: \mu = 0$ vs. $H_1 : \mu \neq 0$. The alternative hypothesis leads to two tailed test. Student's t-statistic based on a sample $x_1, x_2, ... x_n$ from a nomral population N (μ, σ^2), where σ^2 is unknown is,

$$t = \frac{\bar{x} - \mu_0}{\frac{s}{\sqrt{n}}} \qquad \text{... (14.7)}$$

t has $(n - 1)$ d.f.

The value of $\bar{x}$ can be obtained from (14.2.1) and s by the formula (14.6). The value of μ_0 is substituted from null hypothesis. On substituting the value of each term in (14.7), calculated value of t is obtained.

Comparing the value of calculated t with the tabulated value of t for $(n - 1)$ d.f. and α level of significance, the decision is taken about H_0.

If cal $t > t_\alpha$, reject H_0. It implies that accept H_1 and if cal $t < t_\alpha$, accept H_0. it implies that reject H_1.

ASSUMPTIONS ABOUT t-TEST

1. The sample has been drawn from a normal population N (μ, σ^2), where both the parameters are unknown.
2. The sample size is not larger than 30 and smaller than 5.
3. All observations in the sample are independent.
4. Observations are taken and recorded correctly.

Now the application of t test will be illustrated through some example.

Example 14.1. IQ' of 12 drug addict persons who are of the age of 18 years or more in a city area are:

121, 118, 106, 98, 112, 104, 120, 122, 107, 128, 117, 94

Can it believed that in general the average IQ of drug addicts is 110?

Here test, H_0; $\mu = 110$ vs. H_1: $\mu \neq 110$.

To make use of the formula (14.7), following calculations are made.

$$\bar{x} = \frac{1}{12}(121+118+....+117+94)$$

$$= \frac{1347}{12} = 112.25$$

$$\sum_{i=1}^{12} x_i^2 = (121^2 + 118^2 + ... + 117^2 + 94^2)$$

$$= 152407$$

$$s^2 = \frac{1}{11}\{152407 - \frac{(1347)^2}{12}\}$$

$$= \frac{1206.25}{11} = 109.96$$

$$\therefore \quad s = \sqrt{109.96} = 10.47$$

$$t = \frac{112.25 - 110}{\frac{10.47}{\sqrt{12}}}$$

$$= \frac{2.25}{3.02} = 0.745$$

Tabulated value of t for $\alpha = 0.05$ and 11 d.f. from appendix table-4 is 2.201. Since the calculated value of $t = 0.745$ is less than 2.201, H_0 is accepted. It endorses the general notion that the IQ of the drug addicts on an average is 110.

Example 14.2. A drug a adminstered to 15 patients to increase the homoglobin (Hb) in blood. Homoglobin was measured just before administering the drug. Drug was continued for one month and again their homoglobin was tested. Increases in homoglobin in mg was as follows:

Increase in Hb

3.1, 2.5, 1.3, 2.6, 0.6, 1.7, 0.8, – 1.2, 1.5, 1.0, 0.7, 2.7, 2.8, 1.4, 2.3

Is there a significant increase in blood homoglobin as an effect of the drug.

In this problem, one is to test

$H_0 : \mu = 0$ *vs.* $H_1 : \mu > 0$

To apply t-test, proceed as follows:

$$\sum_{i=1}^{15} x_i = 3.1 + 2.5 + \ldots + 1.4 + 2.3$$

$$= 23.8$$

$$\overline{x} = \frac{23.8}{15} = 1.587$$

$$\sum_{i=1}^{15} x_i^2 = 3.1^2 + 2.5^2 + \ldots. + 1.4^2 + 2.3^2$$

$$= 55.76$$

$$s^2 = \frac{1}{14}\left\{55.76 - \frac{(23.8)^2}{15}\right\}$$

$$= \frac{17.997}{14}$$

$$= 1.286$$

$$\therefore \quad s = 1.134$$

$$t = \frac{1.587 - 0}{\frac{1.134}{\sqrt{15}}}$$

$$= \frac{6.149}{1.134}$$

$$= 5.42$$

This is a one tailed test, hence for 5% level of significance, consult t-table for $2\alpha = 2 \times 0.05 = 0.1$ and 14 *d.f.* Table value $t = 1.761$. Since the calculated value of $t = 5.42$ is greater than tabulated value 1.761, H_0 is rejected. This leads to infer that there is significant increase in homoglobin and thus the drug is effective.

LARGE SAMPLE TEST

t-test is based on the assumption that sample size should not be large, *i.e.* not more than 30. If sample size is large, it is presumed that sample variance is almost same as population variance. In this situation, statistic t follows normal distribution. Thus, the test statistic for testing $H_0: \mu = \mu_0$ *vs.* $H_1 : \mu \neq \mu_0$ is,

$$Z = \frac{\bar{x} - \mu}{\frac{S}{\sqrt{n}}} \qquad \text{... (14.8)}$$

All terms in the expression (14.8) are same as in (14.7). Here, S is used in place of s just to show that it is based on large sample. If σ is known on the basis of same previous study, then

$$Z = \frac{\bar{x} - \mu}{\frac{\sigma}{\sqrt{n}}} \qquad \text{... (14.9)}$$

Test procedure remains same as in case of t-test. To decide about H_0, calculated value of Z say 'CZ' is compared with tabulated value of Z for α level of significance. For $\alpha = 0.05$, in case of two tailed test, $Z = 1.96$ and for $\alpha = 0.01$, $Z = 2.58$ and for $\alpha = 0.10$, $Z = 1.64$.

For one tailed test, the value of Z is to be found out from appendix table-4 where area equal to α lies on one tail. For $\alpha = 0.05$, $Z = 1.64$, for $\alpha = 0.01$, $Z = 2.33$ and for $\alpha = 0.10$, $Z = 1.28$

If $|CZ| > Z_\alpha$. table value of z at α level of significance, then reject H_0. Again if $|CZ| < Z_\alpha$, accept H_0. Physical interpretation has to be given in accordance to the problem under investigation.

Example 14.3. A survey was conducted to know the familiarity level of class IX students about the new grading system. A random of 40 students was selected and were rated on the basis of 10 questions schedule. Their familiarity level was as follows:

Familiarity level

2	1	2	3	4	6	1	2	3	2	1	7	5	3	3	2	4	1	8	1
5	2	3	1	3	3	2	2	3	2	2	4	1	6	5	2	3	2	4	2

On an average, the familiarity level of 5 is considered satisfactory. Do the students have satisfactory level of familiarity?

In this problem, one is to test H_0: $\mu = 5$ *vs.* H_1: $\mu \neq 5$, where μ represents the average level of familiarity in the population.

Since $n = 40$, Z -test is to be applied.

Calculations:

$$\bar{x} = \frac{1}{40}(3+1+....4+2)$$

$$= \frac{119}{40} = 2.975$$

$$\sum_{i=1}^{40} x_i^2 = (3^2 + 1^2 + ... + 4^2 + 2^2)$$

$$= 469$$

$$S^2 = \frac{1}{39}\left\{469 - \frac{(119)^2}{40}\right\}$$

$$= 2.948$$

$$\therefore \quad S = 1.717$$

From (14.8), the statistic

$$Z = \frac{2.975 - 5}{\frac{1.717}{\sqrt{40}}}$$

$$= \frac{-2.025}{0.271}$$

$$= -7.47$$

$$|CZ| = 7.47$$

At 5% level of significance, for two tailed test, $Z = 1.96$. Since $|CZ| >$ 1.96, H_0 is rejected. It mean that familiarity level of students is below the average level of familiarity.

Example 14.4. The mean height of 54 policeman is 67 inches with a population standard deviation 3.26 inches. Can it be belived that the average height of policeman is 6.5 feet.

Here the problem is to test, $H_0 : \mu = 66''$ *vs.* $H_1 : \mu \neq 66''$. since σ is known, we make use of statistic (14.9).

Given that $\bar{x} = 67$ $\sigma = 3.26$ and $n = 54$

Thus,

$$Z = \frac{67 - 66}{\frac{3.26}{\sqrt{54}}}$$

$$= \frac{1}{0.44}$$

$$= 2.27$$

Critical value of Z for $\alpha = 0.05$ is 1.96. $|CZ| = 2.27$ is greater than 1.96. Hence, H_0 is rejected. It leads to conclude that average height of policeman is more than 66 inches.

CONFIDENCE LIMITS FOR POPULATION MEAN μ

We have learnt that in point estimation, a single value of the parameter is determined on the basis of sample values. But sometimes, instead of finding a single value, the interest lies in specifying an interval in which the true value of the parameter lies with an assigned probability say, 100 $(1 - \alpha)$%. If $\alpha = 0.05$, then 95 % confidence interval is found out. Such an interval is known as *confidence interval*. The technique of constructing such an interval is called *interval estimation*.

95% confidence internal ensures that any value lying in this interval will be an acceptable value with probability 0.95.

FORMULA FOR CONFIDENCE INTERVAL FOR μ

We noticed that for α level of significance, H_0 is accepted if,

$$-t_\alpha < \frac{\bar{x} - \mu}{\frac{s}{\sqrt{n}}} < t_\alpha \qquad \text{... (14.10)}$$

It means, any value of the test statistic lying between $-t_\alpha$ and t_α, leads to acceptance of H_0.

From inequality (14.10),

$$-t_\alpha \cdot \frac{s}{\sqrt{n}} < \bar{x} - \mu$$

or

$$\mu < \bar{x} + t_\alpha \cdot \frac{s}{\sqrt{n}} \qquad \text{... (14.11)}$$

Similarly,

$$\frac{\bar{x} - \mu}{\frac{s}{\sqrt{n}}} < t_\alpha$$

or

$$\bar{x} - t_\alpha \cdot \frac{s}{\sqrt{n}} < \mu \qquad \text{... (14.12)}$$

Combining the inequalities (14.11) and (14.12), we get

$$\bar{x} - t_\alpha \cdot \frac{s}{\sqrt{n}} < \mu < \bar{x} + t_\alpha \cdot \frac{s}{\sqrt{n}}$$

Thus, the lower confidence limit is $\bar{x} - t_\alpha \cdot \frac{s}{\sqrt{n}}$ and upper confidence limit is $\bar{x} + t_\alpha \cdot \frac{s}{\sqrt{n}}$. In general the confidence limits are writters as,

$$\bar{x} \pm t_\alpha \cdot \frac{s}{\sqrt{n}} \qquad \text{... (14.13)}$$

The difference between upper and lower limits is $2\,t_\alpha \cdot \frac{s}{\sqrt{n}}$, which is known as confidence interval.

If population standard deviation 'σ' is known, then the confidence limits are,

$$\bar{x} \pm Z_\alpha \cdot \frac{\sigma}{\sqrt{n}} \qquad \text{... (14.14)}$$

The expressions for confidence limits clearly reveal that limits are obtained by subtracting and adding the quantity, the product of the standard error of the estimator × critical value of the statistic distribution to the estimate of the parameter. Using this basic concept, confidence limits for any parameters like $(\mu_1 - \mu_2)$, ρ, σ^2 etc. can be constructed.

Example 14.5. For the data given in example 14.1, 95% confidence limits for the mean μ can be found out in the following manner.

As per calculations made in the example 14.1,

$n = 12$, $\bar{x} = 112.25$, $s = 10.47$ and $t_{11}, 0.05 = 2.201$

By the formula (14.13), the confidence limits are,

$$\begin{aligned} \text{Lower limit} &= 112.25 - \frac{10.47}{\sqrt{12}} \times 2.201 \\ &= 112.25 - 6.65 \\ &= 105.60 \\ \text{upper limit} &= 112.25 + 6.65 \\ &= 118.90 \end{aligned}$$

Thus, the confidence limits are (105.60, 118.90).

Example 14.6. 99% confidence limits for μ, given the values, $\bar{x} = 66$, $\sigma = 3.26$, $n = 54$, can be estimated by the formula (14.14).

Value of Z for $\alpha = 0.01$ from the appendix table-4 is 2.58.

$$\begin{aligned} \text{Lower limit} &= 66 - \frac{3.26}{\sqrt{54}} \times 2.58 \\ &= 66 - 1.14 \\ &= 64.86 \\ \text{Upper limit} &= 66 + 1.14 \\ &= 67.14 \end{aligned}$$

99% confidence limits are (64.86, 67.14)

TEST OF EQUALITY OF TWO POPULATION MEAN

Consider two normal populations, $N(\mu_1, \sigma_1^2)$ and $N(\mu_2, \sigma_2^2)$ for the same measurable variable X. One wants to test the null hypothesis,

$$H_0 : \mu_1 = \mu_2 \quad vs. \quad H_1 : \mu_1 \neq \mu_2$$

In case, some prior information is available that μ_1 cannot be less than μ_2 or μ_1 is less than μ_2, then H_0 is tested against $H_1 : \mu_1 > \mu_2$ and $H_1 : \mu_1 < \mu_2$ respectively. As a pratical example, consider two lots of battery cells. Lot-1 produced by an old process with an average life μ_1 hours and lot-2 produced by a new process with an average life μ_2 hours. $H_0 : \mu_1 = \mu_2$ is to be tested under the impression that the new process is superior to the old one in respect of average life of battery. Hence, the alternative hypothesis is to be taken as $H_1 : \mu_1 < \mu_2$.Again if new process is considered inferior than the old one, the alternative hypothesis has to be, $H_1 : \mu_1 > \mu_2$. As a rule of thumb, if there is an inequality sign in H_1, then one tailed test is to be performed and othewise two tailed test is to be applied.

Test of equality of two population means can be carried out in two situations.

Situation-1 : when two populations have same variances, i.e. $\sigma_1^2 = \sigma_2^2$.

Situation-2 : when two population variance are different, i.e. $\sigma_1^2 \neq \sigma_2^2$.

Test under situation-1 : Test of $H_0 : \mu_1 = \mu_2$ *vs.* $H_1 : \mu_1 \neq \mu_2$, based on two independent samples $x_{11}, x_{12}, \ldots, x_{1n_1}$ and $x_{21}, x_{22}, \ldots, x_{2n_2}$ from two normal populations, can be tested by the statistic,

$$t = \frac{\bar{x}_1 - \bar{x}_2}{s_p\sqrt{\frac{1}{n_1} + \frac{1}{n_2}}} \qquad \ldots (14.15)$$

t has $(n_1 + n_2 - 2)$ *d.f*

Since $\sigma_1^2 = \sigma_2^2$, their variance can be pooled and hence, s_p^2, the estimate of the variance of $(\bar{x}_1 - \bar{x}_2)$ can be found out by the formula,

$$s_p^2 = \frac{\sum_{i=1}^{n_1}(x_{1i} - \bar{x}_1)^2 = \sum_{j=1}^{n_2}(x_{2j} - \bar{x}_2)^2}{(n_1 + n_2 - 2)} \qquad \ldots (14.16)$$

$$= \frac{\left\{\sum_i x_{1i}^2 - \frac{\left(\sum_i x_{1i}\right)^2}{n_1}\right\} + \left\{\sum_j x_{2j}^2 - \frac{\left(\sum_j x_{2j}\right)^2}{n_2}\right\}}{n_1 + n_2 - 2} \qquad \ldots (14.16.1)$$

$$= \frac{(n_1 - 1)s_1^2 + (n_2 - 1)s_2^2}{n_1 + n_2 - 2} \qquad \ldots (14.16.2)$$

All notations have their usual meaning. If s_1^2 and s_2^2 are known, ${s_p}^2$ can better be obtained by the formula (14.16.2).

To decide about H_0, compare calculate-t (ct) with tabulated value of t for α level of significance and $(n_1 + n_2 - 2)$ *d.f.* The decision criteria remain same as in case of one sample test.

If H_1 leads to one tailed test, then the test procedure remains the same except that critical value of t is obtained for α level of significance in such a manner that the area of region of rejection on one tail is equal to α. In case of given appendix table-4, one has to consult the table at 2α level.

Test under situation-2 : When $\sigma_1^2 \neq \sigma_2^2$, then the variances of the samples vis-a-vis population can not be pooled. If s_1^2 and s_2^2 are the variances of two samples respectively, then the formula for testing $H_0 : \mu_1 = \mu_2$ against $\mu_1 \neq \mu_2$ can be tested by the statistic,

$$t = \frac{\bar{x}_1 - \bar{x}_2}{\sqrt{\dfrac{s_1^2}{n_1} + \dfrac{s_2^2}{n_2}}} \qquad \text{... (14.17)}$$

In this situation, t is not distributed with $(n_1 + n_2 - 2)$ *d.f.* Hence, to decide about H_0, calculated t is compared with a quantity t^*, where t^* is obtained by the formula,

$$t^* = \frac{t_1 \cdot \dfrac{s_1^2}{n_1} + t_2 \cdot \dfrac{s_2^2}{n_2}}{\dfrac{s_1^2}{n_1} + \dfrac{s_2^2}{n_2}} \qquad \text{... (14.18)}$$

In (14.18), t_1 and t_2 are the critical values of t for level of significance α and $(n_1 - 1)$ and $(n_2 - 1)$ *d.f.* respectively. Other terms are same as in (14.17). Test criteria is, if $|ct| > t^*$, reject H_0 and if $|ct| < t^*$, accept H_0. Rejection of H_0 implies acceptance of H_1 and vice-versa

LARGE SAMPLE TEST

In populations $N(\mu_1, \sigma_1^2)$ and $N(\mu_2, \sigma_2^2)$, the variances σ_1^2 and σ_2^2 are known or S_1^2 and S_2^2 are the estimated variance of σ_1^2 and σ_2^2 based on large samples sizes n_1 and n_2 respectively, then Z-test is applied

To test, $H_0 : \mu_1 = \mu_2$ *vs.* $H_1 : \mu_1 \neq \mu_2$, the test statistic is,

$$Z = \frac{\bar{x}_1 - \bar{x}_2}{\sqrt{\dfrac{S_1^2}{n_1} + \dfrac{S_2^2}{n_2}}} \qquad \text{... (14.19)}$$

If σ_1^2 and σ_2^2 are known, then replace S_1^2 by σ_1^2 and S_2^2 by σ_2^2 in (14.19), to obtain the value of statistic z. To decide about H_0, $|CZ|$ is compared with critical value of Z at α level of siginificance. The decision criteria remain same as in case of one sample test.

Example 14.7. A survey was conducted to test the equality of time devoted by girls and boys in sports. Independent samples of 12 girls and 15 boys were selected. Each of them was asked how many hours they spent on sports per week. The data were as follows:

Time spent per weak (hours)

Girls, (x_1) : 15, 13, 18, 12, 14, 16, 18, 15, 17, 14, 19, 13

Boys, (x_2) : 24, 16, 22, 19, 21, 20, 21, 23, 16, 18, 20, 18, 10, 16, 26

suppose μ_1 is the mean time per week devoted by girls and μ_2 is the mean time per week devoted by boys in their populations. Test of,

$H_0 : \mu_1 = \mu_2$ *vs.* $H_1 : \mu_1 \neq \mu_2$ when $\sigma_1^2 = \sigma_2^2$

can be performed by the statistic (14.15)

calculate the following quantities.

$$n_1 = 12, \sum_i x_{1i} = 184, \bar{x}_1 = 15.33, \sum_i x_{1i}^2 = 2878$$

$$\sum_i x_{1i}^2 - \frac{\left(\sum_i x_{1i}\right)^2}{n_1} = 2878 - \frac{(184)^2}{12}$$

$$= 56.67$$

Similarly

$$n_2 = 15, \sum_j x_{2j} = 290, \bar{x}_2 = 19.33, \sum_j x_{2j}^2 = 5824$$

$$\sum_j x_{2j}^2 - \frac{\left(\sum_j x_{2j}\right)^2}{n_2} = 5824 - \frac{(290)^2}{15}$$

$$= 217.33$$

$$s_p^2 = \frac{56.67 + 217.33}{12 + 15 - 2}$$

$$= \frac{274}{25}$$

$$= 10.96$$

$$s_p = \sqrt{10.96} = 3.31$$

Test statistic

$$t = \frac{15.33 - 19.33}{3.31\sqrt{\frac{1}{12} + \frac{1}{15}}}$$

$$= \frac{-4}{1.28}$$

$$= -3.125$$

Tabulated value of t at $\alpha = 0.05$ and 25 *d.f.* from appendix table-4 for two tailed test is 2.06. Since $|-3.125| > 2.06$, H_0 is rejected. It means that the time devoted per week on an average by girls and boys is different on the basis of mean values, it can be inferred that boys devoted more time on sports than girls.

Example 14.8. For the sake of brevity, we make use of the data and calculations of example 14.7 to test H_0 against H_1 under the assumption $\sigma_1^2 \neq \sigma_2^2$. In this case, test statistic (14.17) is to be used.

Now calculate further-more,

$$s_1^2 = \frac{56.67}{11} = 5.152$$

$$s_2^2 = \frac{217.33}{14} = 15.524$$

Test statistic,

$$t = \frac{15.33 - 19.33}{\sqrt{\frac{5.152}{12} + \frac{15.524}{15}}}$$

$$= \frac{-4}{\sqrt{0.4293 + 1.0349}}$$

$$= \frac{-4}{1.21}$$

$$= -3.306$$

To decide about H_0, t^* has to be worked out.

For $\alpha = 0.05$, $t_{11} = 2.201$ and $t_{14} = 2.145$. Thus,

$$t^* = \frac{2.201 \times 0.4293 + 2.145 \times 1.0349}{0.4293 + 1.0349}$$

$$= \frac{0.9449 + 2.2199}{1.4642}$$

$$= 2.16$$

Now compare t with t^*. Since $|-3.306| > 2.16$, reject H_0, Rest of the interpretation remains same as in example 14.7.

TEST OF SIGNIFICANCE FOR PROPORTIONS

In many situations, measurements are not taken on the subjects rather they are counted whether they possess a particular characteristic or not. This is known as dichotomy. In a dichotomous population, if N_1 is the number of subjects processing a characteristic A out of N subjects, then the proportion of subjects with attribute A is $\frac{N_1}{N} = P$ (say). The proportion of subject not having the characteristic A is $\frac{N - N_1}{N} = 1 - \frac{N_1}{N} = 1 - P = Q$ (say). If we denote proportion P in class C_1 and Q in class C_2, then $P + Q = 1$.

TEST PROCEDURE

Let a population be divided into exhaustive classes C_1 and C_2 on the basis of two attributes. Then each and every unit will belong to either of the two classes. Often the interest lies to confirm whether a population have a preconceived proportion 'P_0' of units in a class say, C_1. This amounts to testing the null hypothesis; H_0: $P = P_0$ *vs.* $H_1 : P \neq P_0$. Such studies are based on a large number of subject selected randomly. Therefore, Z-test is applied. let a random sample of n subjects be drawn from a population of N subjects and out of n subjects, n_1 belong to C_1.

Then, estimated proportion, $\hat{p} = \frac{n_1}{n}$ and $\hat{q} = 1 - \hat{p}$.

Test statistic to test H_0 is,

$$Z = \frac{\hat{p} - \rho_0}{\sqrt{\hat{p}\,\hat{q}/n}} \qquad \text{... (14.20)}$$

The decision about H_0 is taken in the usually manner. If $|CZ| > Z_\alpha$, critical value of Z at α level of significance, then reject H_0. Otherwise accept H_0.

Example 14.9. A survey was conducted by a car servicing company to know whether 70% of its customers are satisfied or not. The company contacted 260 customers and 157 of then showed satisifaction towards the service. Can it be concluded on the basis of data at 5% level of significance that company's expectation is genuinely true.

In this problem one is to test,

$H_0 : P = 0.70$ *vs.* $H_1 : P \neq 0.70$.

Estimate, $\hat{p} = \frac{157}{260} = 0.60$ and thus, $\hat{q} = 1 - 0.60 = 0.40$ statistic Z by the formula (14.20) is,

$$Z = \frac{0.60 - 0.70}{\sqrt{\frac{.60 \times .40}{260}}}$$

$$= \frac{-0.1}{0.03}$$

$$= -3.33$$

For $\alpha = 0.05$, critical value of Z for two tailed test is 1.96. Since $|CZ| >$ 1.96, reject H_0. It means that actually satisfaction level is significantly lower than expected proportion.

TEST OF EQUALITY OF TWO POPULATION PROPORTIONS

There are many situations in which two comparable populations are considered. Then one wants to test that the proportion of subjects or units belonging to similar category or class in the two populations is same or not. In this case, test the hypothesis, $H_0 : P_1 = P_2$ *vs.* $H_1 : P_1 \neq P_2$.

TEST PROCEDURE

Draw two independent random samples, one of size n_1 from population 1 and the other of size n_2 from population 2. let u_1 be the number of subjects out of n_1 that belong to C_1 and u_2 be the number of subjects belonging to C_2. Then the proportion of subjects in the two samples are,

$$p_1 = \frac{u_1}{n_1} \text{ and } p_2 = \frac{u_2}{n_2}$$

H_0 can be test by the test statistic Z, where

$$Z = \frac{p_1 - p_2}{\sqrt{\hat{p}\,\hat{q}\left(\frac{1}{n_1} + \frac{1}{n_2}\right)}} \qquad \text{... (14.21)}$$

where,
$$\hat{p} = \frac{u_1 + u_2}{n_1 + n_2} \text{ and } \hat{q} = 1 - \hat{p} \qquad \text{... (14.22)}$$

To decide about H_0, reject H_0 if $|CZ| > Z_\alpha$ and vice versa.

In case, the alternative hypothesis leads to one tailed test, the critical value of Z_α has to be taken accordingly as explained earlier.

Example 14.10. An education study was carried out to verify whether preference of Xth pass urban and rural students to offer science subjects in same. In a survey of 280 urban students, 137 showed their inclination to science subjects and out of 250 rural students, 108 were inclined towards science subjects. On the basis of data, can it be concluded that urban students have greater interest in science subjects than rural students.

The present problem requires to testing of hypothesis,
$H_0 : P_1 = P_2$ against $H_1 : P_1 > P_2$

Given that $n_1 = 280$, $u_1 = 137$ and hence $p_1 = \frac{137}{280} = 0.489$

Also $n_2 = 250$, $u_2 = 108$ and hence $p_2 = \frac{108}{250} = 0.432$

By the formula (14.22),

$$\hat{p} = \frac{137 + 108}{280 + 250} = \frac{245}{530} = 0.462$$

$$\therefore \quad \hat{q} = 1 - 0.462 = 0.538$$

The test statistic from (14.21) is,

$$Z = \frac{0.489 - 0.432}{\sqrt{0.462 \times 0.538 \sqrt{\frac{1}{280} + \frac{1}{250}}}}$$

$$= \frac{0.057}{\sqrt{0.248 \times 0.0076}}$$

$$= \frac{0.057}{0.0434}$$

$$= 1.31$$

The alternative hypothesis leads to one tailed test. Therefore, for α = 0.05, Z = 1.64. To decide about H_0, compare *CZ* with 1.64. Since *CZ* < 1.64, H_0 is accepted. Hence, it is concluded that urban and rural students are equally proportionally inclined towards offering science subjects.

PAIRED T-TEST

Paired *t*-test is applied when the paired data are from the same subjects often tested in before-after situation across time with some intervention. By intervention we mean some treatment such as diet, testing methods, results from two laboratories, time gap, etc. Also paired *t*-test is used when observations are taken on matched paired subjects. Subjects are paired with such as twins or subjects as alike as possible. Also it is assumed that matched subjects are drawn from a normal population.

The hypothesis to be tested is that the differences say, '*d*' between paired values say, $(x - y)$ are a random sample from a normal population with mean zero.

Let the average of population difference be denoted by $\bar{D}$. The hypothesis under test is,

$H_0 : \bar{D} = 0$ against $H_1 : \bar{D} \neq 0$

To test H_0, the test statistic is,

$$t = \frac{\bar{d}}{\frac{s_d}{\sqrt{n}}} \qquad \text{... (14.23)}$$

t has $(n - 1)$ *d.f.*

where, $\bar{d}$ is the sample mean of the difference 'd_i' of the pairs for $i = 1, 2, ..., n$ and s_d is standard deviation of d's. n is the number of paired observation, *i.e.* sample size. To elucidate further, consider a sample of n paired values (x_i, y_i) for $i = 1, 2, ..., n$ as given below and the differences, d.

Paried values		*Difference*
x	y	$x - y = d$
x_1	y_1	$x_1 - y_1 = d_1$
x_2	y_2	$x_2 - y_2 = d_2$
⋮	⋮	⋮
x_n	y_n	$x_n - y_n = d_n$

As usual,

$$\bar{d} = \frac{1}{n}\sum_{i=1}^{n} d_i \qquad \text{... (14.24)}$$

$$s_d^2 = \frac{1}{n-1}\sum_{i=1}^{n}(d_i - \bar{d})^2 \qquad \text{... (14.25)}$$

$$= \frac{1}{n-1}\left\{\sum_{i=1}^{n} d_i^2 - \frac{\left(\sum_i d_i\right)^2}{n}\right\} \qquad \text{... (14.25.1)}$$

Precautions

1. All difference should be taken in one direction, *i.e.* $(x - y)$ or $(y - x)$. Never larger minus smaller value.
2. While calculating $\bar{d}$ or s_d, the sign of the differences should be taken into consideration.
3. The variable measured for x and y is same and in the same unit of measurement.

To decide about H_0, absolute value of calculated t, *i.e.* $|ct|$ is compared with the critical value of t at α level of significance and $(n - 1)$ degrees of freedom.

Reject H_0, if $|ct| > t_\alpha$, the critical value otherwise accept H_0. Physical interpretation has to be given in accordance with the problem under test.

If alternative hypothesis H_1 leads to one tailed test, then critical value of t is to be consulted from the table such that the area on one tail is equal to α. Rest of the test procedure remains same in all respect.

Example 14.11. A drug was marketed with the claim that it reduces the weight of persons remarkably after its regular use for one month. Initial weights and weights after one month medication of 16 perons were as follows:

Pair No.	*Initial weight in kg. (x)*	*Weight after one month* in kg. (y)	*Difference* $(x - y)$ (d)
1.	85.7	83.4	2.3
2.	85.9	81.6	4.3
3.	88.2	87.4	0.8
4.	76.9	75.1	1.8
5.	81.0	79.2	1.8
6.	74.7	71.7	3.0
7.	69.4	70.8	–1.4
8.	78.9	77.5	1.4
9.	86.3	85.1	1.2
10.	82.5	81.4	1.1
11.	66.7	68.3	– 1.6
12.	73.4	71.9	1.5
13.	77.6	75.8	1.8
14.	80.8	79.1	1.7
15.	77.7	74.4	3.3
16.	82.9	80.6	2.3
Total			25.3

On the basis of the data can it be inferred that the drug reduces the weight significantly, *i.e.* test H: $\bar{D} = 0$ *vs.* $H_1 : \bar{D} > 0$

$$\Sigma d_i = 25.3, \ \bar{d} = \frac{25.3}{16} = 1.581$$

$$\Sigma d_i^2 = (2.3^2 + 4.3^2 + \ldots + 3.3^2 + 2.3^2)$$
$$= 73.59$$

$$s_d^2 = \frac{1}{15}\left\{73.59 - \frac{(25.3)^2}{16}\right\}$$

$$= \frac{33.59}{15}$$

$$= 2.24$$

$$s_d = \sqrt{2.24} = 1.497$$

Statistic,

$$t = \frac{1.581}{\frac{1.497}{\sqrt{16}}}$$

$$= \frac{6.324}{1.497}$$

$$= 4.22$$

Alternative hypothesis indicates to one tailed test. Thus, for $\alpha = 0.05$ and 15 *d.f.*, table value of t is 1.753. Since $ct > 1.753$, H_0 is rejected. Therefore, it is inferred that drug is effective in reducing the body weight of persons significantly.

Example 14.12. Twelve pairs of girls and boys, each pair of the same standard, were tested with regard to their memory. Ten words were spoken and thereafter each of them was asked to write all the words on a sheet of paper provided to them. The number of words that they could write correctly are pairwise recorded below:

Pairs :	A	B	C	D	E	F	G	H	I	J	K	L
Girls (G) :	4	8	5	6	7	3	9	7	6	5	8	4
Boys (B) :	5	6	4	5	7	5	6	8	7	3	5	7

Do the data evince that there is no difference in girls and Boys with regard to memoriszing the words. For the given problem, test the hypothesis,

$$H_0 : \bar{D} = 0 \quad vs. \quad H_1 : \bar{D} \neq 0$$

Find the differences, $G - B = d$

$d : -1, 2, 1, 1, 0, -2, 3, -1, -1, 2, 3, -3$

Calculations,

$$\Sigma d_i = 4, \; n = 12, \; \bar{d} = \frac{4}{12} = 0.33$$

$$\Sigma d_i^2 = 44$$

$$s_d^2 = \frac{1}{11}\left(44 - \frac{4^2}{12}\right)$$

$$= \frac{42.67}{11}$$

$$= 3.8788$$

$$s_d = 1.97$$

To test H_0, test statistic

$$t = \frac{0.33}{\frac{1.97}{\sqrt{12}}}$$

$$= \frac{0.33 \times 3.464}{1.97}$$

$$= 0.58$$

Critical value of t for two tailed test at $\alpha = 0.05$ and 11 *d.f.* is 2.201. Since calculated t is less than 2.201, accept H_0. This evinces that memorizing power of girls and boys is at par in general.

TESTING OF SIGNIFICANCE OF CORRELATION COEFFICIENT

Pearson's population coefficient of correlation, denoted by 'ρ' (rho) is estimated on the basis of sample paired values of the variable X and Y by r as given in chapter 13. It is obvious that the value of r will vary from sample to sample. Sometimes it may come out to be a low value and sometimes a high value. Hence, it is not possible to say whether the correlation between X and Y is significantly high or not. R.A. Fisher propounded that the significance of population correlation coefficient can be tested by student's t-test. This amounts to test, $H_0 : \rho = 0$ *vs.* $H_0 : \rho \neq 0$.

He proved that under H_0, the test statistic is,

$$t = \frac{r\sqrt{n-2}}{\sqrt{1-r^2}} \quad \text{... (14.26)}$$

t has $(n - 2)$ *d.f.*

CONDITIONS FOR VALIDITY OF THE TEST

1. The sample has been drawn from a bivariate normal population.
2. It is necessary that sample size 'n' should be six or more.

On substituting the value of r and n in (14.26), the value of statistic t is obtained. For decision making, compare $|t|$ with the critical value of t for α level of significance and $(n - 2)$ *d.f.* If $|t| > t_\alpha$, the crital value, reject H_0. If $|t| < t_\alpha$, accept H_0. Rejection of H_0 leads to the conclusion that there is significant correlation between the two variables X and Y in the population.

Example 14.13. Test the significant of the correlation coefficient ρ based on the information that for a sample of size 18, the correlation coefficient, $r = 0.54$.

Here we test, $H_0 : \rho = 0$ *vs.* $H_1 : \rho \neq 0$, by the test statistic (14.26).

$$t = \frac{0.54\sqrt{18-2}}{\sqrt{1-(0.54)^2}}$$

$$= \frac{0.54 \times 4}{0.84}$$

$$= 2.57$$

Critical value of t for $\alpha = 0.05$ and 16 *d.f.* from appendix table-4 is 2.12. Since calculated $t = 2.54$ is greater than 2.12, H_0 is rejected. It means that correlation between the two variables is significant. Therefore, it is practically relevant.

CHI-SQUARE (χ^2) TEST OF INDEPENDENCE

Chi-square test of independence is applied when there are two categorical variables from a single population and each variable has two or more categories. The hypothesis under test is whether there is a significant association between these two variables or not. In testing of hypothesis by chi-square test, the data are frequencies. To perform the test, the frequencies are displayed in a contingency table. Before discussing χ^2– test procedure, it seems germane to discuss contingency table.

CONTINGENCY TABLE

It is a sort of cross tabulation in which the frequency distribution of two categorical variables is described simultaneously in a two-way table. A contingency table contain a cell for every combination of the categories of two variables and each cell embodies the frequency of the combination of respective cross categories.

If categorical variable A has m categories say, A_1, A_2, ..., A_m and variable B has p categories say, B_1, B_2, ..., B_p and the corresponding frequencies are denoted by f_{ij} for $i = 1, 2, ..., m$ and $j = 1, 2, ..., p$. A contingency table of order $m \times p$ shall be as displayed below.

Note : It should be checked that the marginal totals of the expected frequencies remain the same as that of observed frequencies.

Table 14.1. Contingency table

A \ B	B_1	B_2 ---------- B_j ---------- B_p	Row Total
A_1	f_{11}	f_{12} ---------- f_{1j} ---------- f_{1p}	R_1
A_2	f_{21}	f_{22} ---------- f_{2j} ---------- f_{2p}	R_2
⋮	⋮	⋮	⋮
A_i	f_{i1}	f_{i2} ---------- f_{ij} ---------- f_{ip}	R_i
⋮	⋮	⋮	⋮
A_m	f_{m1}	f_{m2} ---------- f_{mj} ---------- f_{mp}	R_m
Column Total	C_1	C_2 ---------- C_j ---------- C_p	n

In the above, f_{ij}, is the observed frequency of the cell $A_i\ B_j$.

$$\text{Sample size} = n$$

Also
$$\sum_{i=1}^{m} R_i = \sum_{j=1}^{p} C_j = n$$

Qunatities R_i's and C_j's are called the marginal totals.

CHI-SQUARE TEST

To apply the test, following procedure should be followed.

1. Set up the null and alternative hypothesis.
2. Arrange the observed frequencies in a contingency table.
3. Calculate the expected frequency corresponding to each observed frequency.
4. Use chi-square test statistic.
5. Calculate the value of statistic χ^2
6. Find critical value of χ^2 at α level of significance and corresponding degrees of freedom.
7. Establish the rule(s) for decision making about H_0.

IMPLEMENTATION

1. H_0: Attributes A and B are independent.
   H_1 : Attributes A and B are not dependent.
2. Prepare the contingency table for the problem at hand entering the frequency for each cell as shown in Table 14.1.
3. Under H_0, the expected frequency e_{ij} corresponding to f_{ij} is worked out by the formula,

$$e_{ij} = \frac{R_i \times C_j}{n} \qquad \text{... (14.27)}$$

for all i and j.

4. Pearson's chi-square test statistic is,

$$\chi^2 = \sum_{i=1}^{m} \sum_{j=1}^{p} \frac{(f_{ij} - e_{ij})^2}{e_{ij}} \qquad \text{... (14.28)}$$

x^2 has $(p - 1)(m - 1)$ of *d.f.*

5. Calculate the value of χ^2 by substituting the observed and expected frequency for each cell in the following (14.28).
6. Consult χ^2 Table 5 given in appendix for α level of significance and $(p - 1)(m - 1)$ *d.f.* Let it be denoted by χ^2_α.
7. If $\chi^2_{cal} > \chi^2_\alpha$, reject H_0 and if $\chi^2_{cal} < \chi^2_\alpha$, accept H_0, Rejection of H_0 affirms the association between two attributes. But this association is not causal.

Following the test procedure discussed herefore, null hypothesis can be tested for any problem.

Example 14.14. A company offers three bonus plans to its employees to give their preference to only one of the three plans. A sample of employees was selected and their opinion was obtained. The information gathered from them in accordance to the category of employees is presented in the following contingency table.

Category of employees	*No. of employees favoring* Plan A	Plan B	Plan C	*Total*
Factory workers	75 (65)	55 (54)	20 (31)	150
Clerical staff	50 (52)	42 (43)	28 (25)	120
Technical staff	26 (26.5)	18 (21.5)	16 (12)	60
Executives	19 (26.5)	25 (21.5)	16 (12)	60
Total	170	140	80	390

Can it be belived that the choice of bonus plan is independent of the category of employees.

For the given problem test,

H_0 : Employees' category and bonus plans are independent

vs. H_1 : Employees' category and bonus plans are not independent.

To apply chi-square test, first calculate expected frequencies by the formula (14.7). Expected frequency is worked out for each cell and placed adjacent to the observed frequency in parentheses for the sake of convenience. Calculated frequencics are round to the nearest integer in such a way that the marginal totals remain the same.

$$e_{11} = \frac{150 \times 170}{390} = 65.38, \quad e_{12} = \frac{150 \times 140}{390} = 53.85, \quad e_{13} = \frac{150 \times 80}{390} = 50.76$$

$$e_{21} = \frac{120 \times 170}{390} = 52.30, \quad e_{22} = \frac{120 \times 140}{390} = 43.08, \quad e_{23} = \frac{120 \times 80}{390} = 24.62$$

$$e_{31} = \frac{60 \times 170}{390} = 26.15, \quad e_{32} = \frac{60 \times 140}{390} = 21.54, \quad e_{33} = \frac{60 \times 80}{390} = 12.31$$

$$e_{41} = \frac{60 \times 170}{390} = 26.15, \quad e_{42} = \frac{60 \times 140}{390} = 21.54, \quad e_{43} = \frac{60 \times 80}{390} = 12.31$$

The value of statistic is calculated by the formula (14.28)

$$\chi^2 = \frac{(75-65)^2}{65} + \frac{(55-54)^2}{54} + \frac{(20-31)^2}{31} + \frac{(50-52)^2}{52} + \frac{(42-43)^2}{43}$$

$$+ \frac{(28-25)}{25} + \frac{(26-26.5)^2}{26.5} + \frac{(18-21.5)^2}{21.5} + \frac{(16-12)^2}{12} + \frac{(19-26.5)^2}{26.5}$$

$$+ \frac{(25-21.5)^2}{21.5} + \frac{(16-12)^2}{12}$$

$$= 1.54 + 0.02 + 3.90 + 0.08 + 0.02 + 0.36 + 0 + 0.57 + 1.33 + 2.12 + 0.57 + 1.33$$

$$= 11.84$$

The contingency table is of order 4 × 3. Hence, the degrees of freedom for $\chi^2 = (4 - 1)(3 - 1) = 6$. Critical value of χ^2 for 5% level of significance and 6 *d.f.* from appendix Table 5 is 12.59. Since calculated $\chi^2 = 11.60$ is less than 12.59, H_0 is accepted. It means that preference of bonus scheme is independent of category of employees.

Example 15.14. A car company conducted a survey to know the color choice from 130 males and 120 females of a city. The number of males and females according to their liking for three colors are tabulated below. The company is interested to know whether there is any relation between sex and color choice.

Color of car	*Liking*		*Total*
	Male	*Female*	
Silver white	55 (47)	35 (43)	90
Blue	42 (36)	28 (34)	70
Red	33 (47)	57 (43)	90
Total	130	120	250

Here we test the hypothesis,

H_0 : Linking of color is independent of sex

vs. H_1 : Linking of color depends on sex.

H_0 can be test by χ^2-test. Now calculate the expected frequencies. They are shown in the above contingency table for easiness.

Expected frequencies are estimated by the formula (14.27) and are rounded to the nearest integer.

$$e_{11} = \frac{90 \times 130}{250} = 46.8, \quad e_{21} = \frac{70 \times 130}{250} = 36.4, \quad e_{31} = \frac{90 \times 130}{250} = 46.8$$

$$e_{12} = \frac{90 \times 120}{250} = 43.2, \quad e_{22} = \frac{70 \times 120}{250} = 33.6, \quad e_{23} = \frac{90 \times 120}{250} = 43.2$$

Now the statistic χ^2 by the formula (14.28) is,

$$\chi^2 = \frac{(55-47)^2}{47} + \frac{(35-43)^2}{43} + \frac{(42-36)^2}{36} + \frac{(28-34)^2}{34} + \frac{(33-47)^2}{47} + \frac{(57-43)^2}{43}$$

$$= 1.36 + 1.49 + 1.00 + 1.06 + 4.17 + 4.56$$

$$= 13.64$$

Contingency table is of order 3 × 2. Hence, the degrees of freedom for x^2 is 2.

Critical value of χ^2 for $\alpha = 0.05$ and 2 *d.f.* is 5.99.

Calculated value of $\chi^2 = 13.64$ is greater than 5.99.

Therefore, H_0 is rejected. This leads to the conclusion that liking of color of car is associated with sex.

CHI-SQUARE TEST IN 2 × 2 CONTINGENCY TABLE

Pearson's chi-square statistic (14.28) is applicable for contingency table of any order. But in case of 2 × 2 contigency table, χ^2-value can be obtained without calculating the expected frequencies. Let us consider a 2 × 2 contingency table in general as follows:

Table 14.2. Contingency table of order 2 × 2

B / A	B_1	B_2	*Total*
A_1	a	b	$a + b$
A_2	c	d	$c + d$
Total	$a + c$	$b + d$	n

where $a + b + c + d = n$ (sample size)

Formula for calculating χ^2 directly is,

$$\chi^2 = \frac{n(ad-bc)^2}{(a+b)(c+d)(a+c)(b+d)} \quad \text{... (14.29)}$$

χ^2 has 1 *d.f.*

Decision about H_0 is taken in the usual manner.

Example 14.16. Following table presents the number of patients who turned up for checking to a city hospital. They were checked for symptoms of Asthma and were asked about their habit of smoking.

Symptoms of Asthma	*Ever smoking tabacco* Yes	No	*Total*
Yes	30	20	50
No	25	25	50
Total	55	45	100

The problem is to know whether the occurrence of Asthma is related to smoking.

Here test,

H_0 : Smoking habit is not a cause of Asthma

vs. H_1 : Smoking causes Asthma.

To test H_0, calculate expected frequency for each cell

$$e_{11} = \frac{50 \times 55}{100} = 27.5, e_{12} = \frac{50 \times 45}{100} = 22.5, \text{ similarly } e_{21} = 27.5$$

and $e_{22} = 22.5$

Now the value of χ^2 by the formula (14.28) is,

$$\chi^2 = \frac{(30-27.5)^2}{27.5} + \frac{(20-22.5)^2}{22.5} + \frac{(25-27.5)}{27.5} + \frac{(25-22.5)^2}{22.5}$$

$$= 0.2273 + 0.2778 + 0.2273 + 0.2778$$

$$= 1.01$$

χ^2 has 1 *d.f.* Critical value of χ^2 for $\alpha = 0.05$ and 1 *d.f.* is 3.84. Since $\chi^2_{cal} = 1.01$ is less than $\chi^2_\alpha = 3.84$, H_0 is accepted. It means smoking does not cause Asthma.

χ^2 by the formula (14.29),

$$\chi^2 = \frac{100(30 \times 25 - 20 \times 25)^2}{50 \times 50 \times 55 \times 45}$$

$$= \frac{100 \times 250 \times 250}{50 \times 50 \times 55 \times 45}$$

$$= \frac{100}{99}$$

$$= 1.01$$

Note: The calculation of χ^2 by both the methods has been done to show that the value of χ^2 comes out to be the same.

YATES' CORRECTION FOR CONTINUITY

The distribution of all frequencies in a contingency table is discontinuous. But it is approximated to a continuous distribution-χ^2 considering that a binomial distribution tends to normal distribution when n is large. Therefore, for using χ^2-test it is necessary that sample size should be large and in no case less than 20. All the more, in a 2 × 2 contingency table, if the expected frequency of any cell is less than 5, then the approximation of continuity is strongly violated. In a higher order contingency table if the expected (theoretical) cell frequency is small, i.e. less than 5, than this deficiency is overcome by pooling it with some of the adjacent classes. But in case of a contingency table of order 2 × 2, such a merger of classes is not feasible. Hence, to overcome this lacuna of χ^2 - test, F. Yates in 1934 suggested a correction for continuity in a 2 × 2 contingency table. He proposed that increase the cell frequency less than 5 by $\frac{1}{2}$, *i.e.* (0.5) and adjust other three cell frequencies by adding and substracting $\frac{1}{2}$ in such a manner that marginal totals remain unaltered as they were prior to correction. This correction increases the validity of χ^2-test.

After incorporating the correction in a 2 × 2 contingency table, calculate the value of χ^2-statistic by the formula (14.28) or (14.29) and draw conclusion about H_0 as per procedure.

The botheration of adding and subtracting $\frac{1}{2}$ and then calculating χ^2 by above mentioned formulae can be avoided by amending the formula (14.29) as given below. This formula takes care of Yates' correction.

$$\chi^2 = \frac{n\left(|ad - bc| - \frac{n}{2}\right)^2}{(a+b)(b+d)(a+c)(c+d)} \qquad \text{... (14.30)}$$

$|ad - bc|$ is the absolute value ignoring the sign of the difference. It can easily be verified that the value of χ^2 after yates' correction and by the formula (14.30) is same. Rest of the test procedure remains same.

Example 14.17. The following table provides the result of survey among 30 adults and 20 children about their preference for cookie A and cookie B.

		Preference to cookies		*Total*
		A	B	
Age	Adult	23	7	30
	Child	18	2	20
	Total	41	9	50

Based on data can it be considered that there is an association between the variables age and preference.

In this problem, test

H_0 : There is no association between age and preference

vs. H_1 : The preference varies with age.

The lowest frequency of cell (2, 2) has expected frequency 3.6, *i.e.* less than 5. Hence yates' correction has to be applied. Here the value of χ^2 is calculated by adding and subtracting 0.5 and also by the formula (14.30) to show that both the methods yield the same value of χ^2

Method-1 : After adding and subtracting 0.5, the amended contingency table is,

		Preference to cookie		*Total*
		A	B	
Age	Adult	23.5	6.5	30
	Child	17.5	2.5	20
	Total	41	9	50

Value of χ^2 by the formula (14.29) is,

$$\chi^2 = \frac{50(23.5 \times 2.5 - 17.5 \times 6.5)^2}{30 \times 20 \times 41 \times 9}$$

$$= \frac{151250}{221400}$$

$$= 0.683$$

Method-2 : Now the value of χ^2 by the formula (14.30) is,

$$\chi^2 = \frac{50\left(|23 \times 2 - 18 \times 7| - \frac{50}{2}\right)^2}{30 \times 20 \times 41 \times 9}$$

$$= \frac{151250}{221400}$$
$$= 0.683$$

Critical value, $\chi^2_{0.05,1} = 3.84$. Since the calculated value of $\chi^2 = 0.068$ is less than 3.84, H_0 is accepted. This leads to infer that there is no relationship between age and preference of variety of cookies.

CHI-SQUARE TEST IN ONE WAY CLASSIFICATION

Often a researcher observes the number of subjects or occurrence that falls in two or more groups or classes of a single categorical variable or attribute. Then χ^2 test is employed to test whether the difference between observed frequencies and hypothetical (expected or theoretical) frequencies, as that calculated on the basis of chance probability, is significant or not. This test is also known as *test of goodness of fit*. Also this test is suitable to test whether the observed frequencies support the theoretical ratio in which the frequencies are expected to occur in various classes.

Test procedure is as follows:

1. Establish the null and alternative hypothesis as,
   H_0: The frequencies occur in a theoretical ratio
   $r_1 : r_2 : ...... : r_k$ in k classes.
   H_1 : The theoretical ratio does not hold good.
2. Suppose n sample units occur in k classes such that the observed frequency of the ith class is o_i for $i = 1, 2, ..., k$, i.e.

   classes: $C_1\ C_2\ .....\ C_i\ .....\ C_k$
   obs. frequency: $o_1\ o_2\ .....\ o_i\ .....\ o_k$

   where $$\sum_{i=1}^{k} o_i = n$$
3. Calculate the expected frequency e_i corresponding to o_i for all i. If the theoretical probability p_i of a unit falling in class i is known on the basis of some established distribution, then e_i is equal to np_i. In case, the hypothetical ratio is known based on theory say, $H_0 : r_1 : r_2 : ... : r_k$ and suppose $\sum_i r_i = r$, the expected frequency,

   $$e_i = \frac{n}{r} \times r_i \qquad ... (14.31)$$

   In a way, the quantity $\frac{r_i}{r}$ is the probability of occurrence of a unit to appertain in i^{th} class.

4. Once the theoretical frequencies are worked out, the value of statistic-χ^2 can be calculated by the formula,

$$\chi^2 = \sum_{i=1}^{k} \frac{(o_i - e_i)^2}{e_i} \qquad \text{... (14.32)}$$

χ^2 has $(k-1)$ *d.f.*

5. To decide about H_0, find the critical value of chi-square for α level of significance and $(k-1)$ *d.f.* If $\chi^2_{cal} > \chi^2_{\alpha}$, reject H_0 and if $\chi^2_{cal} < \chi^2_{\alpha}$, accept H_0.
6. Physical interpretation is given as per hypothesis.

Example 14.18. An agricultural scientist might know that in the population of fruit flies, four types of fruit flies say, *A*, *B*, *C*, and *D* appear in the ratio 4 : 3 : 2 : 1. In a sample of 200 fruit flies collected from a orchard, the number of four types of fruit flies was 88, 70, 26 and 16 respectively. Do the observed frequencies approve the theoretical ratio. For the present problem, test

H_0 : The observed frequencies approve the theoretical ratio vs. H_1 : The observed frequencies do not support the theoretical ratio.

Given that

Fruit fly types :	*A*	*B*	*C*	*D*	*Total*
Obs.frequency (*o*) :	88	70	26	16	200
Exp. frequency (*e*)* :	80	60	40	20	200

$n = 200, r = 4 + 3 + 2 + 1 = 10$

$$e_1 = \frac{4}{10} \times 200 = 80, e_2 = \frac{3}{10} \times 200 = 60, e_3 = \frac{2}{10} \times 200 = 40,\ e_4 = \frac{1}{10} \times 200 = 20,$$

*Expected frequencies are shown just below observed frequencies as a facility.

The value of χ^2 by the formula (14.32) is,

$$\chi^2 = \frac{(88-80)^2}{80} + \frac{(70-60)^2}{60} + \frac{(26-40)^2}{40} + \frac{(16-20)^2}{20}$$

$$= 0.8 + 1.67 + 4.9 + 0.8$$

$$= 8.17$$

Calculated value of χ^2 for $\alpha = 0.05$ and 3 *d.f.* is 7.81 since $\chi^2_{cal} = 8.17$ is greater than 7.81, H_0 is rejected. The test affirms that four types of fruit flies do not apper in the postulated ratio.

Example 14.19. Marketing managers in general feel that market of Pepsi and Coke is 50:50. A survey of 500 randomly selected people gave preference to Pepsi and Coke as displayed below.

Pepsi	*Coke*
235	265

Do the data support the mangers' view
Test, H_0: 1 : 1 *vs.* H_1 : H_0 is not true.

Expected frequencies are : $e_1 = \frac{1}{2} \times 500 = 250, \ e_2 = \frac{1}{2} \times 500 = 250.$

Value of χ^2 by the formula (14.32) is,

$$\chi^2 = \frac{(235-250)^2}{250} + \frac{(265-250)^2}{250}$$

$$= \frac{225}{250} + \frac{225}{250}$$

$$= 1.8$$

Table value of χ^2 at $\alpha = 0.05$ and 1 *d.f.* is 3.84. Since $\chi^2_{cal} < 3.84$, accept H_0. This holds the view of the managers that the demand of pepsi and coke is at par.

F-TEST

As discussed with F-distribution in chapter-11, all you require for F-statistic are the values of sample variances of two samples drawn from two normal populations $N(\mu_1, \sigma_1^2)$ and $N(\mu_2, \sigma_2^2)$ respectively. Also the sample sizes n_1 and n_2 are to be known.

Here we test,

$$H_0 : \sigma_1^2 = \sigma_2^2 \ \ vs. \ H_1 : \sigma_1^2 \neq \sigma_2^2$$

The test statistic is,

$$F = \frac{s_1^2}{s_2^2} \qquad \text{... (15.33)}$$

F has (v_1, v_2) *d.f.* where, $v_1 = n_1 - 1$, $v_2 = n_2 - 1$, v_1 is the degrees of freedom for the variance in the numerator and v_2 is the degrees of freedom for the variance in the denominator.

Decision: If calculated value of F is greater than the tabulated value of F at α level of significance and (v_1, v_2) degrees of freedom say, $F_{\alpha,(v_1,v_2)}$, reject H_0. If $F_{\alpha,(v_1,v_2)} > F_{cal}$, accept H_0. Critical values of F can be seen in appendix table-6.

Example 14.20. Fifteen fishes were caught at one coast and twenty on another coast. Their length was measured in centimeters. The measurments were as displayed below.

Coast 1 : 18.8, 20.5, 20.0, 21.0, 17.8, 18.2, 17.8, 19.5, 20.0, 18.2, 18.4, 19.8, 19.8, 20.3, 19.0

Coast 2 : 19.8, 21.0, 20.0, 19.5, 18.9, 18.0, 18.5, 18.2, 20.2, 19.0, 19.2, 20.2 19.2, 17.0, 18.8, 17.6, 18.3, 19.6, 20.2, 18.4

An investigator is interested to test whether the variability in fish size at two coasts is same.

In this problem, he is to test.

$$H_0 : \sigma_1^2 = \sigma_2^2 \quad vs. \quad H_1 : \sigma_1^2 \neq \sigma_2^2$$

To test H_0, first calculate the variance of sample 1 and sample 2 respectively.

$n_1 = 15, \Sigma x_{1i} = (18.8 + 20.5 \; .... + 20.3 + 19.0) = 289.1$

$\Sigma x_{1i}^2 = (18.8^2 + 20.5^2 + ... + 20.3^2 + 19.0^2) = 5586.83$

Similarly, $n_2 = 20, \Sigma x_{2j} = 381.6, \Sigma x_{2j}^2 = 7300.20$

$$\therefore \qquad s_1^2 = \frac{1}{14}\left\{5586.83 - \frac{(289.1)^2}{15}\right\}$$

$$= \frac{14.90}{14} = 1.065$$

$$s_2^2 = \frac{1}{19}\left\{7300.20 - \frac{(381.6)^2}{20}\right\}$$

$$= \frac{19.272}{19} = 1.014$$

To test H_0, the value of F-statistic by the formula (14.33) is,

$$F = \frac{1.065}{1.014}$$

$$= 1.05$$

F has degrees of freedom (14,19).

Critical value of F from appendix table-6 at $\alpha = 0.05$ and (14,19) *d.f.* is 2.25. Calculated value of $F = 1.05$ is less than 2.25. Hence, H_0 is accepted. It means that the variability in fish size at two coasts is same.

Note : Due to certain theoretical reasons, it is advised that larger of the two variances should be taken in the numerator and smaller one in the denominator.

ANALYSIS OF VARIANCE

Analysis of variance (ANOVA) is a technique by which the total variation present in the experimental data is partitioned into components assignable to know sources, so called manipulations, treatments or interventions. But the sum of variation due to specific sources never equals to total variation. The difference is due to uncontrolled or extraneous sources. Such a variation is termed as variation due to error.

ASSUMPTIONS

1. Effects of sources are additive
2. Uncontrolled sources of variation are independent of other sources of variation.
3. Experimental error variances are homogeneous.
4. Experimental errors are distributed normally $N(\mu, \sigma_e^2)$.

HYPOTHESIS

Null hypothesis : k-group mean are equal.

i.e. $H_0 : \mu_1 = \mu_2 = ... = \mu_k$.

Alternative hypothesis, H_1 : At least two means out of k-group means are not equal.

Analysis of variance is peformed by comparing the variance of each group to the variance due to error.

Analysis of variance can be carried out for one or more factors, i.e. multifactors. But in the present text, we will confine to one-way and two way analysis of variance.

ONE-WAY ANALYSIS OF VARIANCE

A one-way analysis of variance is applied when the data are divided into groups according to one factor only.

TWO-WAY ANALYSIS OF VARIANCE

When there are two source of variation and the data can be be arranged in a cross pattern, then two-way analysis of variance is carried out. Usually, one factor is the treatment levels and other is replications or blocks. The interaction of treatments and replications is assigned to error.

ANALYSIS OF VARIANCE TABLE

Analysis of variance table is abbreviated as ANOVA table. The skeleton of ANOVA table in general is as given below.

Source of variation	*Degrees of freedom*	*Sum of square*	*Mean sum of square*	*F-value*
Source or due to	*d.f*	*S.S.*	*M.S.*	*F-value*
A B ⋮ Error				
Total				

Second top row contains column headings in abbreviated form and are always used in this form. *A*, *B*, ... and so on are the factors responsible for the variation due to treatments and other known factors. ANOVA table always contains the two terms, error and total as sources of variation.

In one-way analysis of variance table, there is only one factor *A*. Whereas in two-way ANOVA table, there are two sources of variable factors *A* and *B*. Rest of the table remains same.

Degree of freedom for a factors = Number of factor levels – 1

To calculate sum of square,

Find the sum of all observations = *G*

Calculte a quantity, known as correction factor (C.F.) by the formula,

$$\text{C.F.} = \frac{G^2}{n}$$

where, *n* is the total number of observations.

$$\text{Sum of square due to a factor} = \sum_{i=1}^{k} \frac{T_i^2}{r_i} - C.F.$$

where, T_i is the sum of ith level of factor *A* based on r_i values.

Total sum of square = Sum of the square of each value – C.F.

$$= \sum_{i=1}^{n} x_i^2 - C.F.$$

Error sum of square = Total S.S. – Total of all factors' sum of squares.

Mean sum of square is obtained by dividing the sum of square of a factor by its corresponding degrees of freedom.

F-value for a factor is calculated as the ratio of the factor M.S. to the error M.S.

F has *d.f.* (v_1, v_e), where v_1 is the degree of freedom for the factor and v_e is the *d.f.* for error.

Decision about the significance of a factor is taken by comparing the factor *F*-value with the critical value of *F* at α level of significance, i.e mostly 5% or $\alpha = 0.05$ and corresponding degrees of freedom (v_1, v_e) in the usual manner.

Example 14.21. The following table provides the number of units produced by a factory during three shifts in a day. The data were recorded for one week. But due to some unavoidable circumstances, night shift could not be run on two days and evening shift for one day.

	Shift *Morning* (S_1)	*Evening* (S_2)	*Night* (S_3)
	20	25	19
	23	19	20
	25	22	21
	28	27	19
	32	24	17
	29	23	
	21		
Total	178	140	96
No. of obs.	7	6	5
Mean	25.43	23.33	19.20

This is to test whether the production in there shifts on an average is same.

The problem demands to test the hypothesis,

$H_0 : \mu_1 = \mu_2 = \mu_3$

against H_1 : At least two shifts's average production is not equal.

Analysis of data

Partial calculations have been done and shown below the data table.

Shift total : $s_1 = 178, s_2 = 140, s_3 = 96, \sum_i s_i = 414$

No. of shifts : $n_1 = 7, n_2 = 6, n_3 = 5$ and $\sum_i n_i = 18$

Shift mean : $\bar{s}_1 = \frac{178}{7} = 25.43,\ \bar{s}_2 = \frac{140}{6} = 23.33,\ \bar{s}_3 = \frac{96}{5} = 19.20$

To work out sum of square,

$$\text{C.F.} = \frac{(414)^2}{18} = 9522.00$$

$$\begin{aligned}\text{Sum of square due to } s &= \frac{(178)^2}{7} + \frac{(140)^2}{6} + \frac{(96)^2}{5} - \text{C.F.} \\ &= 4526.28 + 3266.77 + 1843.20 - \text{C.F.} \\ &= 9636.15 - 9522.00 \\ &= 114.15\end{aligned}$$

$$\begin{aligned}\text{Total sum of square} &= 20^2 + 23^2 + \ldots\ldots + 19^2 + 17^2 - \text{C.F.} \\ &= 9800.00 - 9522.00 \\ &= 278.00\end{aligned}$$

$$\begin{aligned}\text{Error sum of square} &= 278.00 - 114.15 \\ &= 163.85\end{aligned}$$

After doing all the required calculations, analysis of variance table is prepared as below.

Source	*d.f.*	*S.S.*	*M.S.*	*F-value*
Shift	2	114.15	57.075	$\frac{57.075}{10.923} = 5.22$
Error	15	163.85	10.923	
Total	17	278.00		

F for shifts has (2, 15) d.f. Critical value of F for $\alpha = 0.05$ and (2, 15) d.f. from appendix table-6 is 3.68. Since the calculated value of F = 5.22 is greater than 3.68, H_0 is rejected. This leads to the conclusion that production level in three shifts is not same.

Example 14.22. The table below presents the grain yield per plant (gms) of seven varieties of maize grown in three complete blocks.

Varieties	*Blocks*			*Total*
	R_1	R_2	R_3	
V_1	79.6	82.1	77.3	239.0
V_2	60.4	65.2	60.0	185.6
V_3	88.8	85.3	91.5	265.6
V_4	74.0	73.1	75.0	222.1
V_5	96.4	94.0	98.8	289.2
V_6	78.2	82.3	75.1	235.6
V_7	52.0	50.0	56.0	158.0
Total	529.4	532.0	533.7	1595.1

At $\alpha = 0.05$, test whether there is a significant difference between yield of varieties and also between blocks.

Analysis of data

Here we test two hypotheses.

1. H_0: $\bar{R}_1 = \bar{R}_2 = \bar{R}_3$ *vs.* H_1 : At least one pair of block means differ significantly.

2. H_0: $\bar{V}_1 = \bar{V}_2 = \ldots\ldots = \bar{V}_7$ *vs.* H_1 : At least two variety means are not equal.

Total of blocks, varieties, grand total have been worked out and displayed in the data table for the sake of convenience.

Each variety has 3 replications. Therefore, $r_1 = r_2 = \ldots\ldots = r_7 = 3$

Each block size = 7.

Total number of observations = 21

$$\text{C.F.} = \frac{(1595.1)^2}{21} = 121159.24$$

$$\text{S.S. due to blocks} = \frac{1}{7}\{529.4^2 + 532.0^2 + 533.7^2\} - \text{C.F.}$$

$$= \frac{848124.05}{7} - \text{C.F.}$$

$$= 121160.58 - 121159.24$$

$$= 1.34$$

$$\text{S.S. due to varieties} = \frac{1}{3}(239.0^2 + 185.6^2 + ... + 235.6^2 + 158.0^2) - \text{C.F.}$$

$$= \frac{375548.13}{3} - \text{C.F.}$$

$$= 125182.71 - 121159.24$$

$$= 4023.47$$

$$\text{Total S.S.} = 79.6^2 + 60.4^2 + ... + 75.1^2 + 56.0^2 - \text{C.F.}$$

$$= 125288.39 - 121159.24$$

$$= 4129.15$$

$$\text{Error S.S.} = 4129.15 - 4023.47 - 1.34$$

$$= 104.34$$

Now ANOVA table can be prepared as follows:

Source	*d.f*	*S.S.*	*M.S.*	*F-value*
Blocks	2	1.34	0.67	0.67/8.70 = 0.08
Varieties	6	4023.47	670.58	670.58/8.70 = 77.08
Error	12	104.34	8.70	
Total	20	4129.15		

F for blocks has (2, 12) d.f. and F for varieties has (6, 12) d.f.
Critical value of F for $\alpha = 0.05$ and (2,12) d.f. is 3.89.
Critical value of F for $\alpha = 0.05$ and (6, 12) d.f. is 3.00.

F-value for blocks in ANOVA is 0.08 which is less than the critical value 3.89. It means that there is difference among blocks.

Calculated F in ANOVA table for varieties is 77.08, which is greater than the critical value 3.00. Hence, H_0 for varieties is rejected. It means that varieties differ significantly in respect of grain yield.

EPILOGUE

Statistical inference deals with estimation, hypothesis testing, decision theory, sequiential analysis, etc. This chapter covers a bit of estimation and succinctly hypothesis testing. The matter is just introductory. Also an effort is made to explicate each topic in a logical and simple manner avoiding mathematical complexities in so far as possible. Still the author is confident that it will fulfil the requirement of most of the students and scientists in applied sciences.

PRACTICE QUESTIONS AND EXERCISES

1. Define and discuss the following terms:
   a. Parameter b. Estimator
   c. Estimate d. Statistic
2. Distinguish between point and interval estimation.
3. Delineate unbiased estimate and its importance.
4. Explain null and alternative hypothesis and their note in testing of hypothesis.
5. What does level of significance imply ?
6. On what basis one decides about one tailed and two tailed test ? What is their implication in testing of hypothesis ?
7. Define student's t-test and also give assumptions undelying it.
8. What hypotheses can be tested by student's t-test ?
9. Develop the expression for estimating confidence limits for population mean μ.
10. What do you understand by large sample tests ? Explain how can you test the equality of two population means in case of large samples.
11. How Z-test can be carried out to test the hypotheses about proportions ?
12. In what situation, a paired t-test is to be used ? Also explain paired t-test.
13. How will you test the significance of correlation coefficient of a bivariate normal population ?
14. Discuss a contingency table and its importance in testing of hypothesis. Also give the test statistic used in case of independence of two attributes.
15. In what situations, chi-square test has to be applied and in what way ?
16. What is yates' correction and its importance ?
17. How can the equality of two population variances be tested ? Explain clearly.
18. What is the purpose of analysis of variance and how can it be carried out in general ?
19. What are the assumptions on which analysis of variance is based ?
20. Give an analysis of variance table and explain how can its entries be worked out ?
21. What is meant by one-way and two-way analysis of variance ?
22. Why do we test null hypothesis by a test statistic ? Why not alternative hypothesis ?
23. Following data presents the levels of fasting serum growth hormone (nanograms per ml) in 12 subjects.

    1.2, 0.2, 0.3, 0.9, 0.7, 1.0, 1.3, 3.0, 2.3, 0.2, 1.5, 2.1

    Test whether the surum growth significant ?

24. Reading scores of 10 ninth-class students before and after a remedial coaching program are given below.

Scores out of 50

Before:	22	28	19	21	24	18	23	32	26	14
After:	24	29	22	23	21	19	25	35	28	22

Test whether the mean difference in scores is significant ?

25. Average rainfall of a city is supposed to be 30 inches per year. The data of last 33 years rainfall are as follows:

Rainfall per year (inches)

32	26	35	23	28	26	31	36	27	28	23
20	31	29	27	25	24	26	28	21	30	32
21	19	24	21	23	27	32	35	33	24	29

Test whether the data support the old claim ?

26. The moisture content in 10 samples of wheat determined by a research laboratory and 11 samples of same wheat by a government laboratory was found to be as presented below.

Res. Lab. : 7.7, 9.4, 6.6, 5.5, 8.1, 5.9, 7.9, 6.9, 9.7, 7.4

Govt. Lab. : 7.5, 9.1, 6.8, 8.0, 6.4, 7.4, 6.5, 9.6, 9.3, 7.7, 8.5

Test the hypothesis that there is no difference in the determinations made by two laboratories with regard to average moisture content.

27. Given the following information,

$n_1 = 18, \quad \bar{x}_1 = 17.67, \quad \sigma_1 = 3.62$

and $n_2 = 15, \quad \bar{x}_2 = 20.44, \quad \sigma_2 = 4.13$

Test the equality of two population means.

28. The running time of seven racers in 400 meter race was as follows:

Running time (seconds)

50.1 49.3 46.2 47.1 46.7 47.9 48.5

i. Can it be taken that average running time is 50 seconds?

ii. Also find 95% confidence limits for population mean running time.

29. 80 students from a rural area appeared in an aptitude test. Only 32 students qualified. Can it be inferred that the success rate of rural students is 50%.

30. Following table gives the number of people who are smokers and non-smokers in relation to lung cancer.

	Lung Cancer	
	Suffering	*Not suffering*
Smoker	62	30
Non-smoker	33	45

i. Test whether the proportion of non-smokers suffering and not suffering from lung cancer is same.

ii. Test, is there any association between smoking habit and occurrence of lung cancer.

31. It is observed that four species of migratory birds reach a particular lake in search of food from distant countries. Number of four species of birds reaching the lake in a season was as follows:

Species of birds:	A	B	C	D
No. of birds:	160	182	154	204

Can it be concluded that four species of birds reach in the same proportion?

32. A survey was conducted in a city to know the liking of 50 elite males and females about Indian and Western music. The results were as follows:

Music	*Liking*		*Total*
	Males	*Female*	
Indian	22	19	41
Western	3	6	9
Total	25	25	50

Is there any reason to believe that sex and liking to two types of music are independent?

33. Mendel conducted an experiment with four crosses to know the genetic effect of colour and shape in the first generation namely, Round and yellow (RY), Round and Green (RG), Wrinkled and Yellow (WY) and Wrinkled and Green (WG). According to his genetic theory, the frequencies in the four crosses should have been in the ratio 9 : 3 : 3 : 1. At the end of the trial, the frequencies in the four crosses were as given below.

Crosses:	RY	RG	WY	WG
Frequency:	315	108	101	30

Do the experimental data justify Mendel's theoretical ratio?

34. A psychometric test was conducted among 150 children of three types, mentally retarted, educationally handicapped and physically handicapped to test their ability. They were rated in three categories, good, poor and bad. Their frequencies in different cells were as displayed below.

Category	*Types of children*			*Total*
	Mentally retarted	*Educationally handicapped*	*Physically handicapped*	
Good	6	14	34	54
Poor	13	28	10	51
Bad	31	8	6	45
Total	50	50	50	150

Test whether there is any relationship between type of deficiency in children and their performance.

35. A company wanted to purchase milling machines. Four brands of machines were tried for five days and their output was recorded. The

machines were operated under uniform conditions. The output in tonnes per day was as tabulated below.

Day	*Machines*			
	A	*B*	*C*	*D*
1.	26.5	28.7	24.6	23.9
2.	27.4	29.8	25.2	22.6
3.	22.8	32.3	21.6	24.7
4.	28.3	30.7	23.2	21.8
5.	24.5	33.9	25.2	23.6

Test whether the machines differ in respect of average production per day.

36. Five drugs were tested on four homogeneous groups of patients suffering from various diseases to control hypertension. Their systolic blood pressure in milimeters of mercury at 8:00 A.M. was recorded as displayed below.

Drug	*Disease A*	*Disease B*	*Disease C*	*Disease D*
D_1	122	140	160	180
D_2	110	130	140	176
D_3	130	128	150	184
D_4	110	145	155	210
D_5	120	160	170	220

Analysis the experimental data to test whether there is any significant difference between drugs and also between diseases as regards the systolic blood pressure.

37. Following data give the price per kg of a standard commodity in two cities. The prices were enquired from a sample of 12 shops in city A and 14 shops in city B.

Rs/kg

City A: 60.5, 71.3, 65.3, 67.8, 61.4, 68.3, 66.0, 64.5, 63.3, 62.8, 69.0, 70.5

City B: 61.4, 58.4, 56.6, 58.3, 54.5, 59.2, 55.5, 53.2, 60.0, 51.8, 53.6, 52.5, 57.4, 52.0

i. Test whether the variability in prices in cities A and B is same.

ii. Using the result of part (i), test whether the average price of the commodity in two cities is at par.

38. Random samples of army-men of two countries revealed the following information will regard to their heights in centimeters.

	Countary-A	*Country-B*
Sample size	500	600
Average height (cms)	173	168
Standard deviation (cms)	8.38	6.55

Test at 1% level of significance, is there significant difference between the average height of army-men of the two counries.

39. The age at marriage of ten pairs of husband and wife was as follows:

	Age in years									
Husband:	23.3	24.5	29.6	25.6	26.3	27.8	22.8	31.6	19.8	28.2
Wife:	21.7	23.3	26.7	22.1	19.9	24.3	21.6	23.9	18.8	21.6

i. Find the correlation coefficient between the age of wife and husband. Also test its significance at $\alpha = 0.05$

ii. Also test the equality of variability in age of wife and age of husband in the population.

40. Throw light on the importance of testing of hypothesis.

OBJECTIVE TYPE QUESTIONS

41. A function of sample variate values is called:
a. An estimate
b. Parameter
c. Statistic
d. Sample

42. In a dichotomous population, the estimate of the variance of population proportion with usual notations is:
a. pq/n
b. $\frac{pq}{n-1}$
c. $\frac{pq}{n(n-1)}$
d. $\frac{pq}{n-1}$

43. The decision whether a test of hypothesis is one tailed or two tailed, depends on:
a. Null hypothesis
b. Alternative hypothesis
c. Researcher
d. Level of significance

44. Level of significance is concerned with:
a. Type I error
b. Type II error
c. Degrees of freedom
d. None of the above

45. Interval estimate for population mean may involve:
a. t-test
b. z-test
c. Both a. and b.
d. Neither a. nor b.

46. t-test is to be applied when:
a. All observations in the sample are independent
b. Sample size lies within the range 5 and 30
c. Sample has been drawn from a normal population
d. All of the above

47. One tailed and two tailed tests affect the test procedure in respect of:
a. Test statistic
b. Degrees of freedom of the test statistic
c. Critical value for decision making
d. Alternative hypothesis

48. Large sample test for population mean utilize:
a. t-test
b. Z-test
c. χ^2-test
d. F-test

49. Test of hypothesis for proportion in a dichotomous population always utilize:
    a. Z-test
    b. t-test
    c. χ^2-test
    d. F-test
50. Paired t-test is used only when the observations are:
    a. On paired units
    b. Equal in the two samples
    c. Discrete
    d. Taken periodically
51. Degrees of freedom for χ^2 statistic in case of 4 × 3 contingency table is:
    a. 12
    b. 9
    c. 6
    d. 8
52. Significance of Pearson's coefficient of correlation can be tested by the statistic:
    a. $t = r\Big/\sqrt{\dfrac{1-r^2}{n-2}}$
    b. $t = \dfrac{r\sqrt{n-2}}{\sqrt{1-r^2}}$
    c. $t = r\sqrt{\dfrac{n-2}{1-r^2}}$
    d. All of the above
53. In a 2 × 2 contingency table, yates' correction is to be applied when:
    a. A cell frequency is less than 5
    b. The expected frequency of a cell is less than 5
    c. A cell frequency is zero
    d. The sample size is less than 20.
54. Yates' correction improves χ^2-test in the sense that:
    a. χ^2-distribution becomes continuous
    b. Lecuna of discontinuity of χ^2-curve is removed
    c. Validity of χ^2-test increases
    d. All of the above
55. chi-square test in one way classification is known as:
    a. The test of goodness of fit
    b. The test of independence
    c. The test of association of attributes
    d. All the above
56. Equality of two population variances can be tested by:
    a. t-test
    b. χ^2-test
    c. F-test
    d. Z-test
57. For a two-way classification with 4 blocks and 5 treatments, degrees of freedom for error are:
    a. 12
    b. 19
    c. 16
    d. 15
58. Analysis of variance is based on the assumption that:
    a. experimental errors are distributed independently and normally
    b. Experimental error is independent of other sources of variation
    c. Effects are additive
    d. All of the above

59. The hypothesis usually tested by analysis of variance is:
    a. Equality of variances of the effects
    b. Equality of means of the effects
    c. Equality of errors of the factors
    d. None of the above
60. Which statistical technique is used to test the equality of treatment effects of an experiment ?
    a. chi-square test of independence
    b. Analysis of variance
    c. Paired t-test
    d. Any of the above

CHAPTER 15

Official Statistics

Statistics is largely used in various sectors and government departments. It can be said that statistics is collected, compiled, analysed and published in all government departments of India, state governments, local bodies, private and public sectors. At the same time statistics has become an inseparable part of all researches. In this chapter a brief description of various statistics used and published by the government and other departments is given. A glimpse of its uses in sciences is also presented.

POPULATION STATISTICS

One of the most important requirements of any government is population statistics. It is oldest in the history of statistics. Population census is conducted at an interval of ten years in India. Population census means the counting of individuals persons under Indian census Act 1948. The census operations are controlled by the office of the Registrar General and Census Commissioner. The information is collected about the number of people in India. Besides census it carries out the job of registering deaths and births. From time to time data are collected about birth rates. The compilation and publication of data is also carried out by the office of Registrar General. Some additional information is also collected during census operations.

AGRICULTURAL AND ALLIED STATISTICS

Statistical data are collected for field crops, fruits, nuts, vegetables, tea and coffee, rubber plantation and growing of trees. The information about these helps to assess the national income and availability of food and other items for human consumption. These data are compiled and published annually by **Directorate of Economics and Statistics** (DES Ag) established under state governments, Ministry of Agriculture.

FORESTRY AND LOGGING STATISTICS

The economic activities considered include forestry and logging, bamboo, sandalwood, charcoal, lac etc. The information about area, out-turn and value of forest products are published in 'Forestry in India' by DES Ag.

FISHING STATISTICS

The activities include commerical fishing in ocean, coastal and off shore waters and also fishing in inland waters like rivers, lakes, tanks, etc. The estimate regarding value of output are collected and published by Central Fisheries Research Institute (CMFRI) and State Fisheries Departments.

MINING AND QUARRYING STATISTICS

This activity covers the extraction of minerals which occur in nature in the form of solids, liquid or gases, e.g. ores, coal, petroleum, natural gas, etc. The data regarding quantity and value of output are published in "Mineral Statistics in India" and 'Bulletin of Mineral Statistics and Information."

MANUFACTURING SECTOR STATISTICS

For the purpose of domestic product estimates, entire manufacturing industry is taken into consideration. Statistical information regarding manufacturing sector and manufactured products are published in a number of journals, magazines and bulletin.

TRANSPORT STATISTICS

This covers information regarding transport by railways, road transport, water and air transport. The data regarding railways are available in **Annual statistical statements** brought out by the Ministry of Railways. Data on volumes of water transport are available in **Merchant Marine Directory** annually.

CENTRAL ORGANISATIONS

There are two main organisations in India working for the Government of India namely—(1) National Sample Survey Organisation, and (2) Central Statistical Organisation.

NATIONAL SAMPLE SURVEY ORGANISATION (NSSO)

This organisation was established in 1950 under the Minstry of Finance. This organisation in cooperation with Indian Statistical Institute, Kolkata, conducts surveys regarding crop production, vital statistics and many other social surveys. NSSO has an all India set-up and it conducts surveys regularly. Sixty seventh round of socio-economic survey started on 25th April, 2010 and is to be conducted during July 2010 to June 2011 in rural and urban areas in India.

CENTRAL STATISTICAL ORGANISATION (CSO)

This organsation was established in 1951 under Cabinet secretariate. Its function is to advise the government of India regarding statistical matters. It is also enstrusted with the task of setting up definitions and to train the personnel for statistical surveys.

STATISTICS IN RESEARCH

Planning of surveys and designing of experiments is a function of statistics. Once, the data are collected by conducting surveys or experiments, the analysis of data is solely a part of statistics. Calculation of mean, variance, correlation coefficient, fitting of regression line, analysis of variance and many other techniques come under the category of analysis of data.

PRACTICE QUESTIONS AND EXERCISES

1. Which organisation governs the census operations and what aspect does it cover?
2. Name various types of statistics collected in India.
3. Describe the role of National Sample Survey Organisation.
4. What are functions of central statistical organisation?
5. Throw light on the need of collecting data?
6. Explain how statistics is useful to researchers?

OBJECTIVE TYPE QUESTIONS

Choose the correct option out of the given four options for each statement.

7. Any government likes to gather information about:
   a. Number of people b. Revenue
   c. Production d. All of the above
8. Census Act was passed in the year:
   a. 1947 b. 1948
   c. 1951 d. 1956
9. Census operation are run under the control of:
   a. National Sample Survey Organisation
   b. Central Statistical Organisation
   c. Registrar General and Census Commissioner
   d. Directorate of Economics and Statistics

10. Central government statistical unit is:
    a. Central Statistical Organisation
    b. National Sample Surveys Organisation
    c. both (a) and (b)
    d. only (a) but not (b)

SUGGESTED BOOKS FOR FURTHER READING

1. Agarwal BL. *Basic Statistics*, 5th ed. New Age International Publishers, New Delhi, 2009.
2. Agarwal BL. *Programmed Statistics*, 2nd ed. New Age International Publishers, New Delhi, 2009.
3. Agarwal BL. *Theory and Analysis of Experimental Designs*. CBS Publishers and Distributors, New Delhi, 2010.
4. Burr IW. *Applied Statistical Methods*. Academic Press, New York, 1974.
5. Collin Rose and Murray DS. *Mathematical Statistics with Mathematica*. Springer, 2000.
6. David Stirzaker. *Elementary Probability*. Cambridge University Press, 2003.
7. Joseph FH. *Statistics*. Thomson Wadsworth, 2004.
8. Kelton G. *Introduction to Survey Sampling*. Sage Publication, Beverley Hill, 1983.
9. Sprott DA. *Statistical Inference in Science*. Springer-Verlag, New York, 2000.
10. Sudman S. *Applied Sampling*. Academic Press, New York, 1974. Vladimir Rotar. Probability Theory. World Scientific, 1998.
11. Vladimir Rotar. *Probability Theory*. World Scientific, 1998.

ANSWERS TO NUMERICAL EXERCISES

CHAPTER 2

8.

Classes	Freq.
18 — 20	4
20 — 22	11
22 — 24	15
24 — 26	6
26 — 28	1
28 — 30	3

9 a.

Class interval	Freq.
0 — 10	4
10 — 20	8
20 — 30	5
30 — 40	12
40 — 50	7
50 — 60	9
60 — 70	2
70 — 80	1

9 b.

cu. freq. distribution Less than type		*cu. freq. distribution More than type*	
Class upper limit or less	*cu. Freq.*	*Class Lower limit or more*	*Cu. Freq.*
10 or Less	4	0 or More	48
20 or Less	12	10 or More	44
30 or Less	17	20 or More	36
40 or Less	29	30 or More	31
50 or Less	36	40 or More	19
60 or Less	45	50 or More	12
70 or Less	47	60 or More	3
80 or Less	48	70 or More	1

22.

Two-way table

	Union member	*Union non-member*	*Total*
Men	3200	300	3500
Women	100	400	500
Total	3300	700	4000

CHAPTER 4

8. A.M. = 92.875 ; $M_d = 93.5$
9. $M_d = 4$
10. $\bar{x} = 140.18$ Rs/day; $M_0 = 14$ Rs/day;
    $Q_1 = 125.8$ Rs/day, $Q_2 = 140.31$ Rs/day, $Q_3 = 155.38$ Rs/day.
11. G.M. = 16.60
14. $f = 10$

CHAPTER 5

9. i. S.D = 2.74 ii. C.V. = 45.67
   iii. Range = 8 or 2 – 10. iv. M.D. about median = 2.22

10. $Q_1 = 7.34$, $Q_2 = 9.25$, $Q_3 = 11.88$;
    i. I.Q.D. = 4.54
    ii. J = 0.158 (By Bowleys's formula) and J = 0.23 (By 5.14)
    iii. $S^2 = 13.2$
    iv. M.D. about mean = 2.827
11. i. Range = 8. 0 or 2 – 10 ii. S.D. , $s = 1.94$
    iii. J = 0.77 (By 5.14). The value of J is small. Therefore, it is concluded that the distribution is slightly positive skew.
12. $CV_A = 42.90$ % and $C.V_{B}. = 26.07\%$.
    Since $C.V_{A}, > C.V_{B}.$, hence series A is more variable.
14. Range = 27 or S – 32. coeff. of range = .73
15. i. I.Q.R = 30 ii. M.D. about median = 13.90
    iii. S.D. $s = 18.534$
16. Two observations are 10, 4.

CHAPTER 6

8. i. $\frac{169}{800}$ ii. $\frac{7}{100}$
   iii. $= \frac{67}{200}$ iv. $\frac{307}{800}$;
   Also $p\ (i) + p\ (ii) + p\ (iii) + p\ (iv) = 1$
9. i. $\frac{3}{20}$ ii. $\frac{97}{120}$ iii. $\frac{1}{24}$
10. i. $\frac{15}{64}$ ii. $\frac{51}{64}$ iii. $\frac{13}{64}$
11. i. $\frac{1}{10}$ ii. $\frac{7}{10}$ iii. $\frac{3}{10}$
12. i. $\frac{7}{15}$ ii. $\frac{1}{3}$ iii. $\frac{2}{15}$ iv $\frac{2}{3}$
13. i. $\frac{7}{30}$ ii. $\frac{11}{50}$ iii. $\frac{7}{75}$ iv. $\frac{4}{75}$
14. i. $\frac{13}{79}$ ii. $\frac{252}{395}$ iii $\frac{78}{395}$
15. i. $\frac{3}{35}$ ii. $\frac{37}{105}$ iii. $\frac{59}{105}$
16. i. $\frac{5}{36}$ ii. $\frac{91}{181}$ iii. $\frac{2}{9}$ iv. $\frac{7}{9}$
17. i. $\frac{8}{45}$ ii. $\frac{3}{10}$ iii. $\frac{7}{10}$ iv. $\frac{43}{90}$

18. i. $\frac{5}{6}$ ii. $\frac{1}{6}$

19. i. $\frac{1}{5}$ ii. $\frac{7}{10}$ iii. $\frac{1}{10}$

20. i. $\frac{4}{5}$ ii. $\frac{1}{5}$

CHAPTER 7

12. i. $\frac{2}{9}$ ii. $\frac{2}{9}$ iii. $\frac{5}{9}$

13. i. $\frac{1}{2}$ ii. $\frac{2}{3}$ iii. $\frac{1}{3}$

14. i. $\frac{1}{2}$ ii. $\frac{1}{8}$ iii. $\frac{3}{8}$ iv. $\frac{3}{8}$

15. i. $\frac{5}{18}$ ii. $\frac{5}{24}$ iii. $\frac{37}{72}$

16. $\frac{441}{5000}$ 17. 13 to 72 18. $\frac{14}{55}$ 19. $\frac{7}{9}$

20. $\frac{7}{8}$ 21. $\frac{1}{2}$ 22. $\frac{1}{7}$

CHAPTER 8

11. i. 4 ii. 15 iii. 120 iv. 1
v. 5 vi. 1 vii. 720 viii. 20
ix 210 x. $\frac{91}{9}$ xi. 1 xii. 1
xiii. 190 xiv. 10 xv. $\frac{1}{52}$

12. $nP_r = nC_r \cdot \underline{|r}$ 13. GGG, GGD, GDG, GDD, DGG, DGD, DDG, DDD.

14. 5, 10, 15, 20, ...

15. HHH, HHT HTH, HTT, THH, THT, TTH, TTT

16. B, C, E.

17. (H, 1), (H, 2), (H, 3), (H, 4), (H, 5), (H, 6) (T, 1), (T, 2) (T, 3), (T, 4), (T, 5), (T, 6)

18. a. $\frac{3}{10}$ b. $\frac{7}{10}$

19. $\frac{278}{343}$

20. a. $\frac{1}{49}$ b. $\frac{1}{343}$ c. $\frac{3}{343}$ d. $\frac{216}{343}$

21. a. $\frac{1}{13}$ b. $\frac{9}{65}$ c. $\frac{47}{91}$ d. $\frac{3}{13}$

e. $\frac{1}{26}$

22. $\frac{7}{282}; D$ 23. $\frac{1}{9}$ 24. $\frac{1}{12}$

25. a. $\frac{1}{216}$ b. $\frac{1}{36}$ c. $\frac{25}{216}$ d. $\frac{35}{36}$

26. $\frac{1}{10}$

27. $\frac{11}{4165}$ [Hint : $P(E) = \frac{4C_4 \times 48C_9}{52\,C_{13}}$]

28. $\frac{5}{396}$ 29. $\frac{1}{6}$ 30. $\frac{8}{25}$

CHAPTER 9

6. $P(A) = P(B)$ 7. $P(A)$

8. a. 1 b. $P(B)$ c. $1 - P(A \cup B)$

d. 1 e. $1(f)\, P(\bar{A})$ or $1 - P(A)$

9. a. False b. True c. False d. True

10. a. True b. False c. True d. False

16. $\frac{35}{3468}; \frac{4}{221}$ 17. 0.1 18. $\frac{1}{2}$ 19. $\frac{3}{5}$

20. $\frac{3}{5}$ 21. $\frac{1}{4}$ 22. $\frac{2}{7}$ 23. $\frac{52}{77}$

24. i. 0.45 ii. 0.55. iii. 0.80 [Hint = use $P(A \cup B \cup C)$]

25. $\frac{7}{13}$ 26. $P(A) = \frac{2}{3}, P(B) = \frac{1}{2}$

27. Check that $P(A) = \frac{1}{2}$, $P(B) = \frac{1}{6}$, $P(C) = \frac{1}{6}$ $P(A \cap B) = \frac{1}{12}$, $P(A \mid B) = \frac{1}{2}$,

$P(B \cap C) = \frac{1}{36}$, $P(A \cap C) = \frac{1}{6}$

28. i. $\frac{1}{10}$ ii. $\frac{17}{20}$ [Hint : $P(A \cap \bar{B}) = P(A) - P(A \cap B)$

and $P(\bar{A} \cup \bar{B}) = 1 - P(A \cap B)$]

29. $\frac{17}{20}$

30. i. 0.37 ii. 0.53 iii. 0.266

[Hint A – Asks for tyres checked, B – Asks for coolant checked. Find $P(A \cup B)$, $P(B \mid A)$ and $P(A \mid B)$]

CHAPTER 10

Section 7.1

13. $\frac{162}{625}$ 14. $\frac{11}{32}$ 15. $\frac{5}{32}$

16. Freq dist.

x :	0	1	2	3	4	
f :	8	32	48	32	8	; $E(x) = 2.0$

17. Freq. dist.

Sucessesses :	0	1	2	3	4	5
Frequency :	3	15	30	30	15	3

Mean = $\frac{5}{2}$; Variance = $\frac{5}{4}$

18. i. 0.151 ii. 0.0082 iii. 0.3555
19. 0.1008 20. 0.2642
21. i. $\left(\frac{5}{6}\right)^5$ or .40187 ii. 0.1608 iii. 0.5981
22. 0.143 23. 0.00952 24. 0.1115 25. $\frac{35}{128}$

CHAPTER 11

11. 0.15731
12. i. 114 ii. 56
 iii. 64 iv. 48 soldiers
13. i. 68.26% ii. 95.44% iii. 99.73%
14. a −2 b. 0 c. 5 d. 8
15. i. Not less than 0.8026 ii. Not more than 0.3829
16. 76.
17. i. 0.001 ii. 0.8314 iii. 0.15866
18. $\mu = 22.11$, $\sigma = 5.56$
19. $\sigma = 14.42$
20. i. 0.72575 ii. 0.27425 iii. 0.17745

CHAPTER 12

8. $s^2 = 8.39$. $s^2 = 20.095$ 11. S.E. $(\bar{x}) = 1.76$
12. S.E $(\bar{x}) = 0.979$ 13. S.E. $(\bar{x}) = 0.556$
19. $s_A = 1.414$, $s_B = 1.496$. since $s_A < s_B$, team A has less variability.

CHAPTER 13

7. Reg. line of y on x; $\hat{y} = 2.02 + 0.57x$
 Reg. line of x on y; $\hat{x} = 1.68y - 2.8$
 corr. coeff.; $r = 0.98$. Almost perfect correlation between x and y.

8. $r_s = 1.0$ 9. $\hat{y} = 5.9 - 0.3x; r = -0.30$

13. No, since the signs of b_{yx}, b_{xy} and r are always the same.

14. $s_y^2 = 39.0625$ 17. $r_s = -0.071$

18. Reg. line of B on A, $\hat{y} = 0.66\, x + 21.74$

Reg. line of A on B, $\hat{x} = 0.32\, y + 28.856$

20. i. $\hat{y} = 21.77 + 0.69\, x$ ii. For $x = 68$, $\hat{y} = 68.69$ inches.

CHAPTER 14

Indicators: * significant at $\alpha = .05$

NS—Non-significant.

23. t = 4.82* 24. t = 2.48* 25. Z = 3.56*

26. t = 0.70 NS 27. Z = – 2.04* 28. (i) t = –3.77*, (ii) (46.65, 49.29)

29. Z = – 1.82 NS 30. (i) Z = –3.28*, (ii) $\chi^2 = 10.77$*

31. $\chi^2 = 8.89$* 32. $\chi^2 = 0.54$ NS 33. $\chi^2 = 0.51$ NS

34. $\chi^2 = 59.78$*

35.

Source	*d.f.*	*S.S.*	*M.S.*	*F-value*
Machines	3	185.72	61.91	F = 1.96 NS
Error	16	505.53	31.60	
Total	19	691.25		

36.

Source	*d.f.*	*S.S.*	*M.S.*	*F-value*
Disease	3	15159.6	5053.2	47.94*
Drug	4	1746.0	436.5	4.14*
Error	12	1264.4	105.4	
Total	19	18170.0		

37. (i) F = 1.24*, (ii) t = 7.52* 38. Z = 10.87*

39. (i) r = 0.70, (ii) t = 2.79*

ANSWER TO OBJECTIVE TYPE QUESTIONS

CHAPTER 1

19. b 20. d 21. d 22. b 23. a 24. b
25. d 26. d 27. a 28. b 29. c 30. c

CHAPTER 2

23. d 24. c 25. b 26. a 27. c 28. d
29. d 30. b 31. d 32. c 33. c 34. a
35. b

CHAPTER 3

19. d 20. c 21. b 22 a 23 b 24. b
25. a 26. d 27. b. 28. a 29. c 30. c

CHAPTER 4

21. d	22. d	23. b	24. c	25. c	26. b
27. c	28. c	29. a	30. d	31. b	32. c
33. d	34. c	35. d	36. b	37. a	38. c
39. b	40. c				

CHAPTER 5

17. d	18. b	19. d	20. d.	21. a	22. b
23. c	24. d	25. a	26. c	27. d	28. c
29. a	30. c	31. a	32. b	33. d	34. c
35. a	36. b	37. c	38. b	39. b	40. c
41. c					

CHAPTER 6

21. c	22. d	23. b	24. d	25. b	26. c
27. a	28. b	29. c	30. c		

CHAPTER 7

23. d	24. b	25. c	26. a	27. c	28 b
29. b	30. d	31. c	32. c		

CHAPTER 8

31. c	32. a	33. d	34. a	35. c	36. c
37. d	38. b	39. c	40. b	41. a	42. b
43. b	44. c	45. d	46. c	47. c	48. b
49. a	50. c				

CHAPTER 9

31. b	32. c	33. d	34. b	35. a	36. d
37. a	38. b	39. b	40. a	41. b	42. a
43. d	44. b	45. d			

CHAPTER 10

26. d	27. a	28. b	29. b	30. c	31. b
32. a	33. c	34. d	35. b	36. b	37 a
38. b	39. c	40. c			

CHAPTER 11

37. d	38. c	39. a	40. b	41. a	42. a
43. b.	44. c	45. c	46. c	47. b	48. d
49. c	50. b	51. d	52. c	53. a	54. c
55. b	56. a	57. b	58. c	59. d	60. c
61. b	62. d	63. a	64. b	65. a	

CHAPTER 12

21. d	22. b	23. c	24. d	25. a	26. c
27. d	28. b	29. c	30. d	31. a	32. c
33. b	34. a	35. b			

CHAPTER 13

21. a	22. b	23. a	24. a	25. c	26. c
27. a	28. d	29. d	30. c	31. b	32. d
33. b	34. c	35. d	36. b	37. d	38. a
39. c	40. c	41. a			

CHAPTER 14

41. c	42. b	43. b	44. a	45. c	46. d
47. c	48 b	49. a	50. a	51. c	52. d
53. b	54. d	55. a	56. c	57. a	58. d
59. b	60. b				

CHAPTER 15

7. d	8. b	9. c	10. c

APPENDIX : STATISTICAL TABLES

Table 1: One digit random numbers

9	8	0	9	5	9	8	1	5	7	1	3	7	3	2	7	1	2	1	9
9	3	8	6	1	4	4	4	5	9	2	9	7	5	8	3	9	4	1	0
9	8	4	4	4	0	2	7	2	0	6	1	4	6	3	0	9	1	4	0
3	4	1	2	1	1	5	4	8	5	7	3	2	3	6	6	9	2	3	0
3	7	5	1	7	6	7	6	7	0	1	5	8	3	0	8	7	6	2	1
0	7	1	9	2	2	3	3	3	9	5	4	1	2	9	7	7	6	1	2
8	4	1	9	2	2	3	3	9	5	9	2	6	1	4	0	0	1	0	1
1	0	9	0	2	6	9	9	2	9	5	7	3	2	8	8	3	5	7	0
0	7	1	3	1	3	1	3	5	8	6	7	9	2	6	1	4	0	0	1
2	4	6	7	2	3	9	0	1	1	7	5	1	7	0	4	9	0	8	6
5	2	7	7	0	5	1	2	0	2	6	9	1	5	9	1	1	6	4	1
9	2	5	7	4	4	2	8	8	9	1	5	3	2	3	3	3	6	9	2
1	3	4	1	5	2	9	9	0	0	9	9	3	9	6	0	5	3	4	1
2	3	7	8	2	7	2	3	8	6	7	1	8	1	4	9	6	1	6	9
7	6	9	8	3	4	3	4	1	3	7	9	0	8	7	0	8	6	7	7
1	7	7	9	9	4	2	0	9	3	6	9	8	2	1	1	2	2	6	3
9	6	8	4	7	2	8	2	2	9	2	6	2	0	9	3	1	3	1	3
3	6	1	2	4	1	9	6	1	3	1	9	3	5	3	4	2	0	4	9
5	1	6	1	3	4	4	7	8	8	5	3	7	5	9	7	7	5	3	6
6	6	0	4	7	1	2	6	2	3	2	5	5	3	8	8	1	4	9	4
9	9	2	7	0	7	4	2	5	0	0	5	9	8	5	7	9	7	2	2
2	6	6	1	2	1	0	3	0	0	3	2	2	5	2	4	0	3	6	1
1	7	7	1	4	6	6	6	5	4	1	2	1	2	2	6	5	1	4	1
1	3	5	0	6	2	1	1	1	1	9	3	7	1	1	4	4	1	1	2
8	8	0	1	6	3	2	0	3	2	6	1	2	6	4	2	5	6	1	7
6	0	3	4	9	6	8	4	3	0	4	8	4	6	9	4	4	5	7	4
6	9	1	4	0	6	0	8	8	3	4	1	1	8	9	8	1	7	8	4
1	9	9	5	1	3	9	0	6	0	9	6	7	9	0	9	5	5	1	6
9	8	5	1	0	6	2	0	5	3	7	6	3	7	2	3	3	2	0	7
8	3	9	1	5	1	7	5	9	3	8	6	2	7	2	4	8	4	4	6

Table 2: Two-digit random numbers

13	31	76	54	08	18	96	35	03	32	73	43	64	16	63	58	00	91	79	97
10	30	01	58	94	10	92	69	19	12	02	91	08	50	33	69	21	79	40	05
20	00	43	15	72	46	23	56	84	19	81	98	29	62	32	10	53	30	15	40
22	43	76	59	00	00	27	53	22	07	32	26	40	30	04	98	17	08	95	74
51	36	38	46	83	70	28	20	98	36	20	34	55	23	02	40	54	30	39	29
97	36	48	20	88	81	84	79	53	02	79	63	51	36	19	99	45	23	53	06
73	33	18	79	84	41	89	19	08	64	26	94	07	75	42	22	95	19	73	40
12	09	40	49	12	80	69	94	62	68	48	63	99	02	98	80	52	61	20	61
76	02	18	21	87	07	42	86	71	40	55	05	45	78	80	32	35	04	04	40
57	26	29	61	70	97	20	14	76	23	56	04	48	17	21	57	48	90	50	78
64	15	38	92	44	63	08	86	25	85	64	39	55	37	90	16	75	38	78	56
18	91	82	36	73	72	37	75	60	17	98	27	54	04	68	15	44	28	42	52
61	31	58	66	32	63	01	05	16	15	38	24	99	10	89	87	83	26	68	14
74	78	49	83	14	04	17	41	71	07	10	01	58	08	30	59	44	03	09	66
00	87	70	95	70	17	14	51	10	17	38	09	85	47	53	33	84	17	04	54
20	54	82	81	84	83	42	49	78	31	01	81	68	41	25	77	29	05	10	12
31	05	62	61	49	14	49	35	38	27	05	76	92	38	67	50	11	50	44	44
18	85	10	42	09	48	33	02	41	73	04	92	80	22	39	67	85	18	40	62
28	32	06	52	05	05	13	47	27	53	16	66	61	45	93	94	15	99	53	66
92	68	77	64	97	51	63	68	06	74	20	50	79	00	17	90	57	01	62	25
55	21	39	44	03	42	41	48	39	44	90	19	66	92	33	11	20	42	95	15
09	83	91	34	27	04	11	23	16	92	44	03	04	94	72	31	65	47	85	04
29	66	20	14	34	97	10	44	95	07	93	03	89	29	20	54	15	61	83	39
89	43	93	48	97	60	02	85	04	58	74	29	44	81	89	58	55	04	64	53
72	56	65	12	16	12	15	81	87	96	76	15	65	84	76	19	19	33	28	35
97	12	69	71	63	29	20	88	95	93	00	37	44	31	10	05	28	58	58	16
03	41	05	12	94	34	02	99	84	78	56	90	81	58	07	12	22	88	93	86
52	85	72	13	48	99	27	80	48	98	61	48	69	80	07	12	78	97	48	46
35	58	53	42	27	69	16	25	80	74	67	67	16	52	08	88	86	51	55	95
61	16	57	20	11	85	07	94	13	55	68	71	75	13	97	90	02	99	49	82
03	41	05	12	94	34	02	99	84	78	56	90	81	58	07	12	22	88	93	86
52	85	72	13	48	99	27	80	48	98	61	48	69	80	07	12	78	97	02	46
35	58	52	42	27	69	17	29	80	74	67	16	52	08	88	86	51	55	95	27
61	16	57	20	11	85	07	94	13	55	68	71	75	13	97	90	02	99	49	32
38	61	18	96	87	33	18	05	71	26	61	34	03	73	59	62	58	86	58	61

(Contd.)

Table 2: (*Contd.*)

83	18	46	07	16	64	02	80	39	64	45	74	74	45	64	94	25	77	90	36
93	05	71	05	24	54	38	76	92	74	85	64	77	73	49	34	69	60	75	80
54	80	77	49	22	86	43	41	12	42	46	08	43	76	58	66	07	27	68	29
65	35	64	56	95	98	62	35	48	52	27	24	54	71	65	69	67	19	03	09
13	40	26	86	73	42	46	61	19	54	71	65	86	58	35	86	45	39	10	52
10	52	72	00	14	99	92	92	70	67	69	00	22	27	08	27	06	22	19	10
65	43	36	81	09	52	22	99	18	03	50	35	21	28	91	24	12	42	66	13
90	20	10	63	14	95	48	76	86	96	47	38	04	13	67	73	89	01	49	97
27	38	16	13	54	85	09	40	65	59	91	27	18	80	90	98	35	54	93	85
52	85	69	14	81	30	69	18	35	19	79	19	12	52	35	54	91	40	56	06
00	06	72	53	99	41	59	14	89	61	77	53	12	56	22	23	08	74	22	71
92	55	56	07	12	40	59	86	57	04	11	37	63	57	32	69	70	86	42	63
42	19	56	67	41	51	10	59	66	20	05	27	75	87	06	69	58	94	97	51
38	00	43	90	75	26	51	59	94	54	35	93	20	22	51	66	83	45	69	74
25	79	15	53	39	99	61	37	19	49	13	35	31	04	75	13	03	49	02	54
03	99	15	77	82	31	03	56	64	11	47	08	60	80	60	08	56	43	05	77
78	93	10	24	14	11	71	95	25	80	67	56	03	79	36	63	26	87	27	88
75	98	65	88	89	26	17	51	25	62	42	72	35	81	02	51	31	98	39	22
67	64	77	59	35	44	12	27	76	90	60	77	31	52	85	17	46	00	58	84
13	36	70	15	79	55	15	69	11	96	02	66	85	20	19	15	93	86	90	77
35	75	73	08	77	52	00	51	08	87	85	48	21	80	25	66	06	81	09	94
80	59	74	35	85	79	24	31	03	74	30	78	68	54	34	55	45	59	70	03
16	28	74	27	69	99	39	82	91	70	01	70	48	62	19	56	88	78	89	52
00	66	54	47	69	26	20	04	67	51	45	32	47	48	46	37	47	53	13	01
28	50	03	74	95	31	52	77	49	07	01	75	60	53	57	70	06	14	35	83

Table 3: Area under the standard normal curve from 0 to Z.

Because the curve is symmetrical, the same table can be used for values going either direction, so a negative 1.45 also has an area of 0.4265, i.e. 42.65 % of the total area under the standard normal curve. Actually one finds area from 0 to σz. Since for a standard normal distribution, σ = 1, it is known as the area under the standard normal curve from 0 to Z

Standard normal curve

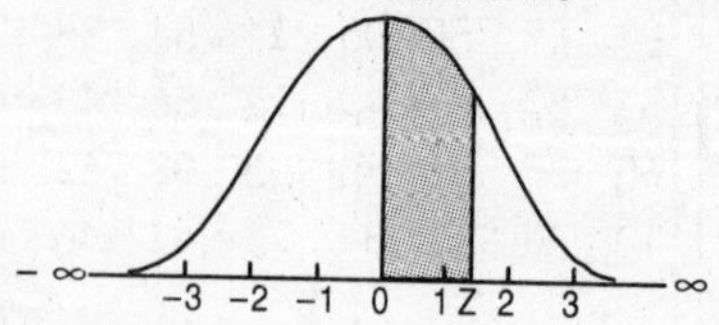

Z	0.00	0.01	0.02	0.03	0.04	0.05	0.06	0.07	0.08	0.09
0.0	0.0000	0.0040	0.0080	0.0120	0.0160	0.0199	0.0239	0.0279	0.0319	0.0359
0.1	0.0379	0.0438	0.0478	0.0517	0.0557	0.0596	0.0636	0.0675	0.0714	0.0753
0.2	0.0793	0.0832	0.0871	0.0910	0.0948	0.0987	0.1026	0.1064	0.1103	0.1141
0.3	0.1179	0.1217	.1255	0.1293	0.1331	0.1368	0.1406	0.1443	0.1480	0.1517
0.4	0.1554	0.1591	0.1628	0.1664	0.1700	0.1736	0.1772	0.1808	0.1844	0.1879
0.5	0.1915	0.1950	0.1985	0.2019	0.2054	0.2088	0.2123	0.2157	0.2190	0.2224
0.6	0.2257	0.2291	0.2324	0.2357	0.2389	0.2422	0.2454	0.2486	0.2517	0.2549
0.7	0.2580	0.2611	0.2642	0.2673	0.2704	0.2734	0.2764	0.2794	0.2823	0.2852
0.8	0.2881	0.2910	0.2939	0.2967	0.2995	0.3023	0.3051	0.3078	0.3106	0.3133
0.9	0.3159	0.3186	.3212	0.3238	0.3264	0.3289	0.3315	0.3340	0.3365	0.3389
1.0	.3413	0.3438	0.3461	0.3485	0.3508	0.3531	0.3554	0.3577	0.3599	0.3621
1.1	0.3643	0.3665	0.3686	0.3708	0.3729	0.3749	0.3770	0.3790	0.3810	0.3830
1.2	0.3849	0.33869	0.3888	0.3907	0.3925	0.394	0.3962	0.3980	0.3997	0.4015
1.3	0.4032	.4049	0.4066	0.4082	0.4099	0.4115	0.4131	0.4147	0.4162	0.4177
1.4	0.4192	0.4207	0.4222	0.4236	0.4251	0.4265	0.4279	0.4292	0.4306	0.4319
1.5	0.4332	0.4345	0.4357	0.4370	0.4382	0.4394	0.4406	0.4418	0.4429	0.4441
1.6	0.4452	0.4463	0.4474	0.4484	0.4495	0.4505	0.4515	0.4525	0.4535	0.4545
1.7	0.4554	0.4564	0.4573	0.4582	0.4591	0.4599	0.4608	0.4616	0.4625	0.4633
1.8	0.4641	0.4649	.4656	0.4664	0.4671	0.4678	0.4686	0.4693	0.4699	0.4706
1.9	0.4713	0.4719	0.4726	0.4732	0.4738	0.4744	0.4750	0.4756	0.4761	0.4767
2.0	0.4772	0.4778	0.4783	0.4788	0.4793	0.4798	0.4803	0.4808	0.4812	0.4817
2.2	0.4821	0.4826	0.4830	0.4834	0.4838	0.4842	0.4846	0.4850	0.4854	0.4857
2.3	0.4893	0.4896	0.4898	0.4901	0.4904	0.4906	0.4909	0.4911	0.4913	0.4916
2.4	0.4918	0.4920	0.4922	0.4925	0.4927	0.4929	0.4931	0.4932	0.4934	0.4936
2.5	0.4938	0.4940	0.4941	0.4943	0.4945	0.4946	0.4948	0.4949	0.4951	0.4952
2.6	0.4953	0.4955	0.4956	0.4957	0.4959	0.4960	0.4961	0.4962	0.4963	0.4964
2.7	0.4965	0.4966	0.4967	0.4968	0.4969	0.4970	0.4971	0.4972	0.4973	0.4974
2.8	0.4974	0.4975	0.4976	0.4977	0.4977	0.4978	0.4979	0.4979	0.4980	0.4981
2.9	0.4981	0.4982	0.4982	0.4983	0.4984	0.4984	0.4985	0.4985	0.4986	0.4986
3.0	0.4987	0.4987	0.4987	0.4988	0.4988	0.4989	0.4989	0.4989	0.4990	0.4990

Table 4: Abridged *t*-table and *Z*-values

	Levels of significance			
Two-tailed test	*0.20*	*0.10*	*0.05*	*0.02*
One-tailed test	*0.10*	*0.05*	*0.025*	*0.01*
d.f. = u				
1	3.078	6.314	12.706	31.821
2	1.886	2.920	4.303	6.965
3	1.638	2.353	3.182	4.541
4	1.533	2.132	2.776	3.747
5	1.476	2.015	2.571	3.365
6	1.440	1.943	2.447	3.143
7	1.415	1.895	2.365	2.998
8	1.397	1.860	2.306	2.896
9	1.383	1.833	2.262	2.821
10	1.372	1.812	2.228	2.764
11	1.363	1.796	2.201	2.718
12	1.356	1.782	2.179	2.681
13	1.350	1.771	2.160	2.650
14	1.345	1.761	2.145	2.624
15	1.341	1.753	2.131	2.602
16	1.337	1.746	2.120	2.583
17	1.333	1.740	2.110	2.567
18	1.330	1.734	2.101	2.552
19	1.328	1.729	2.093	2.539
20	1.325	1.725	2.086	2.528
21	1.323	1.721	2.080	2.518
22	1.321	1.717	2.074	2.508
23	1.319	1.714	2.069	2.500
24	1.318	1.711	2.064	2.492
25	1.316	1.708	2.060	2.485
26	1.315	1.706	2.056	2.479
27	1.314	1.703	2.052	2.473
28	1.313	1.701	2.048	2.467
29	1.311	1.699	2.045	2.462
30	1.310	1.697	2.042	2.457

(Contd.)

Table 4: (*Contd.*)

Levels of significance				
Two-tailed test	*0.20*	*0.10*	*0.05*	*0.02*
One-tailed test	*0.10*	*0.05*	*0.025*	*0.01*
d.f. = u				
31	1.309	1.696	2.040	2.453
32	1.309	1.694	2.037	2.449
33	1.308	1.692	2.035	2.445
34	1.307	1.691	2.032	2.441
35	1.306	1.690	2.030	2.438
36	1.306	1.688	2.028	2.434
37	1.305	1.687	2.026	2.431
38	1.304	1.686	2.024	2.429
39	1.304	1.685	2.023	2.426
40	1.303	1.684	2.021	2.423
45	1.301	1.679	2.014	2.412
50	1.299	1.676	2.009	2.403
55	1.297	1.673	2.004	2.396
60	1.296	1.671	2.000	2.390
65	1.295	1.669	1.997	2.385
70	1.294	1.667	1.994	2.381
75	1.293	1.665	1.992	2.377
80	1.292	1.664	1.988	2.374
85	1.292	1.663	1.990	2.371
90	1.291	1.662	1.987	2.368
95	1.291	1.661	1.985	2.366
100	1.290	1.660	1.984	2.364
Z	1.282	1.645	1.960	2.326

Source: Website and values interpolated by the author.

Table 5: Abridged chi-square table

Critical values of χ_a^2 for a level of significance				
d.f.	$\chi^2_{.100}$	$\chi^2_{.050}$	$\chi^2_{.025}$	$\chi^2_{.010}$
1	2.706	3.841	5.024	7.879
2	4.605	5.991	7.378	9.210
3	6.251	7.815	9.348	11.345
4	7.779	8.488	11.143	13.277
5	9.236	11.070	12.833	15.086
6	10.645	12.592	14.449	16.812
7	12.017	14.067	16.013	18.475
8	13.362	15.507	17.535	20.090
9	14.684	16.919	19.023	21.666
10	15.987	18.307	20.483	23.209
11	17.275	19.675	21.920	24.725
12	18.549	21.026	23.337	26.217
13	19.812	22.362	24.736	27.688
14	21.064	23.685	26.119	29.141
15	22.307	24.996	27.488	30.578
16	23.542	26.296	28.845	32.000
17	24.769	27.587	30.191	33.409
18	25.989	28.869	31.526	34.805
19	27.204	30.144	32.852	36.191
20	28.412	31.410	34.170	37.566
21	29.615	32.671	35.479	38.932
22	30.813	33.924	36.781	40.289
23	32.007	35.172	38.076	41.638
24	33.196	36.415	39.364	42.980
25	34.382	37.652	40.646	44.314
26	35.563	38.885	41.923	45.642
27	36.741	40.113	43.194	46.963
28	37.916	41.337	44.461	48.278
29	39.088	42.557	45.722	49.588
30	40.256	43.773	46.979	50.892
31	41.422	42.557	46.979	52.191
32	42.585	46.194	49.480	53.486

(*Contd.*)

Table 5: (*Contd.*)

Critical values of χ^2_α for a level of significance				
d.f.	$\chi^2_{.100}$	$\chi^2_{.050}$	$\chi^2_{.025}$	$\chi^2_{.010}$
33	43.745	47.400	50.725	54.776
34	44.903	48.602	51.966	56.061
35	46.059	49.802	53.203	57.342
36	47.212	50.998	54.437	58.619
37	48.363	52.192	55.668	59.893
38	49.513	53.384	56.896	61.162
39	50.660	54.572	58.120	62.428
40	51.805	55.758	59.342	63.691
45	57.505	61.656	65.410	69.957
50	63.167	67.505	71.420	76.154
55	68.796	73.311	77.380	82.292
60	74.397	79.082	83.298	88.379
65	79.973	84.821	89.177	94.422
70	85.527	90.531	95.023	100.425
75	91.061	96.217	100.839	106.393
80	96.578	101.879	106.629	112.329
85	102.079	107.522	112.393	118.236
90	107.565	113.145	118.136	124.116
95	113.038	118.752	123.858	129.973
100	118.498	124.342	129.561	135.807

Source: Website and values interpolated by the author.

Table 6: Upper critical values of the F-distribution

Degrees of freedom of the variance in numerator = υ_1

Degrees of freedom of the variance in denominator = υ_2

Level of significance = α

Table is provided for three most commonly used levels of significance, i.e. 10%, 5% and 1%.

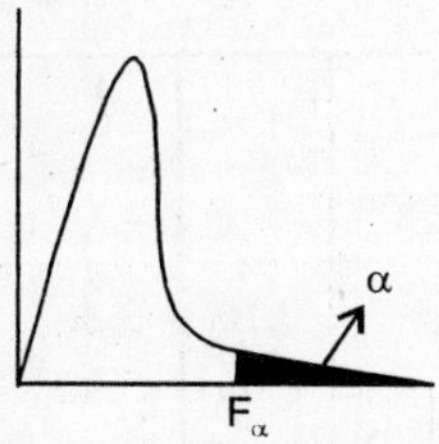

υ_1 / υ_2	α	1	2	3	4	5	6	7	8	9	10
	0.10	39.86	49.50	53.59	55.83	57.24	58.20	58.91	59.44	59.86	60.20
1	0.05	161.45	199.50	215.71	224.58	230.16	233.99	236.77	238.90	240.5	241.90
	0.01	4052	5000	5403	5625	5764	5859	5928	5982	6022	6056
	0.10	8.53	9.00	9.16	9.24	9.29	9.33	9.35	9.37	9.38	9.39
2	0.05	18.51	19.00	19.16	19.25	19.30	19.33	19.35	19.37	19.38	19.40
	0.01	98.50	99.00	99.17	99.25	99.30	99.33	99.35	99.37	99.39	99.40
	0.10	5.54	5.46	5.39	5.34	5.31	5.28	5.27	5.25	5.24	5.23
3	0.05	10.13	9.55	9.28	9.12	9.01	8.94	8.89	8.85	8.81	8.79
	0.01	34.12	30.82	29.46	28.71	28.24	27.91	27.67	27.49	27.35	27.23
	0.10	4.54	4.32	4.19	4.11	4.05	4.01	3.98	3.96	3.94	3.92
4	0.05	7.71	6.94	6.59	6.39	6.26	6.16	6.09	6.04	6.00	5.96
	0.01	21.20	18.00	16.69	15.98	15.52	15.21	14.98	14.80	14.66	14.55
	0.10	4.06	3.78	3.62	3.52	3.45	3.40	3.37	3.34	3.32	3.30
5	0.05	6.61	5.79	5.41	5.19	5.05	4.95	4.88	4.82	4.77	4.74
	0.01	16.26	13.27	12.06	11.39	10.97	10.67	10.46	10.29	10.16	10.05
	0.10	3.78	3.46	3.29	3.18	3.11	3.06	3.01	2.98	2.96	2.94
6	0.05	5.99	5.14	4.76	4.53	4.39	4.28	4.21	4.15	4.10	4.06
	0.01	13.75	10.92	9.78	9.15	8.75	8.47	8.26	8.10	7.98	7.87
	0.10	3.59	3.26	3.07	2.96	2.88	2.83	2.78	2.75	2.72	2.70
7	0.05	5.59	4.74	4.35	4.12	3.97	3.87	3.79	3.73	3.68	3.64
	0.01	12.25	9.55	8.45	7.85	7.46	7.19	6.99	6.84	6.72	6.62
	0.10	3.46	3.11	2.92	2.81	2.73	2.67	2.62	2.59	2.56	2.54
8	0.05	5.32	4.46	4.07	3.84	3.69	3.58	3.50	3.44	3.89	3.35
	0.01	11.26	8.65	7.59	7.01	6.63	6.37	6.18	6.03	5.91	5.81

(Contd.)

Table 6: (*Contd.*)

υ_1 / υ_2	α	1	2	3	4	5	6	7	8	9	10
9	0.10	3.36	3.01	2.81	2.69	2.61	2.55	2.50	2.47	2.44	2.42
	0.05	5.12	4.26	3.86	3.63	3.48	3.37	3.29	3.23	3.18	3.14
	0.01	10.56	8.02	6.99	6.42	6.06	5.80	5.61	5.47	5.35	5.26
10	0.10	3.29	2.92	2.73	2.60	2.52	2.46	2.41	2.38	2.35	2.32
	0.05	4.96	4.10	3.71	3.48	3.33	3.22	3.14	3.07	3.02	2.98
	0.01	10.04	7.56	6.55	5.99	5.64	5.39	5.20	5.06	4.94	4.85
11	0.10	3.22	2.86	2.66	2.54	2.45	2.39	2.34	2.30	2.27	2.25
	0.05	4.84	3.98	3.59	3.36	3.20	3.10	3.01	2.95	2.90	2.85
	0.01	9.65	7.21	6.22	5.67	5.32	5.07	4.89	4.74	4.63	4.54
12	0.10	3.18	2.81	2.61	2.48	2.39	2.33	2.28	2.24	2.21	2.19
	0.05	4.75	3.88	3.49	3.26	3.11	3.00	2.91	2.85	2.80	2.75
	0.01	9.33	6.93	5.95	5.41	5.06	4.82	4.64	4.50	4.39	4.30
13	0.10	3.14	2.76	2.56	2.43	2.35	2.28	2.23	2.20	2.16	2.14
	0.05	4.67	3.81	3.41	3.18	3.02	2.92	2.83	2.77	2.71	2.67
	0.01	9.07	6.70	5.74	5.20	4.86	4.62	4.44	4.30	4.19	4.10
14	0.10	3.10	2.73	2.52	2.39	2.31	2.24	2.19	2.15	2.12	2.10
	0.05	4.60	3.74	3.34	3.11	2.96	2.85	2.76	2.70	2.65	2.60
	0.01	8.86	6.51	5.56	5.04	4.70	4.46	4.28	4.14	4.03	3.94
15	0.10	3.07	2.70	2.49	2.36	2.27	2.21	2.16	2.12	2.09	2.06
	0.05	4.54	3.68	3.29	3.06	2.90	2.79	2.71	2.64	2.59	2.54
	0.01	8.68	6.36	5.42	4.89	4.56	4.32	4.14	4.00	3.90	3.80
16	0.10	3.05	2.67	2.46	2.33	2.24	2.18	2.13	2.09	2.06	2.03
	0.05	4.49	3.63	3.24	3.01	2.85	2.74	2.66	2.59	2.54	2.49
	0.01	8.53	6.23	5.29	4.77	4.44	4.20	4.03	3.89	3.78	3.69
17	0.10	3.03	2.64	2.44	2.31	2.22	2.15	2.10	2.06	2.03	2.00
	0.05	4.45	3.59	3.20	2.96	2.81	2.70	2.61	2.55	2.49	2.45
	0.01	8.40	6.11	5.18	4.67	4.34	4.10	3.93	3.79	3.68	3.59
18	0.10	3.01	2.62	2.42	2.29	2.20	2.13	2.08	2.04	2.00	1.98
	0.05	4.41	3.56	3.16	2.93	2.77	2.66	2.58	2.51	2.46	2.41
	0.01	8.28	6.01	5.09	4.58	4.25	4.02	3.84	3.70	3.60	3.51

(*Contd.*)

Table 6: (*Contd.*)

υ_1 / υ_2	α	1	2	3	4	5	6	7	8	9	10
	0.10	2.99	2.61	2.40	2.27	2.18	2.11	2.06	2.02	1.98	1.96
19	0.05	4.38	3.52	3.13	2.90	2.74	2.63	2.54	2.48	2.42	2.38
	0.01	8.18	5.93	5.01	4.50	4.17	3.94	3.76	3.63	3.52	3.43
	0.10	2.98	2.59	2.38	2.25	2.16	2.09	2.04	2.00	1.96	1.94
20	0.05	4.35	3.49	3.10	2.87	2.71	2.60	2.51	2.45	2.39	2.35
	0.01	8.10	5.85	4.94	4.43	4.10	3.87	3.70	3.56	3.46	3.37
	0.10	2.96	2.58	2.37	2.23	2.14	2.08	2.02	1.98	1.95	1.92
21	0.05	4.32	3.47	3.07	2.84	2.68	2.57	2.49	2.42	2.37	2.32
	0.01	8.02	5.78	4.87	4.37	4.04	3.81	3.64	3.51	3.40	3.31
	0.10	2.95	2.56	2.35	2.22	2.13	2.06	2.01	1.97	1.93	1.90
22	0.05	4.30	3.44	3.05	2.82	2.66	2.55	2.46	2.40	2.34	2.30
	0.01	7.94	5.72	4.82	4.31	3.99	3.76	3.59	3.45	3.35	3.26
	0.10	2.94	2.55	2.34	2.21	2.12	2.05	2.00	1.95	1.92	1.89
23	0.05	4.28	3.42	3.03	2.80	2.64	2.53	2.44	2.38	2.32	2.28
	0.01	7.88	5.66	4.77	4.26	3.94	3.71	3.54	3.41	3.30	3.21
	0.10	2.93	2.54	2.33	2.20	2.10	2.04	1.98	1.94	1.91	1.88
24	0.05	4.26	3.40	3.01	2.78	2.62	2.51	2.42	2.36	2.30	2.26
	0.01	7.82	5.61	4.72	4.22	3.90	3.67	3.50	3.36	3.26	3.17
	0.10	2.92	2.53	2.32	2.18	2.09	2.02	1.97	1.93	1.90	1.87
25	0.05	4.24	3.38	2.99	2.76	2.60	2.49	2.40	2.34	2.28	2.24
	0.01	7.77	5.57	4.68	4.18	3.86	3.63	3.46	3.32	3.22	3.13
	0.10	2.88	2.49	2.28	2.14	2.05	1.98	1.93	1.88	1.85	1.82
30	0.05	4.17	3.32	2.92	2.69	2.53	2.42	2.33	2.27	2.21	2.16
	0.01	7.56	5.39	4.51	4.02	3.70	3.47	3.30	3.17	3.07	2.98
	0.10	2.86	2.46	2.25	2.11	2.02	1.95	1.90	1.85	1.82	1.79
35	0.05	4.12	3.27	2.87	2.64	2.48	2.37	2.28	2.22	2.16	2.11
	0.01	7.42	5.27	4.40	3.91	3.59	3.37	3.20	3.07	2.96	2.88
	0.10	2.84	2.44	2.23	2.09	2.00	1.93	1.87	1.83	1.79	1.76
40	0.05	4.08	3.23	2.84	2.61	2.45	2.34	2.25	2.18	2.12	2.08
	0.01	7.31	5.18	4.31	3.83	3.51	3.29	3.12	2.99	2.89	2.80

(*Contd.*)

Table 6: (*Contd.*)

υ_1 / υ_2	α	1	2	3	4	5	6	7	8	9	10
	0.10	2.82	2.42	2.21	2.07	1.98	1.91	1.86	1.81	1.77	1.74
45	0.05	4.06	3.20	2.81	2.58	2.42	2.31	2.22	2.15	2.10	2.05
	0.01	7.23	5.11	4.25	3.77	3.45	3.23	3.07	2.94	2.83	2.74
	0.10	2.81	2.41	2.20	2.06	1.97	1.90	1.84	1.80	1.76	1.73
50	0.05	4.03	3.18	2.79	2.56	2.40	2.29	2.20	2.13	2.07	2.03
	0.01	7.17	5.06	4.20	3.72	3.41	3.19	3.02	2.89	2.78	2.70
	0.10	2.80	2.40	2.19	2.05	1.96	1.88	1.83	1.78	1.75	1.72
55	0.05	4.02	3.16	2.77	2.54	2.38	2.27	2.18	2.11	2.06	2.01
	0.01	7.12	5.01	4.16	3.68	3.37	3.15	2.98	2.85	2.75	2.66
	0.10	2.79	2.39	2.18	2.04	1.95	1.88	1.82	1.78	1.74	1.71
60	0.05	4.00	3.15	2.76	2.52	2.37	2.25	2.17	2.10	2.04	1.99
	0.01	7.08	4.98	4.13	3.65	3.34	3.12	2.95	2.82	2.72	2.63
	0.10	2.78	2.38	2.16	2.03	1.93	1.86	1.80	1.76	1.72	1.69
70	0.05	3.98	3.13	2.74	2.50	2.35	2.23	2.14	2.07	2.02	1.97
	0.01	7.01	4.92	4.07	3.60	3.29	3.07	2.91	2.78	2.67	2.58
	0.10	2.77	2.37	2.15	2.02	1.92	1.85	1.79	1.75	1.71	1.68
80	0.05	3.96	3.11	2.72	2.49	2.33	2.21	2.13	2.06	2.00	1.95
	0.01	6.96	4.88	4.04	3.56	3.26	3.04	2.87	2.74	2.64	2.55
	0.10	2.76	2.36	2.15	2.01	1.91	1.84	1.78	1.74	1.70	1.67
90	0.05	3.95	3.10	2.71	2.47	2.31	2.20	2.11	2.04	1.98	1.94
	0.01	6.92	4.85	4.01	3.54	3.23	3.01	2.84	2.72	2.61	2.52
	0.10	2.76	2.36	2.14	2.00	1.91	1.83	1.78	1.73	1.70	1.66
100	0.05	3.94	3.09	2.70	2.46	2.30	2.19	2.10	2.03	1.98	1.93
	0.01	6.90	4.82	3.98	3.51	3.21	2.99	2.82	2.69	2.59	2.50
	0.10	2.75	2.35	2.13	1.99	1.90	1.82	1.77	1.72	1.68	1.65
120	0.05	3.92	3.07	2.68	2.45	2.29	2.17	2.09	2.02	1.96	1.91
	0.01	6.85	4.79	3.95	3.48	3.17	2.96	2.79	2.66	2.56	2.47

(*Contd.*)

Table 6: (*Contd.*)

υ_1 / υ_2	α	11	12	13	14	15	16	17	18	19	120
1	0.10	60.47	60.71	60.93	61.07	61.35	61.57	61.74	62.53	62.79	63.06
	0.05	243.0	243.9	244.7	245.4	246.5	247.3	248.0	251.1	252.2	253.3
	0.01	6083	6106	6126	6143	6170	6192	6209	6257	6313	6339
2	0.10	9.40	9.41	9.42	9.42	9.43	9.44	9.44	9.47	9.47	9.48
	0.05	19.40	19.41	19.42	19.42	19.43	19.44	19.45	19.47	19.48	19.49
	0.01	99.41	99.42	99.42	99.43	99.44	99.44	99.45	99.47	99.48	99.49
3	0.10	5.22	5.22	5.21	5.20	5.20	5.19	5.18	5.16	5.15	5.14
	0.05	8.76	8.74	8.73	8.72	8.69	8.68	8.66	8.59	8.57	8.55
	0.01	27.13	27.05	26.98	26.92	26.83	26.75	26.69	26.41	26.32	26.22
4	0.10	3.91	3.90	3.89	3.88	3.86	3.85	3.84	3.80	3.79	3.78
	0.05	5.94	5.91	5.89	5.87	5.84	5.82	5.80	5.72	5.69	5.66
	0.01	14.45	14.37	14.31	14.25	14.15	14.08	14.02	13.75	13.65	13.56
5	0.10	3.28	3.27	3.26	3.25	3.23	3.22	3.21	3.16	3.14	3.12
	0.05	4.70	4.68	4.66	4.64	4.60	4.58	4.56	4.46	4.43	4.40
	0.01	9.96	9.89	9.82	9.77	9.68	9.61	9.55	9.29	9.20	9.11
6	0.10	2.92	2.91	2.89	2.88	2.86	2.85	2.84	2.78	2.76	2.74
	0.05	4.03	4.00	3.98	3.96	3.92	3.90	3.87	3.77	3.74	3.70
	0.01	7.79	7.72	7.66	7.60	7.52	7.45	7.40	7.14	7.06	6.97
7	0.10	2.68	2.67	2.65	2.64	2.62	2.61	2.60	2.54	2.51	2.49
	0.05	3.60	3.58	3.55	3.53	3.49	3.47	3.44	3.34	3.30	3.27
	0.01	6.54	6.47	6.41	6.36	6.28	6.21	6.16	5.91	5.82	5.74
8	0.10	2.52	2.50	2.49	2.48	2.46	2.44	2.42	2.36	2.34	2.32
	0.05	3.31	3.28	3.26	3.24	3.20	3.17	3.15	3.04	3.01	2.97
	0.01	5.73	5.67	5.61	5.56	5.48	5.41	5.36	5.12	5.03	4.95
9	0.10	2.40	2.38	2.36	2.35	2.33	2.31	2.30	2.23	2.21	2.18
	0.05	3.10	3.07	3.05	3.02	2.99	2.96	2.94	2.83	2.79	2.75
	0.01	5.18	5.11	5.06	5.00	4.92	4.86	4.81	4.57	4.48	4.40

(*Contd.*)

Table 6: (*Contd.*)

υ_1 / υ_2	α	11	12	13	14	15	16	17	18	19	120
	0.10	2.30	2.28	2.27	2.26	2.23	2.22	2.20	2.13	2.11	2.08
10	0.05	2.94	2.91	2.89	2.86	2.83	2.80	2.77	2.66	2.62	2.58
	0.01	4.77	4.71	4.65	4.60	4.52	4.46	4.41	4.17	4.08	4.00
	0.10	2.23	2.21	2.19	2.18	2.16	2.14	2.12	2.05	2.03	2.00
11	0.05	2.82	2.79	2.76	2.74	2.70	2.67	2.65	2.53	2.49	2.45
	0.01	4.46	4.40	4.34	4.29	4.21	4.15	4.10	3.86	3.78	3.69
	0.10	2.17	2.15	2.13	2.12	2.09	2.08	2.06	1.99	1.96	1.93
12	0.05	2.72	2.69	2.66	2.64	2.60	2.57	2.54	2.43	2.38	2.34
	0.01	4.22	4.16	4.10	4.05	3.97	3.91	3.86	3.62	3.54	3.45
	0.10	2.12	2.10	2.08	2.07	2.04	2.02	2.01	1.93	1.90	1.88
13	0.05	2.64	2.60	2.58	2.55	2.52	2.48	2.46	2.34	2.30	2.25
	0.01	4.02	3.96	3.90	3.86	3.78	3.72	3.66	3.43	3.34	3.25
	0.10	2.07	2.05	2.04	2.02	2.00	1.98	1.96	1.89	1.86	1.83
14	0.05	2.56	2.53	2.51	2.48	2.44	2.41	2.39	2.27	2.22	2.18
	0.01	3.86	3.80	3.74	3.70	3.62	3.56	3.51	3.27	3.18	3.09
	0.10	2.04	2.02	2.00	1.98	1.96	1.94	1.92	1.85	1.82	1.79
15	0.05	2.51	2.46	2.45	2.42	2.38	2.35	2.33	2.20	2.16	2.11
	0.01	3.73	3.67	3.61	3.56	3.48	3.42	3.37	3.13	3.05	2.96
	0.10	2.00	1.98	1.97	1.95	1.93	1.91	1.89	1.81	1.78	1.75
16	0.05	2.46	2.42	2.40	2.37	2.33	2.30	2.28	2.15	2.11	2.06
	0.01	3.62	3.55	3.50	3.45	3.37	3.31	3.26	3.02	2.93	2.84
	0.10	1.98	1.96	1.94	1.92	1.90	1.88	1.86	1.81	1.78	1.75
17	0.05	2.41	2.38	2.35	2.33	2.29	2.26	2.23	2.10	2.06	2.01
	0.01	3.52	3.46	3.40	3.35	3.28	3.21	3.16	2.92	2.83	2.75
	0.10	1.95	1.93	1.92	1.90	1.88	1.85	1.84	1.75	1.72	1.69
18	0.05	2.37	2.34	2.31	2.29	2.25	2.22	2.19	2.06	2.02	1.97
	0.01	3.43	3.37	3.32	3.27	3.19	3.13	3.08	2.84	2.75	2.66
	0.10	1.93	1.91	1.89	1.88	1.85	1.83	1.81	1.73	1.70	1.67
19	0.05	2.34	2.31	2.28	2.26	2.22	2.18	2.16	2.03	1.98	1.93
	0.01	3.36	3.30	3.24	3.20	3.12	3.05	3.00	2.76	2.67	2.58

(*Contd.*)

Table 6: (*Contd.*)

υ_1 / υ_2	α	11	12	13	14	15	16	17	18	19	120
	0.10	1.91	1.89	1.88	1.86	1.83	1.81	1.79	1.71	1.68	1.64
20	0.05	2.31	2.28	2.25	2.22	2.18	2.15	2.12	1.99	1.95	1.90
	0.01	3.29	3.23	3.18	3.13	3.05	2.99	2.94	2.69	2.61	2.52
	0.10	1.90	1.88	1.86	1.84	1.82	1.79	1.78	1.69	1.66	1.62
21	0.05	2.28	2.25	2.22	2.20	2.16	2.12	2.10	1.96	1.92	1.87
	0.01	3.24	3.17	3.12	3.07	2.99	2.93	2.88	2.64	2.55	2.46
	0.10	1.88	1.86	1.84	1.82	1.80	1.78	1.76	1.67	1.64	1.60
22	0.05	2.26	2.23	2.20	2.17	2.13	2.10	2.07	1.94	1.89	1.84
	0.01	3.18	3.12	3.07	3.20	2.94	2.88	2.83	2.58	2.50	2.40
	0.10	1.87	1.84	1.83	1.81	1.78	1.76	1.74	1.66	1.62	1.59
23	0.05	2.24	2.20	2.18	2.15	2.11	2.08	2.05	1.91	1.86	1.81
	0.01	3.14	3.07	3.02	2.97	2.89	2.83	2.78	2.54	2.45	2.35
	0.10	1.85	1.83	1.81	1.78	1.77	1.75	1.73	1.64	1.61	1.57
24	0.05	2.22	2.18	2.16	2.13	2.09	2.05	2.03	1.89	1.84	1.79
	0.01	3.09	3.03	2.98	2.93	2.85	2.80	2.74	2.49	2.40	2.31
	0.10	1.84	1.82	1.80	1.78	1.76	1.74	1.72	1.63	1.59	1.56
25	0.05	2.20	2.16	2.14	2.11	2.07	2.04	2.01	1.87	1.82	1.77
	0.01	3.06	2.99	2.94	2.89	2.81	2.75	2.70	2.45	2.36	2.27
	0.10	1.79	1.77	1.75	1.74	1.71	1.69	1.67	1.57	1.54	1.50
30	0.05	2.13	2.09	2.06	2.04	2.00	1.96	1.93	1.79	1.74	1.68
	0.01	2.91	2.84	2.79	2.74	2.66	2.60	2.55	2.30	2.21	2.11
	0.10	1.76	1.74	1.72	1.70	1.67	1.65	1.63	1.53	1.50	1.46
35	0.05	2.08	2.04	2.01	1.99	1.94	1.91	1.88	1.74	1.68	1.62
	0.01	2.80	2.74	2.69	2.64	2.56	2.50	2.44	2.19	2.10	2.00
	0.10	1.74	1.72	1.70	1.69	1.65	1.62	1.60	1.51	1.47	1.42
40	0.05	2.04	2.00	1.97	1.95	1.90	1.87	1.84	1.69	1.64	1.58
	0.01	2.73	2.66	2.61	2.56	2.48	2.42	2.37	2.11	2.02	1.92
	0.10	1.72	1.70	1.68	1.66	1.63	1.60	1.58	1.49	1.45	1.40
45	0.05	2.01	1.97	1.94	1.92	1.87	1.84	1.81	1.66	1.60	1.54
	0.01	2.67	2.61	2.55	2.51	2.43	2.36	2.31	2.05	1.96	1.86

(*Contd.*)

Table 6: *(Contd.)*

υ_1 / υ_2	α	11	12	13	14	15	16	17	18	19	120
	0.10	1.70	1.68	1.66	1.64	1.61	1.59	1.57	1.47	1.44	1.38
50	0.05	1.99	1.95	1.92	1.90	1.85	1.81	1.78	1.63	1.57	1.51
	0.01	2.62	2.56	2.51	2.46	2.38	2.32	2.26	2.01	1.95	1.81
	0.10	1.69	1.67	1.65	1.63	1.60	1.58	1.56	1.45	1.42	1.36
55	0.05	1.97	1.93	1.90	1.88	1.83	1.80	1.76	1.61	1.55	1.49
	0.01	2.59	2.53	2.47	2.42	2.34	2.28	2.23	1.97	1.87	1.76
	0.10	1.68	1.66	1.64	1.62	1.59	1.56	1.54	1.44	1.40	1.35
60	0.05	1.95	1.92	1.89	1.86	1.82	1.78	1.75	1.59	1.53	1.47
	0.01	2.56	2.50	2.44	2.39	2.32	2.25	2.20	1.94	1.84	1.73
	0.10	1.66	1.64	1.62	1.60	1.57	1.55	1.53	1.42	1.38	1.33
70	0.05	1.93	1.89	1.86	1.84	1.79	1.75	1.72	1.56	1.50	1.44
	0.01	2.51	2.45	2.40	2.35	2.27	2.20	2.15	1.89	1.79	1.68
	0.10	1.65	1.63	1.61	1.59	1.56	1.53	1.51	1.40	1.36	1.31
80	0.05	1.91	1.88	1.84	1.82	1.77	1.73	1.70	1.54	1.48	1.41
	0.01	2.48	2.42	2.36	2.31	2.23	2.17	2.12	1.85	1.75	1.63
	0.10	1.64	1.62	1.60	1.58	1.55	1.52	1.50	1.39	1.35	1.30
90	0.05	1.90	1.86	1.83	1.80	1.76	1.72	1.69	1.53	1.46	1.40
	0.01	2.45	2.39	2.33	2.29	2.21	2.14	2.09	1.82	1.72	1.60
	0.10	1.64	1.61	1.59	1.57	1.54	1.52	1.49	1.38	1.34	1.28
100	0.05	1.89	1.85	1.82	1.79	1.75	1.71	1.68	1.52	1.45	1.38
	0.01	2.43	2.37	2.31	2.26	2.19	2.12	2.07	1.80	1.69	1.57
	0.10	1.62	1.60	1.58	1.56	1.53	1.50	1.48	1.37	1.32	1.26
120	0.05	1.87	1.83	1.80	1.77	1.73	1.69	1.66	1.50	1.43	1.35
	0.01	2.40	2.34	2.27	2.20	2.15	2.08	2.03	1.76	1.66	1.53

Source: Website and values interpolated by the author.

INDEX